KAPLAN MEDICAL ASSISTANT

Medical Front Office

KAPLAN MEDICAL ASSISTANT

Medical Front Office

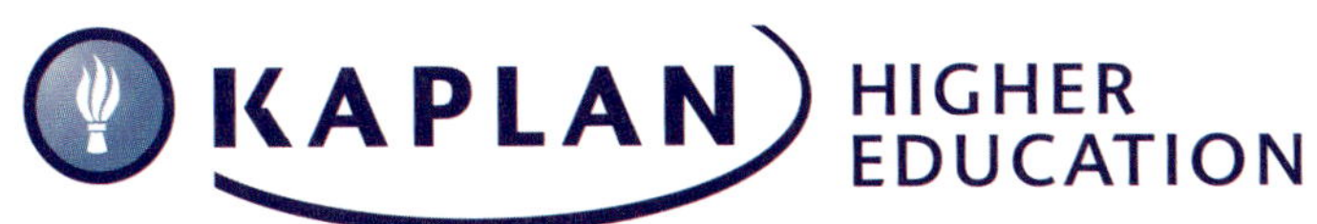

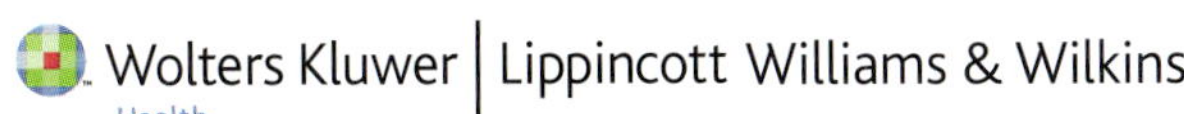

Philadelphia • Baltimore • New York • London
Buenos Aires • Hong Kong • Sydney • Tokyo

All Chapters from Molle EA, et al. *Comprehensive Medical Assisting*, 2nd ed.
Copyright 2005, Lippincott Williams & Wilkins, Philadelphia, Pa.

All study guides and worksheets from West-Stack C and Howe BB.
Study Guide: Comprephensive Medical Assisting, 2nd ed.
Copyright 2005, Lippincott Williams & Wilkins, Philadelphia, Pa.

Publisher: Julie K. Stegman
Acquisitions Editor: John Goucher
Project Manager: Matt Hauber
Production Manager: Eric Branger
Art Coordinator: Jennifer Clements
Cover Design: Armen Kojoyian
Compositor: Aptara, Inc.

351 West Camden Street
Baltimore, Maryland 21201-2436 USA

530 Walnut Street
Philadelphia, PA 19106

Printed in the United States of America

RRW1108

KAPLAN MISSION STATEMENT

Kaplan helps individuals achieve their educational and career goals. We build futures one success story at a time.

ABOUT KAPLAN HIGHER EDUCATION

Kaplan Higher Education offers certificate and degree programs, on campus and online, that prepare students for employment in fields including health care, business, criminal justice, fashion, design and graphic arts, information technology, and paralegal studies. At campuses in the United States and abroad, as well as via online programs through Kaplan University and Concord Law School, we offer educational opportunities that help people advance their careers and improve their lives. Each of our schools is separately accredited by one of several national or regional accrediting agencies approved by the U.S. Department of Education.

Kaplan is responsive to the needs of adult learners, many of whom juggle work, family, and other responsibilities. Our comprehensive support system provides financial aid counseling, academic advising, study skills workshops, time management guidance, and more. Our faculty is committed to ensuring that our students get the maximum value from their experience.

Kaplan, Inc., entered the postsecondary education industry in 2000, with the acquisition of Quest Education Corp., a network of 30 schools. Today, Kaplan Higher Education has become Kaplan's largest business, serving 68,000 students through more than 70 schools in 21 states and online programs in the United States and abroad. The company is market-driven, adding locations and programs in areas that will best serve local employment needs. The company's curricula include programs designed to lead to entry-level employment in many of the country's fastest growing occupations, as projected by the U.S. Department of Labor.

ACKNOWLEDGMENTS

We are pleased to present to you the *Kaplan Medical Assistant* module series, a compilation of materials focusing on fundamental principles that help develop proficient and sensitive medical professionals.

Designed to serve a broad audience of medical, therapeutic, pharmacy, and dental students, this guide offers interdisciplinary readings and activities for academic strategies, medical law, math, health sciences, and complementary medicine.

Primary acknowledgment must go to the many dedicated instructors who continually take on challenges of all shapes and sizes aimed at improving education. The professional literature and journals acknowledge individual contributions, but textbooks cannot adequately pay such tribute. Albert Einstein identified this problem, commenting that although "there are plenty of well-endowed (professionals) . . . it strikes me as unfair to select a few of them for recognition." We are indebted to all these unnamed people.

On a more immediate level, we would first like to thank our consulting editor and publisher, Lippincott Williams & Wilkins, for their expert and exhaustive work. We are especially grateful to Susan Katz, John Goucher, Matt Hauber, Eric Branger, Julie Stegman, Dale Gray, Dana Knighten, and Leigh Wells for their enthusiasm and cooperation in making these books a reality. They have processed a formidable number of materials with dedication, attention to detail, knowledge, and editorial skill.

In addition, we thank the Kaplan Higher Education Faculty Advisory Board for providing educational guidance. They deserve grateful recognition for their indispensable help.

We gratefully acknowledge the following Faculty Advisory Board members:

Anthony Devore, Texas Careers
Denise Gemmel, Technology Education College
Bruce Gilden, Maric College, North County Campus
Mary Hitchens, Maric College
Tereas O'Mara, Professional Careers Institute
Thomas Reynolds, Texas Careers
Lisa Stephens, Professional Careers Institute

CAAHEP COMPETENCIES

Upon completion of this unit, students will be able to demonstrate mastery of the following CAAHEP competencies:

A ADMINISTRATIVE COMPETENCIES
- 1 Perform Clerical Functions
  - a Schedule and manage appointments
  - b Schedule inpatient and outpatient admissions and procedures
- 2 Perform Bookkeeping Procedures
  - a Prepare a bank deposit
  - b Post entries on a daysheet
  - c Perform accounts receivable procedures
  - d Perform billing and collection procedures
  - e Post adjustments
  - f Process credit balances
  - g Process refunds
  - h Post NSF checks
  - i Post collection agency payments
- 3 Process Insurance Claims
  - a Apply managed care policies and procedures
  - b Apply third party guidelines
  - c Perform procedural coding
  - d Perform diagnostic coding
  - e Complete insurance claim forms

B CLINICAL COMPETENCIES
- 4 Patient Care
  - a Perform telephone and in-person screening

C GENERAL COMPETENCIES
- 1 Professional Communications
  - a Respond to and initiate written communications
  - d Demonstrate telephone techniques
- 3 Patient Instruction
  - a Explain general office policies
- 4 Operational Functions
  - a Perform an inventory of supplies and equipment
  - c Utilize computer software to maintain office systems

CONTENTS

UNIT 1

MEDICAL OFFICE PROCEDURES 1

UNIT 2

MEDICAL ACCOUNTING PROCEDURES 91

UNIT 3

MEDICAL INSURANCE AND SOFTWARE 137

Unit I

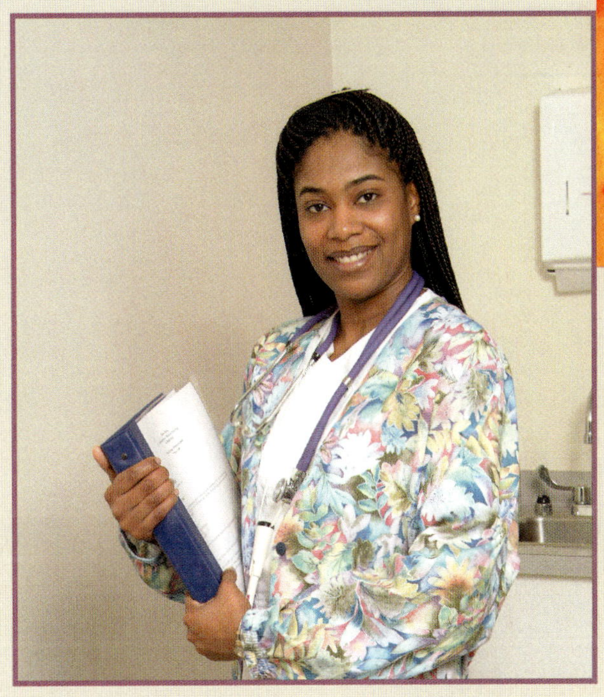

Medical Office Procedures

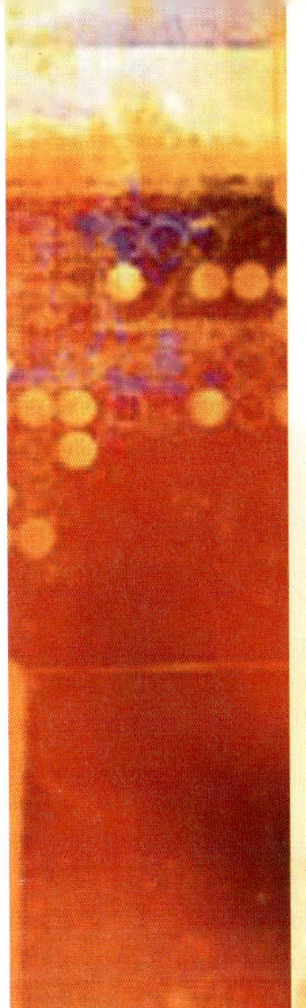

1

The First Contact: Telephone and Reception

CHAPTER OBJECTIVES

In this chapter, you'll learn:

1. To spell and define the key terms.
2. To explain the importance of displaying a professional image to all patients.
3. To list six duties of the medical office receptionist.
4. To list four sources from which messages can be retrieved.
5. To discuss various steps that can be taken to promote good ergonomics.
6. To describe the basic guidelines for waiting room environments.
7. To describe the proper method for maintaining infection control standards in the waiting room.
8. To discuss the five basic guidelines for telephone use.
9. To describe the types of incoming telephone calls received by the medical office.
10. To describe how to triage incoming calls.
11. To discuss how to identify and handle callers with medical emergencies.
12. To list the information that should be given to an emergency medical service dispatcher.
13. To describe the types of telephone services and special features.

KEY TERMS

attude
closed captioning
diction
diplomacy
emergency medical service (EMS)
ergonomic
receptionist
teletypewriter (TTY)
triage

AS A MEDICAL ASSISTANT, YOU are the patient's primary contact with the physician. In certain situations, the patient may spend more time with you than with the physician. Your interaction with the patient sets the tone for the visit and directly influences the patient's perception of the office and the quality of care the patient will receive. Therefore, it is vital that you project a caring and competent professional image at all times. You will have various responsibilities and duties when working as a receptionist. These duties will vary among physician offices. Proper telephone etiquette and use is an essential skill for all medical assistants. You must be able to handle incoming and outgoing calls correctly and efficiently.

PROFESSIONAL IMAGE

Importance of a Good Attitude

An **attitude** is a state of mind or feeling regarding some matter. It can be either positive or negative. Attitudes can be formed by past or present experiences; they can be transmitted from one person to another. How you feel influences how you act; thus, your attitude shapes your behavior. You transmit your attitude to others through your behavior, thereby influencing their attitudes and behaviors.

The medical assistant must be able to transmit a positive attitude to the patient. This requires acceptance of the patient as a unique individual who has the right to be treated with dignity and compassion in a nonjudgmental manner. Ask yourself how you would feel in a similar situation, how you would want to be treated. By demonstrating empathy, interest, and concern, you tell the patient that he or she is important to you and that you care. This exerts a positive influence on the patient's own attitude, behavior, and response.

For example, let's assume that you are working as a receptionist in a busy family practice office. It is the peak of the flu and cold season. Which of the following interactions between the medical assistant and the patient transmits a positive attitude to the patient:

- "I know you feel terrible, Mr. Smith, but so does everyone else in the waiting room. It's the flu season. Just have a seat, and the doctor will see you shortly."
- "I'm sorry you don't feel well. Do you feel well enough to sit in the waiting room for about 10 minutes? The doctor will be ready to see you then."

The second interaction shows the patient that you care about how he feels and reassures him that he will be seen by the physician shortly. In the first interaction, the attitude that was transmitted made Mr. Smith feel like just another sick patient. Your positive attitude will influence the patient's attitude, behavior, and response.

The Medical Assistant as a Role Model

Another way in which you as a medical assistant influence the patient's perception of the medical office is your personal appearance. Good health and good grooming present a positive image to the patient. Taking care of yourself by eating well, exercising regularly, and getting enough rest is important not only for your appearance but also for your job performance. If you are tired or sluggish, you cannot give good patient care.

Pay particular attention to your personal hygiene to avoid offending your patients. A person who is ill is often acutely sensitive to odors, even those normally considered pleasant. A daily bath or shower is essential, followed by an unscented deodorant. Keep your hair clean and styled. Good oral hygiene is important, and during the day you should avoid foods that may give an offensive odor. Keep your fingernails clean and trimmed, with clear or neutral polish. Long nails polished with vivid colors are not appropriate for the medical office. Natural nail tips must be less than a quarter inch long, according to the Centers for Disease Control (CDC). Artificial nails may increase the potential for infection transmission to you and your patients. The CDC recommendation is for health care providers not to wear artificial nails if high-risk patient care is required. If you wear makeup, keep it natural and apply it lightly. Do not wear perfume, cologne, scented lotion, hair spray, or the like.

Most offices have a dress code. Whether you wear a uniform or street clothes, they should be clean, neat, pressed, and in good repair (Fig. 1-1). Wrinkles, missing buttons, split seams, torn hems, and stains project a negative image. Always wear clean, polished shoes. Stockings should be full length, of a neutral shade, and free from runs and holes. Jewelry such as dangling earrings, large rings, long chains, and ornate or multiple bracelets are not appropriate in the health care environment.

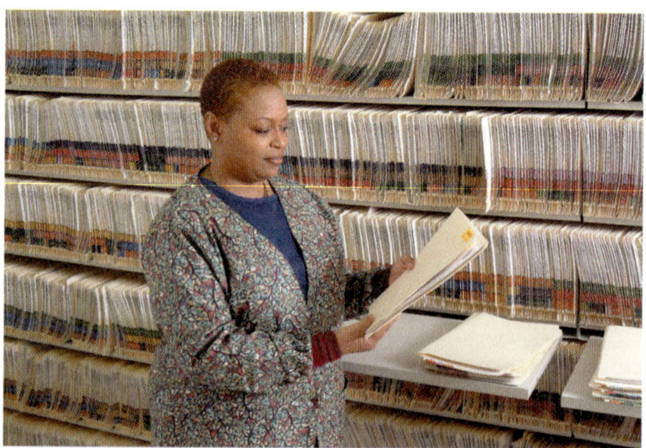

FIGURE 1-1. The properly dressed medical assistant presents a professional and positive image to patients.

Courtesy and Diplomacy in the Medical Office

Being a medical assistant requires excellent human relations skills. In the course of a day you will interact with a variety of personalities in a variety of situations, and you must be able to maintain a positive professional attitude regardless of how difficult the encounter may be. For example, you may have to interact with a person who has done domestic violence to a patient. It is important that you treat him or her with the same courtesy and respect that you offer all patients. Courtesy and diplomacy are fundamental to successful human relations.

Courtesy is based on sensitivity to the needs and feelings of others and demands that everyone be treated with respect and dignity. It is disrespectful to refer to physicians by first name or title only. Always use the title and last name. It is permissible to call a physician by his or her first name outside of clinical areas if the physician so requests. Be courteous to your coworkers as well as your employer and your patients. Do not borrow supplies or use someone else's desk without asking permission. Always knock before entering an office, even if the door is open.

Diplomacy is the art of handling people with tact and genuine concern. Use diplomacy in difficult situations. Patients may be curious about other patients; family members may want to know what the doctor said to the patient—such questions must be met with a polite refusal to disclose confidential information. Pain, worry, and waiting can make a patient unreasonable or irritable. You must exercise self-control and understanding and maintain your professional attitude. Never argue with a patient. Try to calm the patient and communicate your desire to help. Table 1-1 lists three common problems with patients and the diplomatic way to control each situation.

First Impressions

First impressions are lasting. Remember, you have only one chance to make a first impression on patients and other health care professionals. The patient's perception of the medical office is based in part on the impression you make. A negative perception can adversely affect the patient's health. A positive perception contributes to a successful doctor–patient relationship. Patients who feel positive about their relationship with health care providers are likely to follow treatment regimens.

Physician offices must operate as a business to remain financially sound. Patients who are not satisfied with their care may opt to leave the practice. Loss of patients will result in loss of revenue for the practice. As a medical assistant, you play a key role in promoting a positive image for the physician's practice.

Checkpoint Question

1. What are four ways that you can demonstrate a professional image to patients?

RECEPTION

Definition of a Receptionist

The definition of a receptionist will vary greatly among offices. According to the 10th edition of Merriam-Webster's Collegiate Dictionary, a **receptionist** is a person employed to

Table 1-1 DIPLOMACY TABLE

Common Problem	Example of What to Say	Example of What Not to Say
Prolonged Waiting Time "My appointment was for 9:30, and it is now 10. When am I going to be seen?"	"The doctor will see you in about 30 minutes. Would you like to wait or reschedule your visit?"	"We have had some emergencies." "It's flu season. Everyone is sick. Please sit down."
Patient Confidentiality "I am worried about my neighbor. He was seen here yesterday and sent to the hospital by ambulance. What happened?"	"We appreciate your concern, but it is against our office policy to give out patient information."	"He was having some chest pain, but he is fine now." "Yes, we sent him by ambulance because he was very sick."
Patient Discomfort "I am in a lot of pain. I want to see the doctor now!" "I have been vomiting all day. I won't sit in the waiting room. I want to be seen now!"	"I can see that you are in pain. Please have a seat for 1 minute. I will find a room for you to lie down."	"You are going to have to wait your turn. There are three patients ahead of you." "If you need to vomit, the rest room is to your left. You will have about a 20-minute wait."

greet telephone callers, visitors, patients, or clients. In certain physician offices the receptionist may be a non–medically trained professional whose primary task is to greet patients, alert staff members when patients are present, and serve as a telephone operator. This situation is generally found in large, multiphysician practices. If you are working in this type of setting, your role as a medical assistant will be to provide coverage while the receptionist is on break or at lunch.

In other office settings, however, you may work as the receptionist. These offices may also have multiple physicians but choose to have a medically trained person as the receptionist. No matter which type of office you work in, you will need to know and be able to assume the duties and responsibilities of a receptionist.

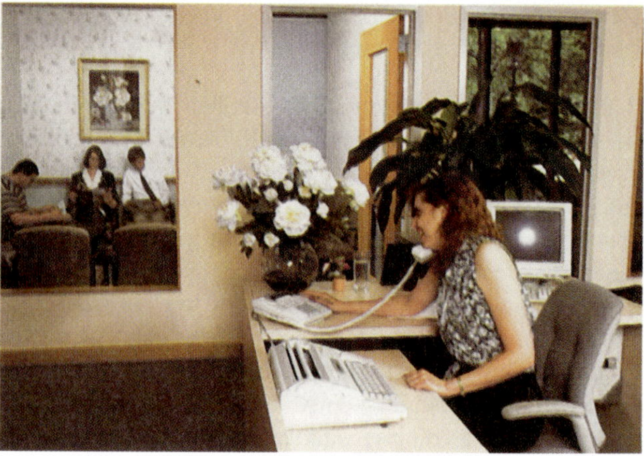

FIGURE 1-2. The receptionist desk and waiting room area must be easily accessible at all times.

Duties and Responsibilities of the Receptionist

The duties of the receptionist begin long before the first appointment of the day. Most offices have the receptionist arrive at least 30 minutes prior to the first appointment. Your first task will be to prepare the office for patient arrivals.

Prepare the Office

As receptionist, you are responsible for preparing the office for patients and for other employee arrivals. These tasks should be done first:

- Unlock doors as appropriate.
- Disengage the alarm system.
- Turn on appropriate lights.
- Turn on computers, printers, copiers, and other electronic devices.
- If the office uses a drop box to leave specimens for evening pickups, check the box to ensure that the specimens were taken.

After those five tasks are done, do a systematic check of the office. The reception area should be clean and tidy. The reception desk should be free from clutter with confidential material safely out of sight (Fig. 1-2). Restock your desk with necessary forms and office supplies before patients arrive. In smaller offices you may be responsible for checking the examination rooms.

This process should not take long. The office should never be left messy or in disarray at the end of the day. Stocking of supplies and cleaning and disinfecting examination rooms should be done before the staff leaves at night. The office should be left in a professional manner.

Retrieve Messages

Another responsibility you may have as a receptionist is to retrieve messages that were left while the office was closed. All physician offices have a method for communicating with their patients after hours. Most offices leave a voice message on their main incoming line that directs patients to call a given number (answering service) for acute medical problems. Usually, this message also instructs patients to leave nonemergency messages on the voice mail.

Messages may be obtained from four sources:

- Answering service
- Voice mail system
- Electronic mail
- Facsimile machine

No matter how a message has been sent, however, all information must be treated confidentially.

Messages should be checked as soon as the office opens, at midday, after breaks, and periodically throughout the day. After retrieving the messages, forward them to the appropriate staff for resolution.

Answering service. Answering services receive calls from patients, hospital staff, and other physicians and communicate the emergency messages to the physician, generally by beeper. Other messages are left for the office staff to obtain the following morning. Examples of messages that could be left here:

- Patients calling the office for a sick appointment (not an emergency) (such as an earache, flulike symptoms)
- Calls from hospitals or skilled nursing facilities about changes in patient status (new wounds or bed sores, patient falls without injury)

Voice mail systems. A voice mailbox is a type of answering machine in which the caller can leave a detailed message. You will need to know the security access code to obtain messages. After you obtain the messages, delete them from the recorder unless otherwise directed by office policy. Examples of messages that could be left here are

- Patients wishing to change or cancel their appointment
- Patients requesting prescription refills

- Family members or patients calling to ask for additional information or clarification about their medical care or test results

Electronic mail. The computer is a vital link for physicians to communicate with all health care professionals. E-mail messages are sent from other physicians, professional organizations, and hospital personnel. Some physician offices provide patients with their E-mail address. Examples of messages left here are

- Memos from professional organizations
- Pharmaceutical representatives' updates or announcements
- Medical staff meeting minutes, announcements from hospital administration
- Upcoming continuing education courses for physicians
- Insurance representatives regarding billing issues

Facsimile machines. All physician offices have a fax machine. The most common messages left here are

- Patient referrals
- Consultation reports
- Laboratory and radiology reports

Checkpoint Question

2. What four locations should you retrieve messages from?

Prepare the Charts

Your next duty will be to gather charts. Gather the charts of all of the patients scheduled to be seen for the day and put them in order by appointment. Review each chart to ensure that it is complete and up to date. Check that adequate clinical data sheets are available for the doctor to record any notes. Test results received since the patient's last appointment and any other new information are placed in the front of the chart for the doctor's review. Make up a chart for each new patient and have the appropriate registration forms ready for the patient to complete. Once the charts are prepared, they are usually kept at the reception desk and given to the doctor or clinical assistant as the patient arrives, although some doctors prefer to have all charts on their desk at the start of the day.

Welcome Patients and Visitors

Make every attempt to greet patients personally and by name, e.g., "Good morning, Ms. Misko." A smile and cheerful greeting promote a positive image and make the patient feel welcome. Try to remember something personal about each patient, such as hobbies, pets, or special interests about which you can ask. Sometimes, you will not be at your desk when a patient arrives. Check the waiting room for new arrivals upon your return. Many offices install a bell or chime on the door and post a sign requesting patients to check in with the receptionist.

Register and Orient Patients

Patients who are new to the office will have to complete a registration form, also called a patient information sheet. On this form the patient provides name, address, and telephone number; the name, address, and telephone number of the insurance company or other party responsible for payment; employer names and addresses; marital status; spouse's name; social security number; and name of the person who referred the patient. Some information sheets include questions

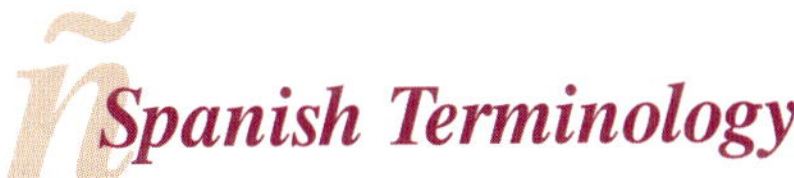

Spanish Terminology

¡Hola!	*Hello!*
¿Cómo se llama usted?	*What is your name?*
¿En qué puedo servirle?	*May I help you?*
¿Cuál es su dirección?	*What is your address?*
¿Cuál es el código postal?	*What is the zip code?*
¿Cuál es su número de teléfono?	*What is your phone number?*
¿Fecha de nacimiento?	*What is your birth date?*
¿Cuántos años tiene?	*How old are you?*
Por favor, sientese en la sala de espera.	*Please have a seat in the waiting room.*
Necesito hacerle unas preguntas.	*I need to ask you some questions.*
Por favor, llene estos papeles.	*Please fill out these papers.*

about medical history. In some cases, you may complete the form while interviewing the patient. Most offices have the patients fill in these forms and ask for your help if questions arise.

After registration, orient the patient to the office. Brochures that give the names of the doctor and staff, office hours, and telephone numbers are helpful. Explain any pertinent office policies or procedures, such as billing procedures, how to make or cancel appointments, and parking. Ask if the patient has any questions. Tell the patient where the water fountain and restrooms are, but caution the patient against using the restroom without checking with you to determine whether a urine specimen is needed. Urine specimens are generally needed for pregnant patients, patients with lower back or abdominal pain or back injuries, and patients being seen for drug or preemployment health examinations. At the appropriate time, you may be responsible for taking patients to the examination room unless another health care worker escorts the patients.

Manage Waiting Time

Patients expect to be seen at the appointed time. They have allotted time in their schedule to see the doctor and do not want to be kept waiting. One of the major complaints of patients is the length of time they must wait to see the physician. Be sure to tell the patients if the doctor is behind schedule. If you expect the wait to be 30 minutes or more past the scheduled time, offer waiting patients some choices. Some choose to leave and come back in an hour, and some choose to reschedule the appointment for another time.

Ergonomic Concerns for the Receptionist

For most of the day you will be sitting at your desk performing these tasks. Occasional lifting of delivery boxes, paper supplies, and so on is required. The duties of the receptionist require you to twist from your primary desk to other areas to reach for files or to answer the telephone. These actions can lead to back injuries and other musculoskeletal disorders. Medical professionals are at high risk for such injuries. Having a good **ergonomic** workstation and good body mechanics, however, can prevent most injuries.

An ergonomic workstation is designed specifically to prevent injuries and often results in increased employee satisfaction and work efficiency. The Occupational Safety and Health Administration (OSHA) has many recommendations for preventing such injuries. Box 1-1 offers workstation recommendations. Here are some other suggestions to prevent injuries:

- Keep items that you must lift at waist level when possible. Keep the load close to the body. Bend at your hips.
- Instruct delivery people to place packages in locations that will not require movement.
- Carry only small loads of paper. Make additional trips as needed.

Box 1-1

ERGONOMIC WORKSTATION RECOMMENDATIONS

The following is a list of recommendations to prevent injuries:

- Your head and neck should be upright, not bent down. All desks should lead you to face forward, not twist. Objects should be within reach to allow your arms to stay close to your body, not extended. Forearms, wrists, and hands should be parallel to the ground. Your thighs should be parallel and your legs perpendicular to the floor.
- Chairs should be appropriate size. The backrest should touch the lumbar area and be strong enough to provide lumbar support. Seats should be cushioned and rounded. The seat should press against the back of your legs or knees. Armrests should support both forearms and not interfere with movement. Your feet should rest flat on the floor or on a stable footrest.
- Desks should be large enough to accommodate all needed equipment. There should be clearance between your thighs and the desk. Nothing should be stored under the desk if it limits your mobility.
- Carpets should be flat and not have a thick pile.
- Upper drawers of file cabinets should not be used if they are above your head and require reaching. Lower drawers should not hold files that require constant access, as this causes excessive bending.

- Place items that you frequently use within easy reach. Moves from side to side are safer than twisting to a desk behind you. Avoid storing charts above chest level to limit reaching over your head. Use a step stool to reach high shelves instead of stretching.
- Telephones with headsets will keep your head upright and allow your shoulders to relax. If you use a stationary phone, a long handset cord can reduce muscle strain. Do not rest the telephone on your shoulder while talking, since this causes neck and back injuries.

Checkpoint Question

3. What is the purpose of having an ergonomic workstation?

The Waiting Room Environment

General Guidelines for Waiting Rooms

The reception area should be designed for the comfort, safety, and enjoyment of all patients. It should be kept clean and uncluttered, with the furniture arranged to allow ample room for walking. A coat rack and umbrella stand should be present. Restrooms and a water fountain should be easily accessible.

Furniture should be aesthetically pleasing, comfortable, and durable. Chairs are preferable to sofas because most people find sharing a sofa with strangers uncomfortable. Chairs allow patients to maintain a degree of privacy and personal space. There should be a variety of soft chairs and firm chairs and chairs with and without arms. Some patients find it hard to stand up from a soft chair; others prefer the comfort. Some need chair arms to push themselves up, and others are more comfortable without chair arms.

A low-key color scheme is advisable. Muted pastels are preferable to bright primary colors, although the latter work well in pediatric offices. Lighting should be bright but not harsh. The room should be well ventilated and kept at a comfortable temperature. Many offices provide soothing background music.

Landscapes, waterscapes, and floral and animal pictures make better wall décor than abstract art. Lamps and plants can add interest to corners. Keep plants in good condition and remove any dead leaves. An office with dead or dying plants does not project a comforting image.

A good selection of reading material should be available. Have a variety of current magazines that are appropriate for your patients. The doctor's professional journals should not be included. The reception area is a good place to set out patient education materials.

Some offices provide television for patients who prefer not to read. Most patients find television relaxing and entertaining, but other patients find it annoying. Television can serve as an education tool. Here are a few tips that you should follow regarding television:

- The volume should be set to allow a group of people to hear the television but not at a distracting volume for the whole waiting room.
- A simple sign placed on the television, "Please do not touch the controls; see the receptionist for channel changes" will prevent patients from selecting inappropriate programs.
- Only family-oriented programs should be shown. It is acceptable to select a news channel. No shows with violence, strong language, or sexual content should be on. Soap operas are not suitable for medical office waiting rooms.
- Some offices leave the television off unless a patient asks to have it on.
- Patients with hearing impairments must be offered the option of **closed captioning** if they choose to watch television. (Closed captioning is the translation of the spoken word into a written format. Most televisions have this capability under their options menu.)

You should check the waiting room several times during the day to make sure it is clean and tidy. Also check the entrance, hallways, and stairs. These areas too must be well lighted and maintained. Liability is a concern if patients slip on ice or snow coming into the office.

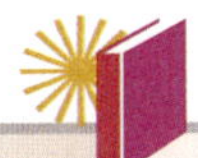

Patient Education

Television as a Teaching Tool

A television in the reception area can entertain patients while they wait for an appointment, but it can also be a patient education tool. By using a television in conjunction with a VCR, you can play a variety of educational videos. Here are some points to keep in mind:

- Be sure all videos have been previewed by the physician.
- Select videos that are geared toward the specialty of the practice (e.g., a video about heart attacks is appropriate for a cardiologist's office but not for a dermatologist's office).
- Carefully assess the graphic nature of certain videos. (A picture of the birth of a child may interest you but be too much for certain patients.)
- Keep in mind the age of the patients and family members who will be in the waiting room. Caution must be used if small children are often in the area. For example, a video about preventing sexually transmitted diseases may provide information appropriate for a family practice office, but it would not be appropriate to show the video in the reception area.

Checkpoint Question

4. What option should you offer hearing impaired patients if they wish to watch television?

Guidelines for Pediatric Waiting Rooms

Pediatric offices tend to be very busy practices with a multitude of reasons for patient visits. Generally, visits to the pediatrician can be divided into three types: well child checks, sick child visits, and follow-up visits. Because of the large volume of sick child visits, most pediatric waiting room areas are broken into two sections, one for well children and the other for sick children. Parents may have to be instructed by you as to which side of the waiting room they should sit in. According to the American Academy of Pediatrics (AAP), no studies document the effectiveness of segregated waiting room areas. The recommendation of the AAP is to move children with a communicable disease into an examination room as quickly as possible. Your employer will provide you with instructions and guidelines for dealing with sick children.

A children's play area must be closely watched and monitored. Toys should be kept away from the general seating area. Here are some guidelines for toys:

- Toys should be simple and easy to clean, without sharp edges.
- A policy must be in place for routine cleaning of these toys.
- Toys should be checked daily to ensure that they are not broken. Toys that are broken must be thrown away. Toys should never be glued or taped together.
- Battery-powered toys that make loud noises are not permissible.
- Toys can be a choking hazard. According to the American Heart Association, small children should never to be given toys that can fit inside a standard toilet paper roll. Although older children would like to play with toys like Legos, these toys should not be present. Older children should be expected to sit quietly while waiting for their appointment.

A good selection of books should be present for parents to read to their children. Books must be checked periodically to ensure that they are clean and no pages have been torn out. A small table and chairs will give children a place to read or color.

Americans with Disabilities Act Requirements

The U. S. Department of Justice is responsible for ensuring that all people are treated without discrimination of any kind. Under this department is the Americans with Disabilities Act (ADA). This act prohibits discrimination on the basis of a person's disability. The ADA Title III act requires that all public accommodations be accessible to everyone. This includes access into medical facilities. It is important that you be aware of the basic concept of the ADA rules. Table 1-2 lists some of the basic facility requirements. Additional information is available on the ADA website.

The existing structural dimensions are not something that you have control of, but you need to ensure that there is a clear path to the physician's office at all times. Here are some steps that you can take to ensure this:

- Check that deliveries are left in a safe place. They must not be left in the waiting area or block the door.
- Keep toys clear of entrance pathways.
- Check that chairs are not moved, creating obstacles that might limit wheelchair accessibility.
- Ensure that doors are not blocked or propped opened with objects.

Table 1-2 SUMMARY OF ADA REQUIREMENTS FOR PUBLIC BUILDINGS

Area	Specifics
Access	Route must be stable, firm, and slip resistant. Route must be 36 inches wide.
Ramps	Ramps longer than 6 feet must have two railings. Railings must be 34–38 inches high. Ramp must be 36 inches wide. Ramps and elevators must be available to all public levels.
Entrance and door	Door must be 32 inches wide. Door handle must be no higher than 48 inches and must be operable with a closed fist. Interior doors must open without excessive force.
Miscellaneous	Carpeting must be no more than 0.5 inch high. Emergency egress system must have flashing lights and audible signals. Space for wheelchair seating must be available. Tables or counters must be 28–34 inches high.
Restrooms	Tactile signs must identify restrooms. Doorway must be at least 32 inches wide. All doors (including stall doors), soap dispensers, hand dryers, and faucets must be operable with a closed fist. Wheelchair stall is required and must be at least 5 feet by 5 feet.

What If

A patient brings in his seeing eye dog and asks, "Can I keep the dog with me in the office?" What would you say?

The Americans with Disabilities Act (ADA) prohibits businesses from banning service animals. A service animal is defined as any guide dog or other animal that is trained to provide assistance to a person with a disability. The animal does not have to be licensed or certified by the state as a service animal. Examples of duties that service animals perform include alerting to sounds patients with hearing impairments, pulling wheelchairs for spinal cord injury patients, picking up items for patients with mobility impairments, sensing smells or auras for seizure patients, and assisting patients with visual impairments. The service animal should not be separated from its owner and must be allowed to enter the examination room with the patient. The ADA law supersedes local health department regulations that ban animals in health care centers. The care of the service animal is the sole responsibility of its owner.

- Limit the amount of stacked papers on counters that may limit the patient's access to you.
- Check the restroom regularly to make sure the entrance is open and not obstructed.

Checkpoint Question

5. What act prohibits discrimination of patients with disabilities?

Infection Control Issues

To prevent the spread of disease, aseptic technique must be used in every aspect of work in the medical office. During the clinical portion of your training, you will learn detailed information about infection control. As a receptionist, however, you need to be aware of a few key points:

- Always follow standard precautions. This means that you must treat all body fluids with precautionary measures.
- Handwashing is the most important practice for preventing the transmission of diseases. You must wash your hands following all direct patient contact (touching the patient) (Fig. 1-3). Since it is not always possible to leave the desk to wash your hands, the CDC has approved the use of alcohol-based antiseptic handwashing solutions for health care providers.
- Patients are often told to bring specimens to the office. Never touch a specimen container without proper gloves and personal protective equipment.
- Patients who arrive coughing and sneezing should be given tissues and instructed to cover their mouth and nose when coughing. Communicate with the clinical staff to have these patients taken directly into examination rooms. Patients who are vomiting, bleeding, or discharging other body fluids must not be left in the waiting room.

Biohazard Waste. All body fluids must be considered infectious and be managed appropriately. All body fluid spills and blood-stained papers must be disposed of in a biohazard container. The spills must be cleaned with an approved germicidal solution. If you have not been trained in handling such waste, do not touch it. Allow the clinical staff to handle the waste. If possible, contain the spill and prevent other patients

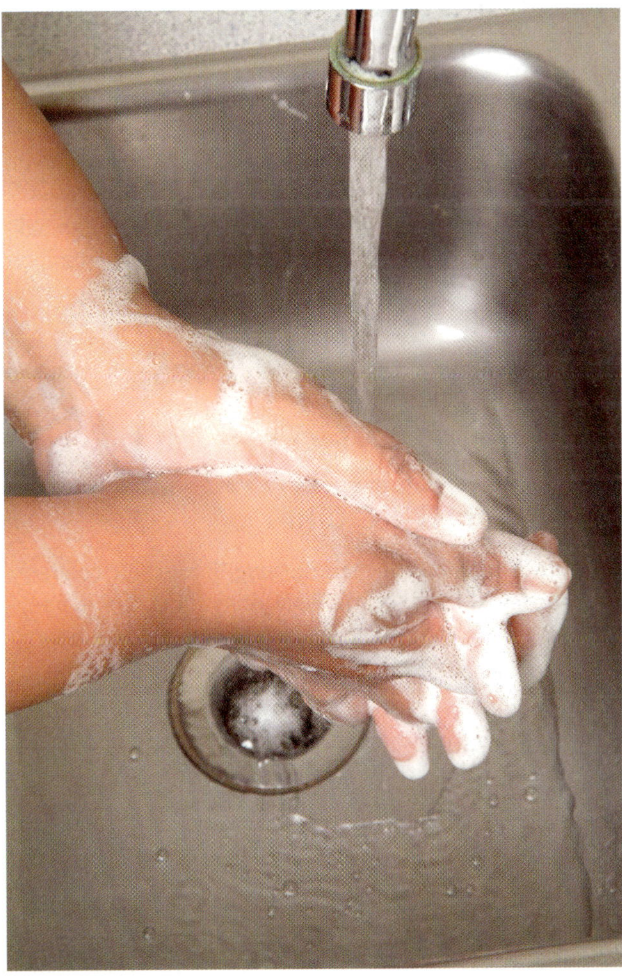

Figure 1-3. Good handwashing skills are essential to prevent disease transmission.

from touching the area. Here are some examples of biohazard waste that you may encounter:

- Dressing supplies with bloodstains from cuts or wounds
- Tissues from patients with acute nosebleeds
- Urine-saturated diapers left in the restroom
- Vomit
- Saturated tissues with sputum

Communicable Diseases. Depending on the type of office you work in, the amount of exposure to communicable diseases will vary. Family practice physicians and pediatricians, for example, treat acute communicable diseases regularly. If you work as a receptionist for a pediatrician, you will need to learn how to look at rashes and determine whether they are contagious.

Good communication between you and the clinical staff is essential to manage patients with communicable diseases. The clinical staff is often aware of patients with such diseases and will communicate it to you. Most infectious diseases can't be transmitted with routine physical contact (handshaking, talking, touching, sharing pencils, using the telephone). Examples of infectious diseases that can't be transmitted by routine physical contact include HIV, hepatitis, and the common cold. Some diseases can be easily transmitted, however, and patients with these diseases should not be left in the waiting room. Box 1-2 lists patients who should not be left in the waiting room.

Patients who have an impaired immune system or are taking medications that hinder their immune system (chemotherapy agents) may require immediate placement in an examination room to prevent exposure to otherwise benign organisms. The clinical staff will alert you to these patients.

Checkpoint Question

6. What is the most antiseptic technique for preventing the transmission of diseases?

The End of the Patient Visit

After physicians have completed the examination or other procedures, they generally direct patients to get dressed and wait for their discharge information. In some offices, physicians provide all discharge instructions, while in other office settings nurses or medical assistants may be assigned to discharge patients. After the medical portion is completed, the patient is escorted to the front desk. It is generally at this time that any fees or copayments are collected by the receptionist. If the doctor has requested a follow-up visit, the appointment should be scheduled. An appointment reminder card is helpful for the patient. You or other administrative personnel may do these tasks. You should bid the patient goodbye in a warm and friendly manner. As patients leave the office, they should feel they have been well cared for by a competent and courteous staff.

Box 1-2

PATIENTS WHO SHOULD NOT BE LEFT IN THE WAITING ROOM

Patients with any of the following diseases or conditions should not be left in the waiting room. These patients should be taken to an examination room as soon as possible:

- Chickenpox
- Conjunctivitis
- Influenza
- Measles and rubella
- Meningitis (or suspected cases)
- Mumps
- Pertussis
- Pneumonia (if patient is coughing)
- Smallpox
- Tuberculosis
- Wounds (if open and draining)

TELEPHONE

Importance of the Telephone in the Medical Office

The medical office is filled with expensive scientific equipment used in the diagnosis and treatment of disease, but one of the most important instruments is the telephone. It allows the patient rapid and easy access to medical care. A patient can schedule an appointment, seek medical advice, request prescription refills, obtain test results, question a bill, or report an emergency simply by picking up the telephone. The telephone also links the physician's office to the rest of the medical community, including hospitals, pharmacies, and other doctors.

You must be able to communicate a positive image of the physician and staff over the telephone without the aid of nonverbal cues such as appearance, facial expressions, body language, and gestures. You must be able to use the tone and quality of your voice and speech to project a competent and caring attitude over the telephone.

Basic Guidelines for Telephone Use

Telephone communication is not effective if either party does not fully understand what is being said. Misunderstandings can be embarrassing, frustrating, or even life-threatening. To have effective telephone communication, you must be able to overcome various obstacles, such as a

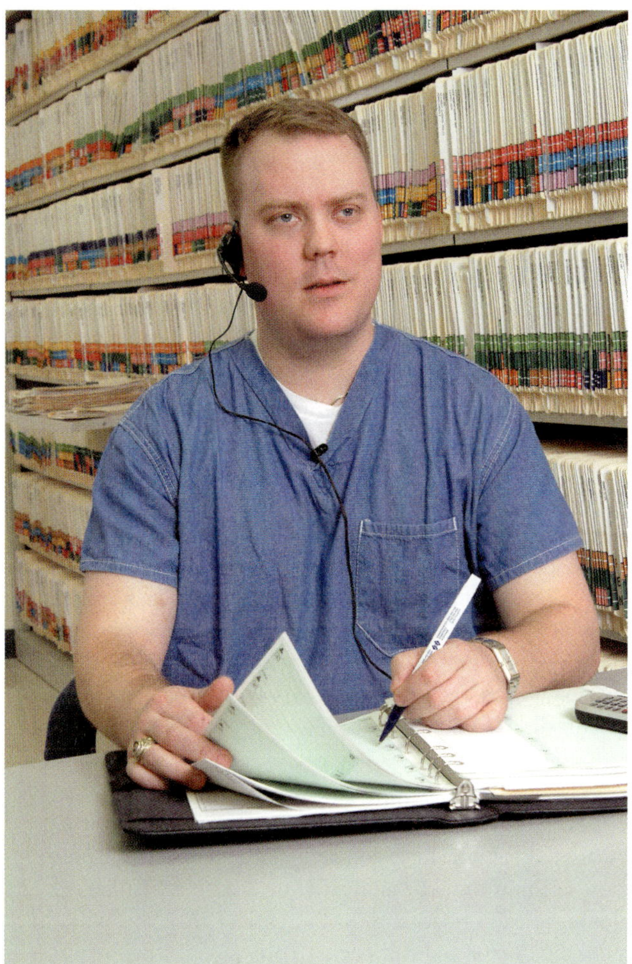

FIGURE 1-4. While speaking on the telephone, be courteous and professional.

noisy environment, a poor telephone connection, a patient's emotional distress, or a patient's hearing or speech impairments (Fig. 1-4).

Diction

Diction refers to how words are spoken and enunciated. You should speak clearly and distinctly. Talk clearly into the mouthpiece; do not prop the handset between your chin and shoulder. Never chew gum or eat while you speak on the telephone. Speak at a moderate pace to avoid slurring your words.

Pronunciation

Make sure you pronounce words correctly to avoid misunderstandings. Avoid using unfamiliar words, slang, and idiomatic expressions. Most patients do not understand medical terminology, so it is best to use lay terms whenever possible. For example, do not ask the patient, "Are you dyspneic?" Instead ask, "Are you having trouble breathing?"

Expression

Put a smile in your voice by sitting up straight and putting a smile on your lips. Speak with a modulated pitch and volume. Use proper inflection to avoid a droning, monotonous speaking style.

Listening

Be an attentive listener. Focus on the conversation and ignore outside distractions. Do not interrupt the speaker. You may have to ask the caller to repeat what was said. Verify your understanding by repeating the message.

Courtesy

Always speak politely and courteously. Address the caller by title and last name. Although many telephone calls interrupt your work, do not allow your voice to betray impatience or irritation. Remember that you are there to help the patient.

Never answer the telephone and immediately put the caller on hold. If you need to answer another line or finish a task before you can engage in conversation, ask if the caller would mind holding. Courtesy demands that you wait for an answer before you place the call on hold. Also of great importance, you must determine whether the call is an emergency. If you are unable to take the call after 90 seconds, check back with the caller and ask whether he or she would like to continue holding. Again, wait for an answer before you place the call on hold. If the hold exceeds 3 minutes, you should apologize to the caller for the delay and offer to return the call as soon as you are available.

If you are already engaged in a telephone conversation and have to answer another line, ask the party with whom you are speaking if he or she would mind holding. Again, wait for a reply before answering the second call. Explain to the second caller that you are on the other line and need to complete that call. Do not handle the second call while the first party waits unless the second call is an emergency, a long distance call that cannot be referred to another worker, or a physician calling to speak with your physician.

Quite often you will find that you are juggling the telephones and patients who are in the office. Exercise your best judgment in balancing the two tasks. If the call is going to take a long time, ask the caller to wait a moment, address the needs of the patient in the office, and then return to the call. Use caution when talking on the telephone in front of patients. Remember, all information about and conversations with patients are confidential.

Checkpoint Question

7. What are the five basic guidelines for telephone use?

Routine Incoming Calls

An incoming call should be given the same courtesy and attention as an arriving visitor. Just as you would not keep a patient waiting without acknowledging his or her presence, so you must acknowledge an incoming call promptly. Answer the telephone by the second ring if at all possible. Identify both the office and yourself to assure the caller that the correct number has been reached, and offer your assistance. The following are examples of common calls that come into a medical office.

Appointments

New patients call to make appointments and established patients call to schedule return visits.

Billing Inquiries

In some offices you may be responsible for handling routine inquiries concerning billing, fees, services, and insurance. You may be asked for specific information concerning the cost of services; do not quote exact prices but tell the patient that costs depend on the type of examination and diagnostic tests performed. Sometimes, third-party callers request information about the patient; remember that no patient information can be given to anyone without a specific release from the patient.

Diagnostic Test Results

Many laboratory and radiology reports are called in to the physician's office before the written copy is sent. Record the information and post it on the front of the chart for the physician to review. If the results are needed at once, bring the information to the physician's attention immediately upon receiving the report. Having at hand a blank laboratory slip or specially designed forms listing the most frequently ordered reports for your office will save time and make it easier to accurately record the results as they are relayed from the laboratory or radiology department. Administrative personnel will place a written copy of test results in the patient's chart.

Routine and Satisfactory Progress Reports

At the end of an office visit a patient may be told to call in a progress report within a few days. If the patient says he or she is feeling better or getting stronger or the symptoms have resolved, take down the information, record it in the patient's chart, and place it on the physician's desk for review. You may also handle routine progress reports from hospitals, home health agencies, and other allied health professionals. For example, a home care nurse may call and report that a patient's blood pressure is now within normal limits, or a physical therapist may call the office and to say that a patient's range of motion is improving. Again, record the information and place it on the physician's desk for review.

Test Results

Patients often call for their test results, and many doctors allow the medical assistant to report favorable test results to patients. Your office will have a specific policy for handling these calls. It is illegal to give information to anyone other than the patient without the patient's specific consent.

Unsatisfactory Progress Reports and Test Results

The doctor must speak with patients whose progress or test results are unsatisfactory. The urgency of the patient's condition determines whether the call requires the physician's immediate attention. The physician will discuss serious unsatisfactory test results with the patient. In less serious cases, the physician may ask you to speak with the patient. Never discuss unsatisfactory test results with a patient unless the doctor directs you to do so.

Prescription Refills

As a medical assistant, you can handle requests for prescription refills if they are indicated on the chart. If there is any doubt, tell the pharmacy or the patient that you will check with the doctor and call back.

Other Calls

Other calls you ordinarily handle include requests for referrals to other physicians, clarifying instructions for patients, and calls concerning routine administrative matters.

Ask the physician which calls he or she prefers to have transferred immediately and which calls can be returned later. Calls from other physicians should be directed to the physician immediately or according to office policy. Physicians also receive personal calls. Your employer will tell you which calls should be put through immediately. Otherwise, take a message and tell the caller that the doctor will return the call.

Challenging Incoming Calls

Unidentified Callers

Sometimes, callers who ask to speak with the physician refuse to state their name or the nature of their business. In such instances you should politely but firmly tell the caller that you can't interrupt the physician and politely explain that you would be happy to take a message. If the caller persists, ask the caller to call back at a specific time when the physician will be available. Alert the physician that there will be a call for him or her at the specified time. Unidentified callers may be sales representatives.

Irate Patients

When a caller is angry, you must be careful to keep your own temper in check. Try to calm the patient and offer assurance that you want to help. Listen carefully and take notes. If you cannot resolve the situation, let the patient know you must consult with the physician and offer to call back. The physician will probably want to speak with the patient personally. Always tell the physician about complaints regarding fees or care.

Medical Emergencies

As a medical assistant, you must be able to differentiate between routine calls and emergencies. To do this, first try to calm the caller and ask specific questions concerning the patient's condition. Severe pain, profuse bleeding, respiratory distress, chest pain, loss of consciousness, severe vomiting or diarrhea, and a temperature above 102.08F are all emergencies, and you should immediately put the call through to the physician or an appropriate health care professional. In some offices, nurses will be assigned to handle these calls.

Determine the patient's name, location, and telephone number as quickly as possible in case you are disconnected or the patient is unable to continue the conversation. This will allow you to direct emergency personnel to the patient's aid. The office should have a policy for handling emergency calls when the doctor is not in the office. Most policies advise you to direct patients to go to the nearest emergency room or walk-in center.

Ask the physician to list instances that might constitute an emergency in his or her specialty and to describe how they should be handled. For example, if you work for a cardiologist, most of your emergency calls will be patients with chest pain and trouble breathing. The cardiologist may instruct you to ask the patient standard questions, have you instruct patients to take certain medications, and then instruct the patient to dial for an ambulance. If you are working for an obstetrician, your emergency calls will be related to patients who have labor concerns or sudden onset of bleeding. Most obstetricians have precise recommendations for when patients in labor should go to the hospital (e.g., contractions lasting more than 1 minute with a frequency of every 5 minutes). Once you have the list of the most common calls and what your response should be, put the list in a prominent place near the telephone.

Triaging Incoming Calls

Usually the office telephone has multiple lines, and frequently several patients call at the same time. You must be able to **triage** (sort) them into a priority order. How would you sort these four calls?

- Line 1: Caller wants to make an appointment for her son, who has a 101.3°F fever.
- Line 2: Caller wants to see the doctor this afternoon because he is having chest pain.
- Line 3: Caller is upset because she has been disconnected 3 times and has a question about her bill.
- Line 4: Caller needs a prescription refill.

Who would you take first? Why? Last? Why?

Any patient with a potentially life-threatening problem needs to be taken first. Therefore, talk first to caller 2. Follow your office policy for emergencies. Sometimes, a nurse will further assess the emergency or the patient may be directed to call 911. The caller on line 3 needs attention next. The longer she waits, the more upset and difficult to please she will be. Explain to the patient that you have to get the bill and chart, and ask for a phone number where you can call her back. Make the appointment for the caller on line 1. Again, follow your office policies regarding patient care issues. Caller 4 is last. Remember, you need to get back to caller 3 promptly. Do not leave messages unresolved.

Taking Messages

Taking messages for the physician or other health care professionals will be a large part of your daily responsibilities. Taking messages is easier using notepads designed for this task. Office supply companies have an assortment of pads, or your physician may choose to design his or her own. Carbonless copies give you a record of the messages taken during the day and the action taken.

The minimum information needed for a telephone message includes the name of the caller, date and time of the call, telephone number where the caller can be reached, a short description of the caller's concern, and the person to whom the message is routed.

Before you end the call, tell the patient when to expect a return call. Callback times vary from office to office. Some physicians return calls only at the end of the day, while others return calls randomly. Learn the policy of the office in which you are working.

The patient's chart must document all calls. If you return the call to the patient, document your conversation in the medical record. Some message pads are designed to be added to the progress note on the patient's chart when the call is complete.

Checkpoint Question

8. What is the minimum information needed for taking messages?

Outgoing Calls

General Guidelines for Outgoing Calls

You will make outgoing calls as well as receive incoming calls. You should prepare for your calls carefully; have all information gathered and know what you want to say before you dial the number. If you are calling a patient to reschedule an appointment, be able to explain why the change is necessary and be prepared to offer a new appointment time.

At times you may have to make long distance calls. Keep in mind the difference in time zones; if you do not know the time zone of the city you are calling, check the front of the telephone directory. Long distance calls should be dialed directly, without operator assistance. If you dial a wrong number or become disconnected during the call, notify the long distance operator immediately to avoid charges.

Your employer may ask you to place a conference call, which connects three or more people. Notify all parties of the date and time the call will be made to ensure that everyone will be available to participate. Participants should be given the access phone number and the access code in advance of the scheduled call.

Calling Emergency Medical Services

Some patients will need immediate transport to a hospital. When emergencies occur in the physician's office, the clinical staff will be busy providing lifesaving procedures to the patient. As a receptionist, you will be directed to call the local **emergency medical service (EMS)** for transport. In most areas of the United States, the emergency number is 911. Prior to placing the call, obtain the following information:

- Patient's name, age, and sex. (Age is important, especially if the patient is a newborn or child. This will allow the dispatcher to send the most appropriate responders.)
- Nature of the medical problem (chest pain, abdominal pain, bleeding).
- Type of service the physician is requesting. Generally, there are two levels of care: basic and advanced life support. Types of services will vary from community to community.
- Any specific instructions or requests the physician may have. Generally, patients are taken to the nearest hospital; the physician may have made arrangements for the patient to be admitted at a specific hospital, however, because of a condition or diagnosis. For example, a patient with a high-risk pregnancy may be sent to a hospital with an appropriate newborn nursery instead of the community hospital. It is important that this information be told to the dispatcher so the appropriate team can be sent.
- The location of the office and any specific instructions for access, e.g., 92 Main Street, Medical Office Group, third floor, last door on the left.

After gathering the information, dial the emergency medical service number. Speak in a slow, calm voice to the dispatcher. Give the information. If the dispatcher has additional questions, answer them. Ask the dispatcher the approximate arrival time for the ambulance. Do not end the call until instructed to do so by the dispatcher.

After placing the call, alert the staff to the approximate arrival time and any other pertinent information. Ensure that the path for the ambulance personnel is unobstructed and accessible. Reassure other patients in the waiting room. If the patient has any family members present, offer them assistance and reassurance.

Checkpoint Question

9. What patient information should you know before calling emergency medical services?

Services and Special Features

The telephone system that is used for physician offices should be large enough to serve the needs of the office. For example, if you are working for a single dermatologist, two incoming phone lines may be enough. If you are a receptionist for a large family practice with multiple physicians and other practitioners, however, the number of incoming lines will be greater. Most offices also have unpublished incoming numbers or lines. Staff members, families, and other physicians primarily use these private lines. In addition, most offices have a direct line to the local hospital. A wide variety of communication equipment is available today, and communications consultants can help determine the appropriate services and equipment for your office. At minimum, the phone system should have recall, volume control, intercom, call forwarding, and caller identification. Cordless headsets prevent neck injuries and allow for mobility.

Most physicians have a cellular telephone. This number should never be given to anyone, although it should be readily accessible for staff members. Physicians and other health care professionals also have pager systems. Most pager systems allow you to send typed messages to the recipient via the computer. These messages are displayed on the pager, e.g., "Kate Larke's blood sugar was 420," or "Please call Dr. Harrison about Patrick Burke." Typing messages directly into a pager system is good time management.

Telecommunication Relay Systems

Patients with hearing or speech impairments often have difficulty communicating with a standard telephone. The ADA requires that telephone companies have telecommunication relay systems (TRS) available 24 hours a day (Fig. 1-5). A relay system allows the caller to type messages into a special telephone that transmits the message across the lines to the

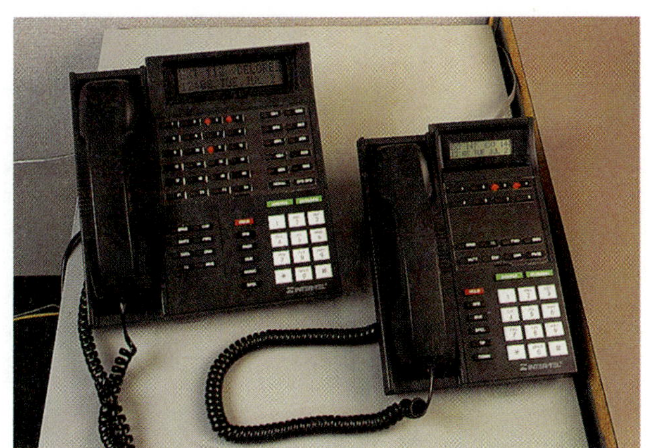

FIGURE 1-5. Various telephone systems.

other party. The other party reads the message and types a response. The communication continues through written messages. A telephone with an attachment for typing messages is called a **teletypewriter** (TTY). If the other party does not have the capabilities to read the message, an operator can be used to translate the message. Most physician offices have a TTY phone or access to one. The Federal Communication Commission has set minimum standards for TRS and TTY systems for public buildings. These standards can be found on their website.

Procedure 1-1

Handling Incoming Calls

Equipment/Supplies

- Telephone
- Telephone message pad
- Writing utensil (pen or pencil)
- Headset (if applicable)

Steps	Purpose
1. Gather the needed equipment.	Ensures that all materials are available and ready for use.
2. Answer the phone within two rings.	Demonstrates professionalism and courtesy to the caller.
3. Greet caller with proper identification (your name and the name of the office).	Demonstrates professionalism and courtesy to the caller.
4. Identify the nature or reason for the call in a timely manner.	Allows the call to be appropriately managed.
5. Triage the call appropriately.	Prompt identification of emergency calls is important for good patient care.
6. Communicate in a professional manner and with unhurried speech.	Demonstrates compassion and caring for the patient. An unhurried speech pattern is reassuring to the patient.
7. Clarify information as needed.	Prevents errors in communication.
8. Record the message on a message pad. Include name of caller, date, time, telephone number where the caller can be reached, description of the caller's concerns, and person to whom the message is routed.	Promotes good communication between you and the recipient of the message.
9. Give the caller an approximate time for a return call.	Provides reassurance to the patient that the call will be handled promptly and timely.
10. Ask the caller whether he or she has any additional questions or needs any other help.	Confirms that the patient's needs have been met.
11. Allow the caller to disconnect first.	Ensures that the caller has completed the communication.
12. Put the message in an appropriate place.	Ensures that the call will be handled correctly and the intended recipient gets the information.
13. Complete the task within 10 minutes.	Ensures that the call is handled promptly and efficiently.

Procedure 1-2

Calling Emergency Medical Services

Equipment/Supplies

- Telephone
- Writing utensil (pen, pencil)
- Patient information

Steps	Purpose
1. Obtain the following the information before dialing: patient's name, age, sex, nature of medical condition, type of service the physician is requesting, any special instructions or requests the physician may have, your location and any special information for access.	Information is necessary for quick and correct dispatch of EMS personnel. Certain types of patients require special teams for transport.
2. Dial 911 or other EMS number.	Call can't be placed if number is not dialed correctly.
3. Calmly provide the dispatcher with the above information.	Allows information to be communicated quickly and professionally.
4. Answer the dispatcher's questions calmly and professionally.	Allows dispatcher to obtain any additional information and verify the message.
5. Follow the dispatcher's instructions, if applicable.	Following instructions provides good patient care.
6. End the call as per dispatcher instructions.	Ensures that all communication needs have been met.
7. Complete the task within 10 minutes.	Prompt access to EMS promotes good patient care and is essential for good outcomes.

RESPONSIBILITY FOR SCHEDULING and managing the flow of patient care in a medical office or clinic is one of the most important duties assigned to a medical assistant. As appointment manager, you make the first, last, and most durable impression on the patient and **providers**. Depending on your demeanor and actions, that impression can be favorable or unfavorable. A properly used appointment system helps maintain an efficient office. If improperly used, it can mean confusion and chaos; more important, it can waste precious time for the patient, the provider, and the staff.

To use the office facilities and the physician's availability most efficiently, determine which patients will be seen, when they will be seen, and how much time to allot to each of them, depending on their problems. Of course, every practice will have occasional delays and emergencies. Your responsibility is to manage all of this while maintaining a calm, efficient, and polite attitude.

APPOINTMENT SCHEDULING SYSTEMS

There are two systems of appointment scheduling for outpatient medical facilities: the manual system, which uses an appointment book, and a computerized scheduling system. The choice of systems will depend on the size of the practice, how many providers' schedules must be managed, and the preferences of the staff responsible for the daily schedule. Whether a medical office uses a manual or computerized system, many of the guidelines for effectively scheduling the workday discussed in this chapter are the same.

Manual Appointment Scheduling

Medical offices may choose to use a manual appointment scheduling system even if the other administrative functions in the office are computerized.

The Appointment Book

If your medical office uses a manual system of scheduled appointments for patient office visits, you will need an appointment book. An appointment book provides space for noting appointments for an entire year. It may have a single sheet for each day and a separate page for each provider or show an entire week on two facing pages. Some offices prefer an appointment book with pages showing only one day at a time; others may want to see a whole week at a glance. A different color page for each day may also be desired.

The more information required for scheduling, the larger the pages should be. Make sure the book has enough space for all pertinent information (e.g., patient's name, telephone number, reason for visit), is divided into time units appropriate for your practice (e.g., 10- or 15-minute intervals), can open flat on the desk where it will be used, and fits easily into its storage place when not in use.

Establishing a Matrix

Before you begin using the appointment book, you will have to set up a **matrix**. A matrix is established by crossing out times that providers are unavailable for patient visits (Fig. 2-1). For example, the physician may have a breakfast meeting and not be in the office until 10:00 A.M. This is indicated by crossing out the blocks from 8:00 to 10:00 A.M. Write in the reason for crossing off the space (e.g., vacation, meeting, hospital rounds). Some practices reserve specific times or even days for certain activities, such as physical examinations and surgery. Also, it is advisable to block off 15 to 30 minutes each morning and afternoon to accommodate emergencies, late arrivals, and other delays. Some physicians want their professional or personal obligations noted on the appointment schedule so that patients are not booked immediately before these times.

Once you have acquired and prepared an appointment book, it is not enough to schedule a time and date for a patient visit and hope everything will run smoothly. Before actually making an appointment, you should review the schedule carefully, evaluating the needs of each patient and considering the physician's preferences and availability of the office facilities. At the beginning of each day, copies of the schedule should be distributed to all staff members. Along with the notations in a patient's chart, the

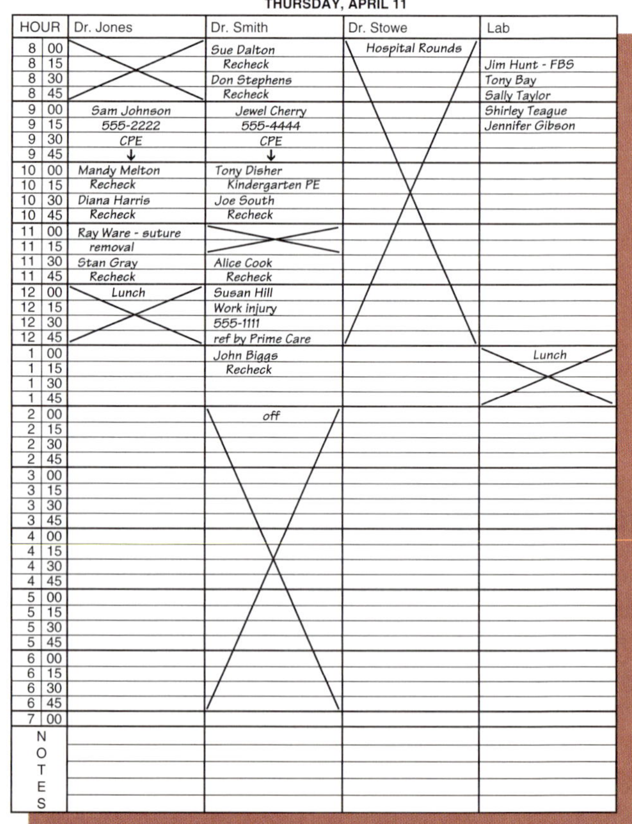

THURSDAY, APRIL 11

HOUR	Dr. Jones	Dr. Smith	Dr. Stowe	Lab
8 00		Sue Dalton	Hospital Rounds	
8 15		Recheck		Jim Hunt - FBS
8 30		Don Stephens		Tony Bay
8 45		Recheck		Sally Taylor
9 00	Sam Johnson	Jewel Cherry		Shirley Teague
9 15	555-2222	555-4444		Jennifer Gibson
9 30	CPE	CPE		
9 45	↓	↓		
10 00	Mandy Melton	Tony Disher		
10 15	Recheck	Kindergarten PE		
10 30	Diana Harris	Joe South		
10 45	Recheck	Recheck		
11 00	Ray Ware - suture			
11 15	removal			
11 30	Stan Gray	Alice Cook		
11 45	Recheck	Recheck		
12 00	Lunch	Susan Hill		
12 15		Work injury		
12 30		555-1111		
12 45		ref by Prime Care		
1 00		John Biggs		Lunch
1 15		Recheck		
1 30				
1 45				
2 00		off		
2 15				
2 30				
2 45				
3 00				
3 15				
3 30				
3 45				
4 00				
4 15				
4 30				
4 45				
5 00				
5 15				
5 30				
5 45				
6 00				
6 15				
6 30				
6 45				
7 00				
NOTES				

FIGURE 2-1. Sample page from manual appointment book.

```
Visual PRO/5
Settings  Edit  Print  Help
PRINT APPOINTMENT SCHEDULES                                  DATE 06/17/03

ENTER:  99-CANCEL   CR-MORE
—
                      <LEONARD H. MCCOY, MD - 18-Jun-03>
 Time  TOA  Patn# Patient Name                 Phone#        Alt.ID#        STS.ID
------------------------------------------------------------------------------------
09:00a OV   5020 JOHNSON, CARMEN L.            336/768-5348 []                 .SS
09:00a
09:15a OV   5024 JENKINS, RHONDA L.            336/768-5348 []                 .SS
09:30a OV   2030 MABE, DONNA NELSON            919/765-8912 [ ]                .SS
09:45a OV   2056 WRIGHT, HENRY SIMON           919/765-8574 [HMO - B1]         .SS
10:00a WI   2235 SMITH, ASHLEY                 003/456-7889 [345]              .SS
10:15a OV   5004 SMITH, WILLIAM                336/768-5348 []                 .SS
10:30a NP   2776 SIMPSON, MARJORIE             336/768-5348 []                 .SS
10:45a OV   5080 BUNNY, GREY                   336/768-5348 []                 .SS
11:00a
12:00p
01:30p NP   2777 COLTRANE, COURTNEY            336/768-5348 []                 .SS
01:45p OV   2060 THOMAS, JEFFERY LEE           919/768-4110 [2060]             .SS
01:45p WI   5024 JENKINS, RHONDA L.            336/768-5348 []                 .SS

— MORE —
```

```
Visual PRO/5
Settings  Edit  Print  Help
PRINT APPOINTMENT SCHEDULES                                  DATE 06/17/03

ENTER:  99-CANCEL   CR-MORE
—
                      <LEONARD H. MCCOY, MD - 18-Jun-03>
 Time  TOA  Patn# Patient Name                 Phone#        Alt.ID#        STS.ID
------------------------------------------------------------------------------------
02:00p CPE  5006 EVANS, RUSSELL                336/768-5348 []                 .SS
02:15p CPE  5006 EVANS, RUSSELL                336/768-5348 []                 .SS
02:30p OV   2768 MORRISON, JAMES               336/768-5348 []                 .SS
02:45p
03:00p OV   2496 BOWERS, MILLIE E              919/475-2401 [LEXNE]            .SS
03:15p NP   2778 SAMUEL, MICHAEL               336/768-5348 []                 .SS
03:45p OV   2015 CARTER, ROY LEE               919/378-2589 [HMO/AMA - B1]     .SS
04:00p RC   2518 CARPENTER, PETER              919/760-0408 []                 .SS
04:10p RC   2545 ZUCKER, CELIA                 910/765-8414 [12487]            .SS
04:15p
04:30p OV   2038 RAGEN, ARTHUR CHARLES         919/765-8524 [MCD - B5]         .SS


— END OF DAY —
```

FIGURE 2-2. A computer-generated appointment schedule with space for all providers of care. (Courtesy of MICA Information Systems, Winston-Salem, North Carolina.)

pages of the appointment book provide documentation of a patient's visits and any changes, such as cancellations and rescheduled appointments. This provides further legal documentation to protect the physician and the patient in case of a dispute.

Computerized Appointment Scheduling

Medical management software designed to assist with administrative functions includes systems for appointment scheduling. Computerized scheduling often saves time. Information used to establish a matrix (e.g., hospital rounds 7:30–8:30, lunch 12:30–1:30) has to be entered only once.

Any medical office software will have an appointment toolbar that requires one click to add a patient, add to the waiting list, see a calendar, or search for available times. Many software packages offer an advanced search that defines the resources required for a certain type of appointment.

This quick method allows you to search for available appointment times. Typically, you enter the desired date, and the computer displays the schedule for that day, showing any available time slots. Another feature allows you to search the appointment database for the next available time slot. For example, a patient is instructed to return in 3 months and has a preference for the time of day. You can search for the first available afternoon appointment with that particular provider.

Depending on the specific software, you can also print numerous documents, such as the daily or weekly appointment schedule, appointment reminders, or billing slips. Once the daily schedule is printed, this important document is referred to as the daily activity sheet or the day sheet and is the guide for everyone involved in the flow of patient care. Figure 2-2 shows a computer-generated daily activity sheet.

An important advantage to computerized appointment scheduling is the easy access to billing information. For example, a patient may call for an appointment, and the medical assistant can inform the patient that he needs to pay his balance due of $32 when he comes in to be seen.

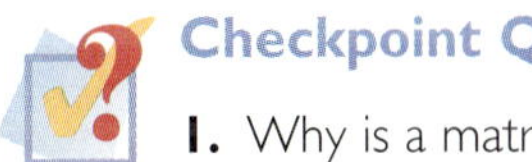

Checkpoint Question

1. Why is a matrix established?

TYPES OF SCHEDULING

Structured Appointments

Most medical offices use a system of structured or scheduled appointments for office visits. Each patient is assigned a time on the schedule and allotted a specific period for examination and treatment. Box 2-1 shows examples of time allotment. The advantages of this system include good time management and optimum use of the office facility. Additionally, a daily schedule may be developed and charts may be prepared in advance of patient arrival.

Box 2-1

HOW MUCH TIME DO I ALLOT?

Every outpatient medical facility has variables that determine the time allotted for each service. Factors like the number of providers, the number of examination rooms, and the size of the office must be considered when establishing the appointment scheduling guidelines. This partial list of typical outpatient services shows an estimate of the time needed for each.

Complete physical examination	1 hour
School physical	30 minutes
Recheck	15 minutes
Dressing change	10 minutes
Blood pressure check	5 minutes
Patient teaching	30 minutes–1 hour

A disadvantage of this system is that a patient may need more of the physician's time than you have scheduled. Therefore, it is important that you ask the proper questions at the time the appointment is made to anticipate the time needed. Such questions might include "Why do you need to see the doctor?" The patient's reply will tell you how many issues will be addressed. "Do you have a form to be completed for your physical?" The answer to this question will tell you whether this is a school physical or a complete physical.

The practice of adding **buffer** time to the schedule gives extra time to accommodate emergencies, walk-ins, and other demands on the provider's daily time schedule that are not considered direct patient care. Such tasks include returning phone calls, reviewing records, and transcribing reports. For example, you may cross off 30 minutes at the beginning and end of the daily schedule to be used as a buffer.

Methods of scheduling patients include clustering, wave, modified wave, stream, and double booking.

Clustering

Clustering is grouping patients with similar problems or needs. For example, an obstetrics and gynecology practice may see all pregnant patients in the morning and other patients in the afternoon. A pediatrician may schedule vaccinations on certain days of the week. Special tests like sigmoidoscopies may be scheduled one morning a week. Advantages to clustering include maximum use of special equipment, ease in maintaining control of the schedule, the ability to provide many patients with information about their particular situation at the same time, and efficient use of employees' time.

Wave and Modified Wave

Outpatient medical facilities may use the **wave scheduling system** or modify the wave system in ways that work for their particular specialty. With the wave system, several patients are scheduled the first 30 minutes of each hour. They are seen in the order that they arrive at the office. The second half of each hour is left open. This technique works well in large facilities with several departments giving medical care. For example, several patients may arrive for a 9:00 appointment, be seen by the physician, be sent to the laboratory for blood work, and return to the physician 20 minutes later. The physician has the second part of the hour to see these patients after their testing. That second half of each hour is used as a buffer or extra time that can be used for emergencies, walk-ins, returning phone calls, and tasks other than direct patient care. Modifications to this system may include seeing new patients who will have complete physical examinations on the hour with three or four rechecks scheduled on the half hour. For example, a 75-year-old man being seen for a complete physical would be scheduled at 9:00 A.M., with a 22-year-old being seen for a follow-up of strep throat and a 6-year-old being seen for recheck of an ear infection scheduled at 9:30 A.M.

Fixed Scheduling

Fixed scheduling is the most commonly used method. It divides each hour into increments of 15, 30, 45, or 60 minutes. The reason for each patient's visit will determine the length of time assigned. Patients who are late or do not report for their appointment can cause major problems in the flow of the day. It is helpful to schedule chronically late patients at the end of the day. Another tactic is to tell the patient to arrive 30 minutes prior to the time you schedule.

Streaming

Streaming is a method that helps minimize gaps in time and backups. Appointments are given based on the needs of the individual patient. If a patient is being seen for a complete physical, 1 hour may be allotted. The next patient seen may need a blood pressure recheck, which would be allotted a 15-minute slot. Although this method ensures a smooth work flow, the medical assistant scheduling the appointment must understand the procedures and guidelines for deciding the time that should be allotted. Box 2-1 outlines examples of services and their probable time allotments.

Double Booking

With **double booking** two patients are scheduled for the same period with the same physician. This works well when patients are being sent for diagnostic testing because it leaves time to see both patients without keeping either one waiting unnecessarily.

Flexible Hours

Offices that operate with flexible hours are open at different times throughout the week. For example, Monday, Wednesday, and Friday office hours might be from 8 A.M.to 5 P.M., and Tuesday and Thursday office hours might be from 8 A.M. to 8 P.M. Some offices may also be open on Saturdays for all or part of the day. Patients still have scheduled appointments, but this greater range of available appointment times better accommodates work and family schedules. Your main challenge with flexible hours is to determine which patients really need to be scheduled for these special times. For example, Saturday appointments may be reserved only for patients whose work schedules do not permit weekday appointments. Flexible hours are most often used by clinics, group practices, and family physicians.

Open Hours

A medical office that operates with open hours for patient visits is open for specified hours during the day or evening. Patients may arrive at any time during those hours to be seen by the physician in the order of their arrival; there are no scheduled appointments. This system is commonly seen in emergency walk-in clinics and eliminates patient complaints such as "I had an appointment at 2 P.M. but had to wait until 3 P.M. to be seen." Open-hour scheduling, however, has some clear disadvantages:

- Effective time management is almost impossible.
- The facilities may be overloaded at some times and empty at other times.
- Charts must be pulled and prepared as each patient arrives.

So that patients are seen in the order in which they arrive, some offices use sign-in sheets. Some sign-in sheets require that patient's record the reason for their visit. The use of sign-in sheets is prohibited under the Health Insurance Portability and Accountability Act of 1996 regulations. Effective April 2003, sign-in sheets are considered a breach of confidentiality, since patients signing the sheet can see the names and medical conditions of other patients.

Checkpoint Question

2. What are the three systems that can be used for scheduling patient office visits?

FACTORS THAT AFFECT SCHEDULING

Patients' Needs

People express their needs in varied ways. A patient might be feeling uncertainty, embarrassment, shyness, or fear. With a patient in an emotional state, even the slightest real or imagined miscommunication can lead to negative response from the patient. Be courteous and maintain your professionalism.

Before scheduling an appointment, you should determine:

- Why the patient wishes to see the physician
- How long the patient has had the symptoms
- Whether the problem is **acute** (abrupt onset) or **chronic** (longstanding)
- The most convenient time for the patient to come in (e.g., early morning or evenings)
- Any special transportation services the patient requires (community or hospital van services operate only during certain hours)
- Whether the patient needs to see other office staff
- Any third-party payers' constraints
- Receipt of necessary documentation for referrals when the patient is enrolled in a program that requires such documentation

Control of the appointment schedule is your responsibility. Strive to accommodate a patient's requests whenever possible, but not if it will overload the schedule. For example, if a patient requests a 2 P.M. appointment this Tuesday and you already have patients in that time slot, politely explain that you cannot schedule the appointment then unless you have a cancellation. You might offer a later time on Tuesday or on another day at 2 P.M.. You can also ask if the patient wishes to be put on a move-up list to be notified if an earlier appointment opens up. In other words, you control the schedule. Do not let it control you.

Providers' Preferences and Needs

The management of the practice depends on the desires and requirements of the providers working in it. Providers in a medical practice may include the physician, nurse practitioner, or physician's assistant. Some providers often run behind schedule; others are extremely punctual. Recognize your providers' habits and communicate any problems to a supervisor. The physician may allow you to adjust the schedule to accommodate his or her habits. If you are employed to assist the physician with clinical duties (e.g., removing sutures, performing electrocardiograms, giving injections), the schedule can be adjusted to accommodate a larger number of patients while still allowing the provider enough time to give each patient personal attention.

As discussed earlier, the physician also needs time to receive and return telephone calls, review laboratory and pathology reports, dictate chart notes or correspondence, and so on. If your physician is on the staff of a teaching hospital, you may also have to block off time for clinic conferences and other teaching duties.

The physician will need time to meet with unscheduled office visitors other than patients. Such visitors might include other physicians and sales representatives from medical supply or pharmaceutical companies. You should determine in advance how the physician wants you to handle these visitors. For example, the physician may want to be notified immediately if another physician comes to the office. With salespersons or pharmaceutical representatives, however, the physician may have another staff member meet with them or may request that an appointment be scheduled for a more convenient time.

Physical Facilities

The physical facilities available in the medical office will affect the management of the appointment schedule. Consider these points: How many providers use the facility? How many examination rooms are there? Is it necessary to resterilize instruments between procedures, or is more than one set of instruments available? You would not want to schedule two sigmoidoscopies at the same time, for example, if the office has only one appropriately equipped examination room. You must thoroughly understand the requirements for procedures to be performed in the office to schedule appointments accurately.

Checkpoint Question

3. What are three factors that can affect appointment scheduling?

SCHEDULING GUIDELINES

Whether the patient is making an appointment by telephone or in person, be pleasant and maintain a helpful attitude. Always write the patient's telephone number on the schedule when making appointments. Emergencies and delays are unavoidable, and schedule corrections can be made quickly if the telephone number is handy. Leave some time slots open during each day, perhaps 15 to 20 minutes in the morning and in the afternoon. Invariably problems will arise (e.g., late patients, emergencies) and disrupt the regular appointment schedule. These open blocks can allow the schedule to catch up. Also, patients calling for appointments will not appreciate being told that no time is available for 2 or 3 weeks. Open slots can be used to schedule brief appointments as needed. Procedure 2-1 describes the steps for scheduling appointments for new patients.

New Patients

Most appointments for new patients are made by telephone. The information you exchange at this encounter is crucial, and entering the patient's data accurately is imperative. The first encounter with a new patient is discussed in Procedure 2-1.

An office brochure can be mailed to the patient in advance of the appointment. Some offices send new-patient forms to be filled out and brought in at the appointment. When scheduling an appointment for a new patient, follow these guidelines:

1. Allow an adequate amount of time for the appointment. To do so, obtain as much information as possible from the patient:
   - Full name and correct spelling
   - Mailing address
   - Day and evening telephone numbers
   - Reason for the visit
   - Name of the referring physician or individual
   - Responsible party and third party payer (insurance plan)
2. Explain the office's payment policy. Most offices require full or partial payment at the time of an initial visit, and patients must understand this policy. Instruct patients to bring all pertinent insurance information.
3. Be sure patients know your office location; if needed, give them concise directions. You may also want to tell patients how long they can expect to be at the office.
4. Some patients are sensitive about messages left on an answering machine or given to a coworker. To avoid violating confidentiality, ask the patient if it is permissible to call at home or at work and include this information in the patient's chart.
5. Before ending the call, confirm the time and date of the appointment. You might say, "Thank you for calling Mr. Brown. We look forward to seeing you on Tuesday, December 10, at 2 P.M."
6. Always check your appointment system or book to be sure that you have placed the appointment on the correct day in the right time slot.
7. If the patient was referred by another physician, you may need to call that physician's office in advance of the appointment for copies of laboratory work, radiology and pathology reports, and so on. Remember, the patient must give authorization to release medical documents. Give these reports to the physician prior to the patient's appointment.

Established Patients

Established patients will be given return appointments when necessary. Most return appointments are made before the patient leaves the office. Procedure 2-2 describes the steps for scheduling a return appointment.

When making a return appointment, follow these guidelines:

1. Carefully check your appointment book or screen before offering an appointment time. If a specific examination, test, or x-ray is to be performed on the return visit, avoid scheduling two patients for the same examination at the same time.
2. Offer the patient a specific time and date. For example, you might say, "Mrs. Hernandez, I have next Tuesday, the 15th, available at 3:30 P.M." (Avoid asking the patient when he or she would like to return, as this can elicit indecision.) If the offered appointment is not convenient, offer another specific time and date.
3. Write the patient's name and telephone number in the appointment book or enter in the information on the appointment screen.
4. Transfer the pertinent information to an appointment card and give it to the patient. Computerized systems print an appointment card. Repeat aloud the appointment day, date, and time to the patient as you hand over the card (Fig. 2-3).

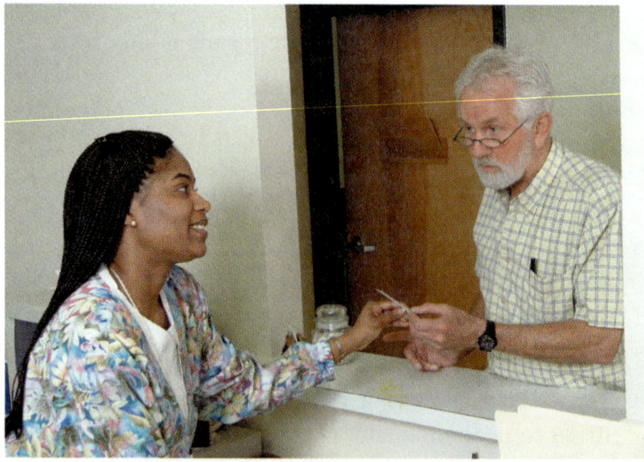

FIGURE 2-3. Photograph of a medical assistant handing a patient an appointment card.

5. Double-check your book or screen to be sure you have not made an error.
6. End your conversation with a pleasant word and a smile.

PREPARING A DAILY OR WEEKLY SCHEDULE

In most offices, as medical assistant you are responsible for preparing a daily and weekly schedule of appointments. Make a copy for the providers and other office staff members. When there are changes in the schedule, ensure that corrections are made on all copies. Place the next day's schedule on the physician's desk before he or she leaves for the day. Give the next week's schedule to the physician before he or she leaves on Friday. Schedules should include not only patients' appointments but also hospital rounds, surgeries, meetings, and any personal engagements on the schedule. Computer systems print a daily or weekly schedule, but you must remember to make changes manually as the day progresses.

PATIENT REMINDERS

Offices use various kinds of reminders to tell a patient about an appointment that should be made or to remind them that an appointment has been made on a specific date and time. These reminders are the appointment card, the telephone call, and the mailed card.

Appointment Cards

An appointment card is given to the patient when he or she leaves the office. It should have the following information:

- Patient's name
- Day, date, and time of the return visit
- Physician's name and telephone number

If the patient requires a series of appointments, try to make them on the same day of the week and at the same time of day. This will make it easier for the patient to remember the appointments. Unless your appointment card allows you to list the complete series of appointments, however, give the patient a card for the next appointment only and repeat this procedure after each subsequent visit. When the patient has to save several cards, they can easily be lost or cause confusion. If using a manual system, write on the card with ink so that it cannot be altered. Computer appointment scheduling software provides appointment cards that can be printed on special perforated paper.

Telephone Reminders

All new patients and patients with appointments scheduled in advance should receive a telephone reminder the day before their appointment. Computer systems can place the call to the programmed number and remind the patient of the appointment with a prerecorded message. Remember, do not call a patient at work or leave a message unless you have been given permission to do so. Make the telephone reminder simple. Identify your office, yourself, and state the date and time of the appointment. For example, you might say, "This is Ms. Palmer from Dr. Reid's office. I'm calling to confirm your appointment for tomorrow, Thursday, February 10, at 3:30 p.m." Unless the patient has a question, then say, "Thank you and good-bye." This reminder helps jog the patient's memory, and if the patient must cancel or reschedule an appointment, you will have time to fill the slot. Keep a list with the names and phone numbers of patients who have asked to be called or who need to be seen sooner than their next appointment. This list may be called a cancellation list, a waiting list, or a move-up list. Make a notation on the appointment schedule, such as confirmed, left message, or no answer.

Mailed Reminder Cards

Some offices send reminder cards instead of making phone calls. Reminder cards are also used to remind patients who could not be reached by phone that it is time to keep an upcoming scheduled appointment. These should be mailed at least a week before the date of the appointment. In addition, reminder cards are sent after a set period since a patient's last appointment. Reminder cards are often used to alert patients to the need for annual examinations (e.g., Pap smears, mammograms, prostate examinations).

To handle this kind of reminder, keep a supply of preprinted postcards in the office (Fig. 2-4). The cards should have a simple one- or two-sentence message, such as, "According to our records, you are due for your annual physical. If you would kindly call the office, we will be glad to arrange an appointment for you." The physician's name, address, and telephone number should be printed on the card. Place the card in a tickler file (Box 2-2) and mail it at the appropriate time. Some medical management software packages produce a list that can be used to alert patients of necessary services.

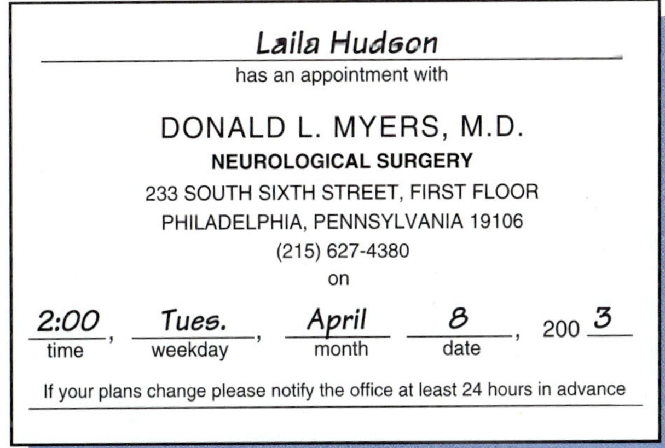
Laila Hudson
has an appointment with
DONALD L. MYERS, M.D.
NEUROLOGICAL SURGERY
233 SOUTH SIXTH STREET, FIRST FLOOR
PHILADELPHIA, PENNSYLVANIA 19106
(215) 627-4380
on
2:00, Tues., April 8, 200 3
time weekday month date
If your plans change please notify the office at least 24 hours in advance

FIGURE 2-4. Sample reminder postcard.

Box 2-2

A TICKLER FILE CAN TICKLE YOUR MEMORY

A **tickler file** helps remind you to do something by a certain time in the future. It can be something as simple as a card file box (like a recipe box) or an accordion folder with insert guides in chronological order. The guides may be in weekly or monthly divisions. Put patient appointment reminder cards in the appropriate location in the file. Check the file each week or month, depending on the divisions, then mail the reminders.

Medical office computer software often offers help with patient reminders. With a search of the database, a report of every female patient over age 50, for example, could be generated. Some systems even generate patient reminders based on preprogrammed criteria.

Box 2-3

WHEN DOES THE PATIENT NEED TO BE SEEN NOW?

When the patient calls with any of the following complaints:

- Shortness of breath
- Severe chest pain
- Uncontrollable bleeding
- Large open wounds
- Potential accidental poisoning
- Bleeding in a pregnant patient
- Injury to a pregnant patient
- Shock
- Serious burns
- Severe bleeding
- Any symptoms of internal bleeding (dark, tarry stools; discoloration of the skin)

Note: Remember to check with the physician for proper procedures concerning triage.

Checkpoint Question

4. What are the three types of patient reminders?

ADAPTING THE SCHEDULE

Emergencies

When a patient calls with an emergency (Fig. 2-5) , your first responsibility is to determine whether the problem can be treated in the office. The office should have a policy for evaluation of the situation. The word **STAT** is used in the medical field to indicate that something should be done immediately (Box 2-3). You also should have a list of appropriate questions to ask the patient, such as "Are you having chest pain? Are you having difficulty breathing? How long have you had the symptoms?" (Box 2-4). When several symptoms occur together, they may indicate a particular problem. This group of complaints is referred to as a **constellation of symptoms**. One group of symptoms found to indicate a certain disorder is severe right lower quadrant pain, nausea, and fever. A physician who sees this constellation of symptoms considers appendicitis.

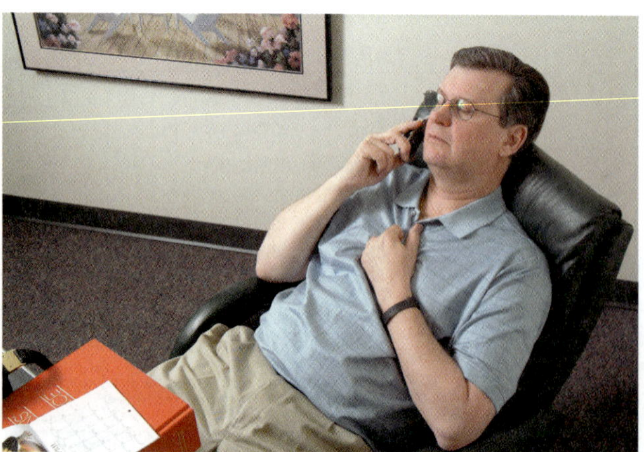

FIGURE 2-5. Patient at home making an emergency call.

Patients Who Are Acutely Ill

Patients who are acutely ill often have serious though not life-threatening conditions. These patients need to be seen as soon as possible but not necessarily on that same day. Obtain as much information about the patient's medical problem as you can so your message to the physician will allow him or her to decide how soon the patient should be seen. Place the chart with a note in the location selected by the

Box 2-4

COULD IT BE A HEART ATTACK?

When a patient calls complaining of the following constellation of symptoms, you should assume that this is a potential heart attack:

- Shortness of breath
- Chest pain
- Arm or neck pain
- Nausea and/or vomiting

Studies have shown that in women, early symptoms of a heart attack are different from those in men. These symptoms include jaw, neck, and back pain and severe fatigue. Keep this in mind when questioning the patient.

Call 911 and stay on the line with the patient. Do not advise the patient to drive to the hospital. Follow office policies for such an emergency.

physician, and tell the patient you will call back as soon as the physician makes a decision.

Walk-in Patients

Walk-in patients are those who arrive at the office without a scheduled appointment and expect to see the physician that day. Typically, the physician will have a set protocol, or prescribed list of steps, for handling such situations. In general, you must first determine the reason for the walk-in. Patients with medical emergencies need to be seen immediately. Other patients can be asked to have a seat in the waiting room while you inform the physician of the patient's presence. The physician can then make the decision to see the patient or not.

If the patient is to be seen, explain that you will work him or her into the schedule as soon as possible for a brief examination. When the patient leaves the office, you might apologize for the delay, then ask the patient to schedule an appointment for the next visit.

If the physician decides not to see a walk-in patient, you will have to ask the patient to schedule an appointment and to return later.

Late Patients

Patients who are late cause problems in the schedule. You should gently but firmly apologize for any delay but tell the patient, "You were late and Dr. Wooten is seeing another patient now. The doctor should be able to see you in about 15 minutes." Patients who are routinely late should be politely advised that "according to our office policy, patients who are more than 15 minutes late will have to be rescheduled." Some offices have found that scheduling the habitually late patient at the end of the day is helpful. In addition, ask patients to call the office if they know ahead of time they are going to be late.

Physician Delays

Of course, sometimes the physician calls in to say he or she has been delayed and will be in the office later. If office hours have not yet begun, call patients with appointments scheduled early, and give them the option of coming in later in the day or rescheduling the appointment for another day. If patients are waiting in the office, inform them immediately if the physician will be delayed. For example, you might say, "Dr. Franklin has been delayed and will probably be 20 to 30 minutes late. Would you like to wait, or would you prefer to reschedule for another time?" Always keep your patients informed; most people will understand if they know you have not ignored or forgotten them. Most patients appreciate the fact that the physician would also be available to them in an emergency. If you reschedule an appointment, note in the patient's chart the reason for the cancellation or rescheduling.

Missed Appointments

A missed appointment, or no-show, occurs when a patient neglects to keep an appointment and does not notify the office. When this happens, call the patient to try to determine why the appointment was missed and to reschedule for another time. If you are unable to reach the patient by telephone, send a card asking the patient to call the office to reschedule. Note in the patient's chart the missed appointment and that you have either rescheduled the appointment or mailed a card to schedule another appointment. Even if the facility does not routinely remind patients of appointments, be sure to call and remind habitually late patients the day before the appointment.

Continued failure to keep appointments should be brought to the attention of the physician, who may want to call the patient personally (particularly if the patient is seriously ill) or send a letter expressing concern for the patient's welfare. In extreme cases, the physician may choose to terminate the physician–patient relationship. Notations of all actions and copies of any letters sent to the patient should become a permanent part of the individual's medical record. Box 2-5 is a sample of a chart note.

CANCELLATIONS

Cancellations by the Office

You may have to cancel a patient's appointment if the physician is ill, has an emergency, or has personal time off. Patients who must be rescheduled need not be told the specific reason for the physician's absence. These cancellations should be noted in the patient's medical record.

When you have advance notice, write a letter to patients with appointments you must cancel, indicating that the physician will be away from the office but will return by a certain date. Patients should be alerted to cancellations a week before their appointments. Ask the patient to call the office to reschedule. If you have to cancel on the day of the appointment, call the patient and explain. For example, you

Box 2-5

CHARTING EXAMPLE

05/12/03–1530

Mrs. Parrish was called regarding missing scheduled appointment for today at 9:30A.M. Patient said she forgot about the appointment. Appointment was rescheduled for 05/14/03 at 10:00A.M. Patient was advised of the need to have regular prenatal checkups. Patient verbalized understanding. Dr. Wong was notified that appointment was missed and rescheduled.—Norreen Brooks, CMA might say, "Dr. Flora has been called out of the office unexpectedly. Would it be convenient to reschedule your appointment for sometime next week?" If the patient arrives at the office before you can contact him or her, apologize and politely explain the situation. Most patients will be understanding. When a physician is unavailable for an extended period, another physician must cover the practice or be on call. Everyone in the office should have a list of names and addresses of on-call physicians, and you should give this information to your patients, according to your office policy. When a locum tenens, or substitute physician, is employed, the office appointments will not be interrupted.

Cancellations by the Patient

When a patient cancels an appointment, ask the reason for the cancellation and mark it on your appointment schedule and in the patient's chart. Offer to reschedule at another time. If the patient is being seen for a continuing problem, be sure he or she understands the necessity for the follow-up visit. If the patient wants to call back for an appointment, make a note to yourself to check on the call-back in a few days. If a patient cancels appointments frequently, bring this to the physician's attention.

If a patient cancels an appointment and you have a full schedule, no action is needed. If your schedule is light, however, refer to your move-up list to try to fill the vacancy.

MAKING APPOINTMENTS FOR PATIENTS IN OTHER FACILITIES

Referrals and Consultations

When the provider requests assistance from another physician in **consultation** or makes a **referral** to another physician for the patient, make certain that the referral meets the requirements of any third-party payers. Managed care companies like HMOs have strict requirements regarding **precertification** and documentation for referrals to specialists and other facilities. Be sure the physician you are calling is on the preferred provider list for the patient's insurance company. Patients should be given a choice when being referred to a specialist.

When calling another physician's office for an appointment for your patient (Procedure 2-3), provide the following information:

- Physician's name and telephone number
- Patient's name, address, and telephone number
- Reason for the referral
- Degree of urgency
- Whether the patient is being sent for consultation or referral (see Box 2-6 for an explanation of the terms referral and consultation)

> **Box 2-6**
>
> **REFERRAL OR CONSULTATION?**
>
> It is important to know the difference between a referral and a consultation. According to the coding guidelines in the *Current Procedural Coding Terminology*, a consultation is a request for the opinion of a colleague. A letter is provided to the referring physician by the consultant and contains the consulting physician's impression and recommendations for the patient, but the patient returns to the referring physician for treatment. For example, an orthopedist may send a patient with rheumatoid arthritis to a rheumatologist for medication management, but the orthopedist will continue the patient's care based on the rheumatologist's recommendations.
>
> A referral usually involves a specialist and requires that the patient's care be transferred to that specialist. For example, a patient may see a physician for an ingrown toenail but be referred to a podiatrist for care.

Record in the patient's chart the time and date of the call and the person who received your call. Tell the person you are calling that you wish to be notified if your patient does not keep the appointment. If this occurs, be sure to tell the physician and enter this information in the patient's record.

Write the name, address, and telephone number of the referral doctor on your office stationery and include the date and time of the appointment. Give or mail this information to your patient. The patient may call the referring physician to make his or her own appointment. If this is the situation, ask the patient to call you with the appointment date and document it in the chart.

Diagnostic Testing

Sometimes, patients are sent for diagnostic testing or treatment at another facility. Such testing includes laboratory tests, radiology, computed tomography, magnetic resonance imaging, and nuclear medicine studies. These appointments are usually made while the patient is still in the office. Before scheduling, determine the exact test or tests the physician requires and how soon the results are needed. (Be sure to indicate to the facility if the results are needed immediately, or STAT.) Also, check with the patient for any time restrictions he or she may have. Give the facility the patient's name, address, telephone number, the exact test or tests required, and any other special instructions from the physician. Give the patient a laboratory or x-ray referral slip with the time and date of the appointment and the name, address, and telephone number of the outside facility.

Some laboratory studies or x-ray tests require advance preparation by the patient. Give your patient a written and verbal explanation of the required preparation, and be sure he or she understands the importance of following the instructions. On the patient's chart, note the name of the outside facility and the date and time of the appointment. Also place a reminder in your tickler file or on your appointment schedule to be sure the test results are received as requested.

Surgery

You also assist with the scheduling of procedures in a hospital operating room or an outpatient surgical facility. Determine the patient's need for precertification with the insurance carrier. You may have to call the number on the back of the patient's insurance card for a precertification number. Call the participating facility chosen by the patient and specify the time and date the physician has requested. The operating facility will need to know the exact procedure, the amount of time needed, the type of anesthesia required, and any other special instructions your physician may have. The facility will also need the patient's name, age, address, telephone number, insurance information, and the precertification number if required.

If the hospital has supplied your office with preadmission forms, give a copy to the patient and make sure he or she understands the need to complete and return the form in a timely manner. Follow the policies of the surgical facility regarding preadmission testing, which may include laboratory studies, x-rays, or autologous blood donation (donation of a person's own blood in advance). Write down all appointment dates, times, and locations for the patient and be certain he or she understands where to go and when.

Finally, note in the patient's record the name of the operating facility and the date and time the surgery is scheduled. You may also need to arrange for hospital admission by providing the same information to the hospital admitting department.

Spanish Terminology

¿A qué se debe su visita?	Why do you need to see the doctor?
¿Desde cuándo se siente mal?	How long has this being going on?
¿Prefiere la cita en la mañana o en la tarde?	Would you prefer morning or afternoon?
Llamo para recordarle su cita.	I am calling to remind you of your appointment.
Le daré una cita para que vea al Doctor nuevamente.	I will give you an appointment to return to see the doctor.
Para su próxima visita, por favor traiga su tarjeta del seguro y todas las medicinas que esté tomando.	Please bring your insurance card and medicine bottles with you for your appointment.

Días de la semana	Days of the week	Horas del día	Times of the Day
Domingo	Sunday	A la una	One o'clock
Lunes	Monday	El medio pasado uno	1:30
Martes	Tuesday	Dos en punto	2:00
Miércoles	Wednesday	Son las dos y media	2:30
Jueves	Thursday	Tres en punto	3:00
Viernes	Friday	Son las tres y media	3:30
Sábado	Saturday	Siete en punto	7:00
		Son las siete y media	7:30
		Ocho en punto	8:00
		Son las ocho y media	8:30
		Nueve en punto	9:00
		Son las nueve y media	9:30

Checkpoint Question

5. What information should be readily available when calling to schedule a patient for surgery in another facility?

WHEN THE APPOINTMENT SCHEDULE DOES NOT WORK

No appointment schedule runs smoothly all the time, and an occasional glitch is to be expected. If, however, you find that your schedule is chaotic nearly every day, you should determine the cause. Evaluate the schedule over time, generally 2 to 3 months. For example, make a list of all patients seen, their arrival times, the amount of time they spent with the physician, the time they left, and the amount of time needed to perform each examination or treatment. Since the work flow of the office affects every staff member, involve all employees in your study.

Office meetings are an ideal way to identify scheduling problems. Your evaluation may reveal that many of your patients are arriving late or that you have not allotted enough time for certain procedures. Sometimes, a habitually delayed physician is the problem. You may find that too many staff people are making appointments. If this is the case, you can assign only one staff person to handle all scheduling. Some problems may never be completely solved. If they are identified, however, you can often make adjustments to avoid causing frustration for both patients and office personnel.

Procedure 2-1

Making an Appointment for a New Patient

Steps	Reason
1. Obtain as much information as possible from the patient, such as: • Full name and correct spelling • Mailing address (not all offices require this) • Day and evening telephone numbers • Reason for the visit • Name of the referring person	To stay on schedule, you must allow enough time for the appointment. This information will help determine appointment needs and save time at the first visit.
2. Explain the payment policy of the practice. Most offices require payment at the time of an initial visit. Instruct patients to bring all pertinent insurance information.	Patients must understand this policy if they are to follow it
3. Be sure patients know your office location; give concise directions if needed. You may also want to give patients an idea of how long they can expect to be at the office.	Helps patients arrive on time and lets them budget their time.
4. To avoid violating confidentiality, ask the patient if it is permissible to call at home or at work.	Some patients are sensitive about messages left on an answering machine or given to a coworker.
5. Before ending the call, confirm the time and date of the appointment. Say, "Thank you for calling, Mr. Brown. We look forward to seeing you on Tuesday, December 10, at 2 P.M."	Repeating the appointment time will ensure that effective communication has taken place and increase the likelihood that the patient will be there on time.
6. Always check your appointment book to be sure that you have placed the appointment on the correct day in the right time slot.	Failure to record every appointment in the proper location can cause overbooking, frustrated physicians and staff, and irate patients.
7. If the patient was referred by another physician, you may have to call that physician's office before the appointment for copies of laboratory work, radiology and pathology reports, and so on. Remember, the patient must give authorization to release medical documents. Give this information to the physician prior to the patient's appointment.	Having the necessary information will eliminate ordering of tests that have already been done and will give the physician the tools to care for the patient.

Procedure 2-2

Making an Appointment for an Established Patient

Steps	Reason
1. Determine what will be done at the return visit. Check your appointment book or computer system before offering an appointment.	If a specific examination, test, or scan is to be performed, you will want to avoid scheduling two patients for the same examination at the same time.
2. Offer the patient a specific time and date. Avoid asking the patient when he or she would like to return, as this can cause indecision.	Give the patient a choice, and if neither time is convenient, offer another specific time and date. Giving a patient a choice is good practice. "Mrs. Chang, we can see you next Tuesday, the 15th, at 3:30 P.M. or Wednesday, the 16th, at 9:00 A.M."
3. Write the patient's name and telephone number in the appointment book or enter it in the computer.	Writing the phone number in the appointment book or making a notation in the computer will give you a quick reference if you need to call the patient to change the appointment.
4. Transfer the pertinent information to an appointment card and give it to the patient. Repeat aloud the appointment day, date, and time to the patient as you hand over the card (Fig. 2-4).	Repeating the information reinforces the patient's memory and helps ensure that the appointment will be kept.
5. Double-check your book or computer to be sure you have not made an error.	Errors in appointments waste the patient's, staff's, and physician's time.
6. Whether in person or on the phone, end your conversation with a pleasant word and a smile.	A smile always feels good to a patient who may be apprehensive about needing to return to the doctor.

Procedure 2-3

Making an Appointment for a Referral to Another Provider

Steps	Reason
1. Make certain that the requirements of any third-party payers are met.	Some third-party payers require that referrals be precertified. Preexisting conditions may not be covered for referral. Most companies require that only the patient's primary care physician (PCP) or gatekeeper make referrals. It is important to research each situation. Telephone numbers for precertification and questions will be printed on the back of the insurance card.
2. Refer to the preferred provider list for the patient's insurance company. Allow the patient to choose a provider from the list.	Managed care companies have strict requirements for precertification and documentation for referrals. If there is more than one provider with the same qualifications, the patient should always be given a choice.
3. Have the following information available when you make the call: • Physician's name and telephone number • Patient's name, address, and telephone number • Reason for the call • Degree of urgency • Whether the patient is being sent for consultation or referral	The referred or consulting physician's office needs to know these things to serve the patient well.
4. Record in the patient's chart the time and date of the call and the name of the person who received your call.	This is necessary for proper documentation of the patient's care.
5. Tell the person you are calling that you wish to be notified if your patient does not keep the appointment. If this occurs, be sure to tell your physician and enter this information in the patient's record.	This is necessary for proper documentation of the patient's care.
6. Write down the name, address, and telephone number of the doctor you are referring your patient to and include the date and time of the appointment Give or mail this information to your patient.	It is important that the patient have a reminder so the appointment will be kept.
7. If the patient is to call the referring physician to make the appointment, ask the patient to call you with the appointment date, then document this in the chart.	Recording the appointment information in the patient's chart completes the transaction and proves that the physician's order was carried out.

SUMMARY

The outpatient medical facility can be chaos without an efficient appointment system. Moving patients through the facility while treating each person equally and thoroughly is one of the biggest challenges in the medical office. It is difficult for a busy practice to run smoothly all of the time. You need structure, but you must be flexible. Available times, equipment and room usage, and personnel coverage must be considered when finding just the right formula for a well-run and efficient office.

The goals of the outpatient medical facility are to provide quality patient care and maintain financial stability. To reach those goals, an office must have a plan for the efficient scheduling and carrying out of the daily activities. Appointment scheduling systems include manual systems using appointment books and computerized systems that render helpful reports and daily activity sheets. The size of a practice, the number of physicians, the types of services, and so on are considered when establishing an appointment scheduling system. Sick patients calling to make appointments should be given priority, and there are established guidelines for determining the urgency of a patient's problem. Other functions, such as phone calls, reviewing records, and lunch breaks, are also scheduled into the daily activities of the office. An established protocol or list of steps should be in place to handle pharmaceutical representatives and other visitors to the office. As the medical assistant at the front desk, you will be one of the most important factors in the daily operation of the outpatient medical facility. As a medical assistant, you will make appointments, document encounters with patients that deal with appointments, and make referrals to other health care facilities. Learning the issues involved in successful appointment scheduling will help you make sure your facility runs smoothly.

Critical Thinking Challenges

1. Assume that you are the office manager in a physician's office. Create a policy and procedure for scheduling patients.
2. Sign-in sheets can cause a breach in patient confidentiality. What other methods could you use that would limit the potential for invasion of patient privacy?
3. You notice that patients typically wait 30 to 45 minutes past their scheduled appointment times because of the physician. How would you approach a physician who chronically runs late?

Answers to Checkpoint Questions

1. A matrix is established to indicate times of each day that are not available for patient appointments.
2. The three systems that can be used for patient office visits include scheduled appointments, flexible hours, and open hours.
3. The three factors that can affect scheduling are patients' needs, physicians' preferences, and the physical facilities.
4. The three types of reminders are appointment cards, telephone reminders, and mailed reminder cards.
5. When scheduling a patient for surgery, the following information is needed: demographic and insurance information, the patient's name, age, address, telephone number, precertification number (if required), diagnosis, surgery planned, and any special instructions.

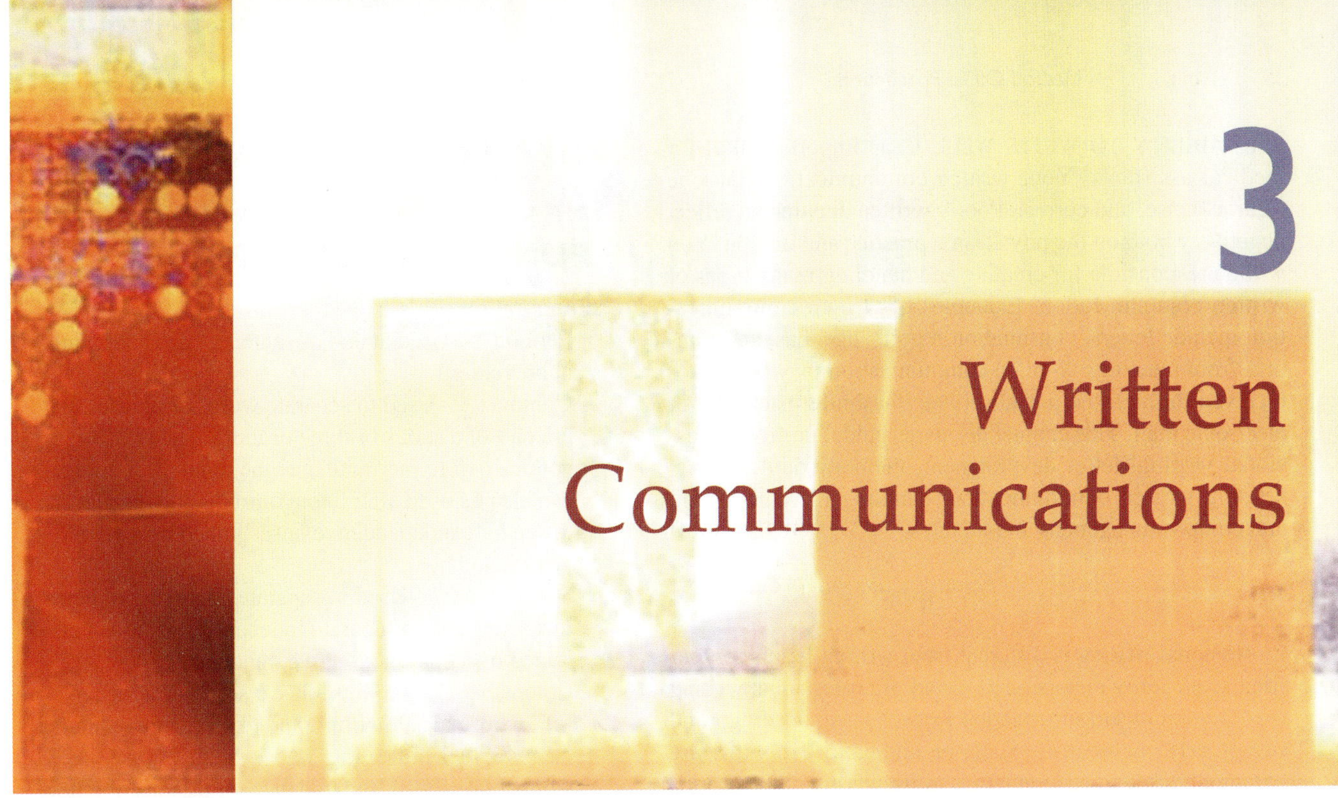

3 Written Communications

CHAPTER OBJECTIVES

In this chapter, you'll learn:

1. To spell and define the key terms.
2. To discuss the basic guidelines for grammar, punctuation, and spelling.
3. To describe six key guidelines for medical writing.
4. To discuss the eleven key components of a business letter.
5. To describe the three steps to writing a business letter.
6. To describe the process of writing a memorandum.
7. To discuss the various mailing options.
8. To identify the types of incoming written communication seen in a physician's office.
9. To list the items that must be included in an agenda.
10. To identify the items that must be included when typing minutes.

PERFORMANCE OBJECTIVES

In this chapter, you'll learn:

1. To write a business letter.
2. To write a memorandum.
3. To address and send written communication.
4. To open and sort mail.

KEY TERMS

agenda
annotation
BiCaps
block
enclosure
font
full block
intercaps
margin
memorandum
proofread
salutation
semiblock
template

THE ABILITY TO WRITE WELL IS an important skill for medical assistants. Your written communication must be clear, concise, and correct. Poorly written documents reflect negatively both on the physician's practice and on you. You will be responsible for creating and handling many types of written communication. Examples of written communication include letters, consultation reports, agendas, and minutes from meetings. Written communication may be sent or received through the postal service, facsimile machines, or electronic mail. This chapter discusses guidelines for professional writing, letter development, memorandum writing, sending written communication, handling incoming mail, and composing agendas and minutes.

PROFESSIONAL WRITING

Professional writing is different from writing letters to your friends or family members. The goal of professional writing is to communicate information in a concise, accurate, and comprehensible manner. Slang or idiomatic terms that are commonly used in writing letters to friends are not appropriate for business letters. For example, "Drop by and say hi" is not suitable for a professional letter, even if you know the recipient personally.

Basic Grammar and Punctuation Guidelines

Grammatical rules seem to be an endless maze of twists and turns! And each rule comes with numerous exceptions. You must be familiar with these rules and be able to apply them to your writing. Key rules of punctuation and grammar are listed in Box 3-1.

Basic Spelling Guidelines

Good spelling skills take time to acquire. Box 3-2 gives you basic tips for spelling. Many words sound exactly alike but are spelled differently and have different meanings. Be very careful with these words. Which of the following sentences has a spelling error?

- Wound cultures were taken from the left lower leg site.
- Wound cultures were taken from the left lower leg cite.

The first sentence is correct. Site and cite sound alike, and both are spelled correctly, but in the second sentence, the wrong word was used. These types of errors occur as a result of poor word usage and poor spelling. Appendix E lists words that are most likely to be misused or misspelled.

Guidelines for Medical Writing

Writing letters to medical professionals follows many of the standard guidelines. There are, however, some specific guidelines about which you need to be aware. They are discussed next.

Box 3-1

BASIC GRAMMAR AND PUNCTUATION TIPS

Punctuation

- Period (.)—Used at end of sentences and following abbreviations.
- Comma (,)—Used to separate words or phrases that are part of a series of three or more. The final comma before the "and" may be omitted. A comma can also be used after a long introductory clause or to separate independent clauses joined by and, but, yet, or, and nor.
- Semicolon (;)—Used to separate a long list of items in a series and to separate independent clauses not joined by a conjunction (e.g., and, but, or).
- Colon (:)—Used to introduce a series of items, to follow formal salutations, and to separate the hours from minutes indicating time.
- Apostrophe (')—Used to denote omissions of letters and to denote the possessive case of nouns.
- Quotation marks (" ")—Used to set off spoken dialogue, some titles (e.g., journal articles, newspaper articles, television and radio program episodes), and words used in a special way.
- Parentheses [( )]—Used to indicate a part of a sentence that is not part of the main sentence but is essential for the meaning of the sentence. Also used to enclose a number, for confirmation, that is spelled out in a sentence.
- Ellipsis (. . .)—Used in place of a period to indicate a prolonged continuation of a conversation or list. Also used to display individual items or to connect phrases that are loosely connected.
- Diagonal (/)—Used in abbreviations (c/o), dates (2003/2004), fractions (3/4), and to indicate two or more options (AM/FM).

Sentence Structure

- Avoid long, run-on sentences.
- A verb must always agree with its subject in number and person.
- Ensure that the proper pronoun (he or she) is used.
- Adjectives should be used when they add an important message. Don't overuse adjectives or adverbs. Remember, double negatives used in one sentence make the sentence positive.

Capitalization

- Capitalize the first word in a sentence, proper nouns, the pronoun "I," book titles, and known geographical names.
- Names of persons, holidays, and trademark items should be capitalized.
- Expressions of time (a.m. and p.m.) should not be capitalized.

Box 3-2

BASIC SPELLING TIPS

When in doubt about the spelling of a word, always use a dictionary or a spell check. Keep in mind that a computer spell check will check for spelling but will not alert you to inappropriate word usage.

- Remember this rhyme: I comes before e, except after c, or when sounded like a as in neighbor and weigh. Examples: achieve, receive. (The exceptions are either, neither, weird, leisure, and conscience.)
- Words ending in -ie drop the e and change the i to y before adding -ing. Examples: die, dying; lie, lying.
- Words ending in -o that are preceded by a vowel are made plural by adding s. Example: studio, studios; trio, trios. Words ending in o that are preceded by a consonant form the plural by adding es. Examples: potato, potatoes; hero, heroes.
- Words ending in -y preceded by a vowel form the plural by adding s. Examples: attorney, attorneys; day, days. Words ending in -y that are preceded by a consonant change the y to i and add es. Examples: berry, berries; lady, ladies.
- The final consonant of a one-syllable word is doubled before adding a suffix beginning with a vowel. Examples: run, running; pin, pinning. If the final consonant is preceded by another consonant or by two vowels, do not double the consonant. Examples: look, looked; act, acting.
- Words ending in a silent -e generally drop the e before adding a suffix beginning with a vowel. Examples: ice, icing; judge, judging. The exceptions are dye, eye, shoe, and toe. The e is not dropped, however, in suffixes beginning with a consonant unless another vowel precedes the final e. Examples: pale, paleness; argue, argument.
- For all words ending in -c, insert a k before adding a suffix beginning with e, i, or y. Examples: picnic, picnicking; traffic, trafficker.

Accuracy

Many of the medical documents or letters that you will write contain information that requires precision, accuracy, and careful attention to details. Inaccurate information in some letters can lead to injury of a patient and lawsuits and can harm the physician's practice. Some of your letters will be placed in the patient's permanent medical record. Most letters will start with the physician asking you to draft a letter. He may or may not give you some notes to follow. Either way, your responsibility in typing the letter is to be as accurate as possible and to question anything about which you are unsure. Here are some examples of inaccuracy:

- You wrote, "The patient was started on the MVP chemotherapy regimen." The physician, however, had written "MVPP." These are two completely different regimens. MVP is used for treating lung cancer, and MVPP is used for Hodgkin's lymphoma.
- The physician wrote, "Patient was told to take Dristan Cold tablets." You rearranged the sentence, however, and wrote "The patient had a cold and was told to take Dristan tablets." Dristan Cold contains an antihistamine medication that plain Dristan does not. Never edit a physician's sentence unless you are sure that it will not affect the meaning.
- The physician wrote, "There is no reason for him to start radiation therapy at this time." You wrote, however, "There is reason for him to start radiation therapy at this time." The simple elimination of the word "no" completely changes the meaning of the sentence and can lead to errors in patient care.
- The physician wrote, "Hospitalization is needed because the patient continues to be violent." You typed, however, "Hospitalization is needed because the patient continues to be violet." The meaning of the sentence has been changed by the elimination of one "n" in violent.

Checkpoint Question

1. What are three consequences that could arise from inaccurate information in a business letter?

Spelling

Spell check in word processing programs can be a great asset, but it has limitations. Medical terminology spell check software should be added to your computer and be updated frequently.

You can add medical terms into your computer's spell check dictionary, but make sure that any word you add is spelled correctly! Spell checks can never be 100% stocked with all the needed terms, especially in the medical profession, as new technologies, medications, and treatments arise daily. Remember, spell check will not recognize words that are spelled correctly but misused. Which of the following sentences has a spelling error?

- The patient's mucus was yellow.
- The patient's mucous was yellow.

Mucus (noun) refers to a sticky secretion. Mucous is a type of membrane that secretes mucus. The second sentence is wrong. Here is another example:

- The physician received a plague.
- The physician received a plaque.

There is a big difference between plaque (commemorative item) and plague (bacterial disease)! Box 3-3 lists some commonly used medical words that can easily be misspelled or misused.

Box 3-3

COMMONLY MISUSED OR MISSPELLED MEDICAL TERMS

- anoxia and anorexia
- aphagia and aphasia
- bowl and bowel
- emphysema and empyema
- fundus and fungus
- lactose and lactase
- metatarsals and metacarpals
- mucus and mucous
- parental and parenteral
- postnatal and postnasal
- pubic and pubis
- rubella and rubeola
- serum and sebum
- uvula and vulva

Capitalization

Pay particular attention to how words, names, and abbreviations are capitalized. Words or phrases with unusual capitalization are called intercaps or **BiCaps**. Never change how a word is capitalized unless directed to do so. Ask for clarification and mark the proof letter with a question mark for the physician to answer. For example m-BACOD is a very different medication regimen from M-BACOD. Here are some other common medical intercaps: pH, RhoGam, rPA, ReoPro, aVR.

Abbreviations and Symbols

Abbreviations and symbols can save time in long handwriting and with typing. Use abbreviations sparingly. When typing professional letters, you should spell out all abbreviations that are not universally accepted (e.g., p.m.). Become familiar with the abbreviations and symbols that are used where you work. Most offices have a policy listing their approved ones. Following are some ways abbreviations can be misinterpreted:

- The physician wrote, "The patient had good BS." You assumed that BS meant bowel sounds, so you typed "The patient had good bowel sounds," but the physician meant the abbreviation BS to mean breath sounds.
- Do not change < or > signs to *less than* or *greater than* unless you are sure of what the statement is saying. For example, "The patient will not be admitted to the hospital until her hemoglobin is less than 13." If you made a mistake and typed "greater than 13," confusion could occur.
- The symbols for male (♂) and female (♀) are commonly used in handwritten notes, but you should replace these symbols with words when writing a business or professional letter.

Plural and Possessive

Converting words to plural or possessive form can be tricky in English. Refer to your medical terminology book or a dictionary when you are unsure. Which of the following sentences is correct?

- The patient had multiple bullas.
- The patient had multiple bullae.

The second sentence is correct. *Bullae* means multiple blisters; *bulla* is one blister.

Numbers

In general, numbers one to ten should be spelled out, except when used with units of measurement (e.g., 5 mg), and those over 10 may be expressed as a numeral. Here are some important tips you will need to remember about numbers:

- Numbers referring to an obstetrical patient's medical history are not written out: "The patient is a gravida 3, para 2." Do not convert these numbers.
- Watch decimal point placement. There is a huge difference in medication between 12.5 mg and 1.25 mg.
- Double-check that you have not transposed numbers. For example, you typed, "The patient's red blood cell count was 5.1," but it was actually 1.5. A red blood cell count of 1.5 is incompatible with life.

WHAT IF

You are writing a letter and can't find out how to spell a word. What should you do?

Begin with your computer's spell check software. Spell check is generally under the heading Tools at the top of the screen. Most programs offer suggestions for the misspelled word. Be very careful that you do not select the wrong word on the suggestion list. You may also either look up the word in a dictionary or use an online dictionary. Two Web addresses that offer online dictionaries are given in this chapter. You may ask a colleague for spelling assistance. An option is to exchange the word for another word from a thesaurus. Be sure that the meaning of the sentence does not change if you use a different word. If these steps do not work, print the letter, mark the word with a question mark, and leave it for the physician. Never mail a letter with a spelling error.

- Roman numerals should never be changed to words. For example, "lead II of the patient's electrocardiogram" should never be changed to "lead two of the patient's electrocardiogram."
- Many health care professionals use military time. Time that is written in military style does not have to be changed if the recipient of the letter is familiar with it (doctors, nurses). If the letter is going to a patient or other person who may not be able to interpret it, however, either convert the time or express the standard time in parenthesis; for example, "The patient's next appointment is at 1430 hours (2:30 P.M.)." No colons are used in military time.
- Temperatures must always have the correct symbol for Celsius or Fahrenheit included (98.6°F or 37°C).
- Telephone numbers should include the area code in parentheses or followed by a hyphen, then the number with a hyphen. Add extensions to the number by placing a comma after the last digit of the number, then type Ext. and the number: (800) 555-0000, Ext. 6480. Periods may replace hyphens and parentheses: 800.555.0000.

LETTER DEVELOPMENT

Writing effective business letters is a skill that requires practice and careful attention to detail. To write a professional business letter, you must:

- Understand the components of a letter
- Use the correct letter format
- Ensure that the message is clear, concise, and accurate

These skills are described in the following sections.

Components of a Letter

A typical business letter has 11 components. We will explore each one, beginning at the top of the page. For easy reference, Figure 3-1 displays a sample business letter with these components marked.

1. *Letterhead.* The letterhead consists of the name of the practice or physician, address, telephone number, fax number, and sometimes the company logo. The letterhead is often embossed in color and centered on the top of the page. The letterhead may also be preset into a **template**. (Templates are discussed later in the chapter).
2. *Date.* The date includes the month, day, and year. It should be positioned two to four spaces below the letterhead. The date must be typed on only one line and abbreviations should not be used.
3. *Inside address.* The inside address refers to the name and address of the person to whom the letter is being sent. A nine-digit zip code should be used if available. The inside address is placed four spaces down from the date unless the letter is being mailed with a window envelope and it will not be aligned correctly. Never abbreviate city or town names. States can be abbreviated. Never abbreviate business titles (e.g., President, Chief Executive Officer). Here are some other points to remember:
   - If the letter is going to a business, type the name of the addressee, followed by his or her title, name of the business on the next line, then the address.
   - If the letter is being addressed to two or more people at different addresses, type the individual address block one line space under the other or place the addresses side by side.
   - If the letter is going to two people at the same address but with different last names, type the woman's name on the first line, man's name on the second line, then the address. If the sexes are the same, do them in alphabetical order, followed by the address.
4. *Subject line.* The subject line, an optional component, is used to state the intent of a letter or to indicate what the letter is regarding. It is placed on the third line below the inside address and is written as Re: (an abbreviation for regarding) followed by the subject. For example, Re: Blood tests.
5. *Salutation.* The **salutation** is the greeting of the letter. It is placed two spaces down from the inside address or the subject line. Capitalize the first letter of each word in the phrase and end the phrase with a colon. It is permissible to eliminate the salutation if the letter is informal or if a subject line has been used. When writing to a physician, write out the word doctor. Here are some recommendations when writing salutations:
   - If the letter is going to one person and the gender is known write, Dear Mr. Rogers.
   - If the letter is going to one person and the gender is *not* known, write, Dear Pat Smith (use the person's first name).
   - If the letter is going to a woman and a man with different last names, always address the woman first: Dear Ms. Ray and Mr. Oscar.
   - If the letter is going to several people, place them in alphabetical order: Dear Mr. Andersen, Mr. Cats, Ms. Dart, and Mr. Raymond.
   - To Whom It May Concern, Dear Sir, or Dear Madam should not be used.
6. *Body of the letter.* The body of the letter contains the message. It should be single-spaced with double spacing between the paragraphs. Here are some guidelines for writing the body of the letter:
   - If the letter is more than one page long, try to avoid dividing a paragraph at the end of a page. If you must, leave at least two sentences at the

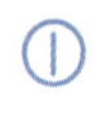

Benjamin Matthews, M.D.
999 Oak Road, Suite 313
Middletown, Connecticut 06457
860-344-6000

February 2, 2003

Dr. Adam Meza
Medical Director
Family Practice Associates
134 N. Tater Drive
West Hartford, Connecticut 06157

Re: Ms. Beatrice Suess

Dear Doctor Meza:

Thank you for asking me to evaluate Ms. Suess. I agree with your diagnosis of rheumatoid arthritis. Her prodromal symptoms include vague articular pain and stiffness, weight loss and general malaise. Ms. Suess states that the joint discomfort is most prominent in the mornings, gradually improving throughout the day.

My physical examination shows a 40-year-old female patient in good health. Heart sounds normal, no murmurs or gallops noted. Lung sounds clear. Enlarged lymph nodes were noted. Abdomen soft, bowel sounds present, and the spleen was not enlarged. Extremities showed subcutaneous nodules and flexion contractures on both hands.

Laboratory findings were indicative of rheumatoid arthritis. See attached laboratory data. I do not feel x-rays are warranted at this time.

My recommendations are to continue Ms. Suess on salicylate therapy, rest and physical therapy. I suggest that you have Ms. Suess attend physical therapy at the American Rehabilitation Center on Main Street.

Thank you for this interesting consultation.

Yours truly,

Benjamin Matthews, MD

Benjamin Matthews, MD

BM/es

Enc. (2)

cc: Dr. Samuel Adams

FIGURE 3-1. Components of a business letter. This letter is done in full block format and contains these elements: (1) letterhead, (2) date, (3) inside address, (4) subject line, (5) salutation, (6) body, (7) closing, (8) signature and typed name, (9) identification line, (10) enclosure, (11) copy.

bottom of the first page. Use the widow and orphan control feature of your word processor program to prevent orphan lines from appearing.

- Tables and graphs should not be broken. They should appear on one page only.
- Web addresses and e-mail addresses should fit on one line and never be continued to another page.
- If the letter is more than one page long, page numbers should be used.
- Use a bulleted format to highlight key points for the reader. For example, "The possible side effects of this medication are:" (then list them vertically with a bullet symbol).
- Letterhead is used only on the first page of the letter. The second page should be the same quality paper as the letterhead. Start the second page with a continuation line (name of person the letter is going to and the date of the letter). Continue the letter two lines down from the continuation line. Your margins must be the same as those on page 1. Most templates type the continuation line for you.

7. *Closing*. The closing concludes the letter. Some common closings are: Sincerely, Yours truly, Regards, Respectfully, and Cordially yours. Only the first word is capitalized and a comma follows the phrase. Closings are placed two spaces down from the end of the letter. Never put the closing alone on a page.
8. *Signature and typed name*. The name of the person sending the document is typed four spaces below the closing, with the person's title typed directly below. The physician will read and sign the letter above the typed name. If you are instructed to sign the letter, sign the physician's name followed by a slash mark and your name, e.g., Susan James, MD/Raymond Smith, RMA.
9. *Identification line*. The identification line, an optional component, indicates who dictated the letter and who wrote it. It consists of abbreviations only. The initials of the person who dictated the letter are capitalized (generally the physician); the initials of the writer of the letter are in lower case (generally these will be yours). The identification line can also be called the reference line.
10. *Enclosure*. An **enclosure** is something that is included with a letter. It is abbreviated Enc. and is placed two spaces down from the identification line. The number of documents included is placed in parentheses; if only one document is included, just the abbreviation Enc. is used.
11. *Copy*. The abbreviation c is used to indicate that a duplicate letter has been sent. It is typed two spaces below the enclosure line. Usually, letters are copied to managers, supervisors, or to the physician who requested that the given information be dispersed.

Checkpoint Question

2. Whose address is typed as the inside address? What is the purpose of the salutation? What is the purpose of the identification line?

Letter Formats

There are three basic types of letter formats: *full block*, *semiblock*, and *block*. Office policy or the physician preference's will dictate which format you use.

Full Block

In **full block** format, each line is flush left. Full block is the most formal format and is most commonly used for professional letters. Figure 3-1 shows a letter in full block format.

Block

In **block** format, the date, subject line, closing, and signatures are flush right. All other lines are flush left (Fig. 3-2).

Semiblock

In **semiblock** format, the first sentence of each paragraph is indented five spaces, if done on a typewriter, or is tabbed, if done on a computer (Fig. 3-3). Semiblock is also referred to as modified block.

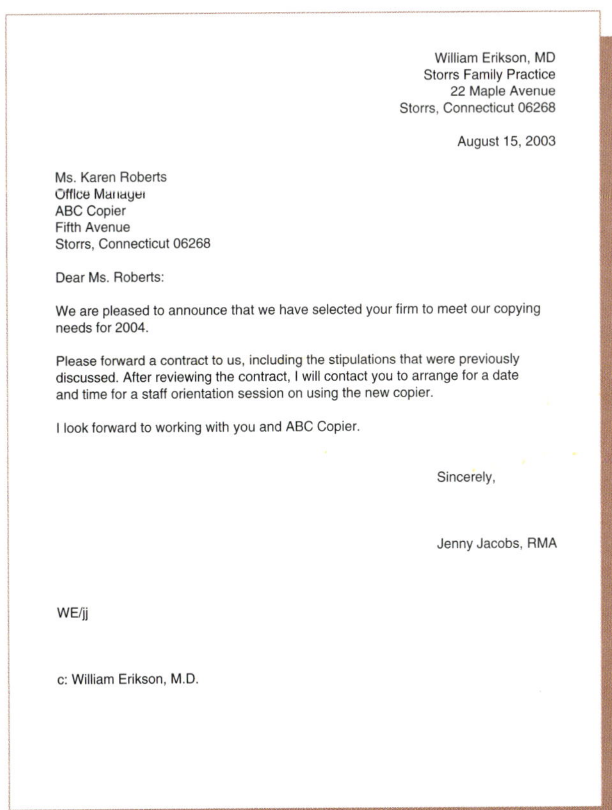

William Erikson, MD
Storrs Family Practice
22 Maple Avenue
Storrs, Connecticut 06268

August 15, 2003

Ms. Karen Roberts
Office Manager
ABC Copier
Fifth Avenue
Storrs, Connecticut 06268

Dear Ms. Roberts:

We are pleased to announce that we have selected your firm to meet our copying needs for 2004.

Please forward a contract to us, including the stipulations that were previously discussed. After reviewing the contract, I will contact you to arrange for a date and time for a staff orientation session on using the new copier.

I look forward to working with you and ABC Copier.

Sincerely,

Jenny Jacobs, RMA

WE/jj

c: William Erikson, M.D.

FIGURE 3-2. Sample block letter.

Elizabeth Jones, M.D.
750 East Street, Suite 205
Hialeah, Florida 33013
305-311-2666

June 12, 2003

Margaret Trent
18 Cambridge Street
Hialeah, Florida 33013

Dear Ms. Trent:

As per our phone conversation, your blood glucose level remains elevated. It is essential that we stabilize your blood sugar level.

In order to achieve normal blood sugar levels, you must follow the enclosed diet. A meeting with a Registered Dietitian can be arranged for you to discuss any dietary concerns you may have.

I am also enclosing patient education instructions for the use of a glucometer. You must test your blood sugar every morning and keep a diary of your results. Glucometers can be purchased from any pharmacy. If you need assistance in using the glucometer, please contact Raymond Smith, CMA, at 555-6423.

Presently, I do not wish to prescribe any medications. If we are unable to get your blood sugar under control, I will prescribe an oral diabetic medication.

Please call my office and schedule an appointment for the week of June 20 for a blood draw and a follow-up visit.

Sincerely,

Elizabeth Jones, M.D.

EJ/rs

enc. (2)

FIGURE 3-3. Sample semiblock letter.

Writing a Business Letter

To create a professional business letter, follow these three steps: preparation, composition, and editing. Box 3-4 gives you some guidelines for starting to write a letter.

Preparation

Good preparation is a key element in writing professional business letters. Preparation consists of planning the content and the mechanics of the letter.

Mental Preparation. Before you begin to compose a letter, mentally prepare your message. You might start formulating the message by envisioning yourself talking to the person to whom you are sending the letter. Preparation offers three benefits:

1. It helps eliminate writer's block.
2. It gets you to focus on the message, not the mechanics (e.g., spelling, grammar, punctuation).
3. It enhances your organization.

Using cue cards or note cards will help ensure all the necessary information is covered in the letter.

Mechanics of the Letter. Before you begin to type the letter, select the appropriate *template*, *margin*, and *font*. A template

Box 3-4

HOW TO START WRITING A LETTER

By determining the answers to these four questions, you can better prepare the message of your letter.

1. Who is my reader?
   It is very important that you use proper gender identification. Be especially careful with names that can be used for males or females (eg, Sam, Kelly, Ronnie, Alex, Tracy). Determine the reader's comprehension level. Letters to physicians will be more technical and will use medical terminology. Letters to patients will be less technical and use medical terminology sparingly.
2. What do I want my reader to do?
   This is your call to action; make it clear and specific. For example, you might write, "Please complete the enclosed insurance form (2 pages). Be sure to include all necessary information and sign your name. Place the form in the enclosed envelope and return it to our office by June 15, 2003." Avoid using "at your earliest convenience"; include a date for the required action. If possible, include a response mechanism, such as a self-addressed, stamped envelope.
3. What do I want to say?
   Briefly list the necessary information. To help you remember all of the necessary information, ask yourself who, what, where, when, why, and how.
4. How will I organize my message?
   Here are three basic ways that you can organize your message:
   - *Chronological:* Discuss items in a sequential manner, beginning with the earliest date and proceeding to the most recent date. For example, when discussing the physician's career, list his or her earlier experiences before the most recent career achievements.
   - *Problem oriented:* Let the reader know about a specific problem and provide instructions for correcting the problem. For example, if a patient's blood work came back with abnormal findings, a letter would be sent, identifying the problem (e.g., low hematocrit) and advising the patient on the possible causes, treatments, and follow-up procedures.
   - *Comparison:* Evaluate the effectiveness of two or more items. For example, as an office manager, you may have to write to the physician comparing two service contracts or two sample computer software packages.

Box 3-5

FONTS

Here are fonts that would be suitable for a business letter:

- This is 12-point Times New Roman.
- This is 10-point Times New Roman.
- This is 12-point Garamond.
- This is 12-point Arial.

Here are fonts and sizes that would not be appropriate:

- This is 8-point Times New Roman.
- **This is 12-point Colossalis Black.**
- THIS IS 12-POINT COTTONWOOD.
- This is 12-point Tekton.
- **This is 12-point impact.**

provides you with the skeleton of the letter. The key elements are already set and spaced correctly, so you just type in the pertinent information. Most computers have numerous letter templates or a letter wizard. These programs will make the process of letter writing easy, fast, and professional. You may use macros in your template to make repetitive tasks faster.

The **margin** is the blank space around the letter. A 1-inch margin is used for both left and right sides of the letter and the bottom. Margins are used to center the components of the letter in a standarized manner. If you select a template, your margins will be set for you.

Next, select the font. A **font** is the typeface; it affects the way words look and how easy it will be to read the letter. **Choose a font that is easy to read and that is appropriate in size.** Avoid cute or elegant fonts that can be difficult to read or see. The most common fonts used in business letters are Times New Roman, Garamond, and Arial. Box 3-5 gives you some examples of fonts and their sizes.

Checkpoint Question

3. Before you begin to type a letter, name three mechanics that you need to select.

Composition

The goal of composition is to ensure that your message is transmitted clearly, concisely, and accurately to your reader. As you did during preparation, focus on the message, not on the mechanics.

A clear message ensures that your reader knows precisely what is expected; an unclear message leaves room for doubt.

Unclear: Please contact me.
Clear: Please contact me by Thursday, October 1.
Unclear: You need to make an appointment for blood work.
Clear: Call Temple Hospital laboratories (555-4010) and make an appointment for a blood glucose test on March 13.

A concise message is short and to the point. Wordy phrases with many adjectives should not be used.

Not concise: Please enclose a check in an envelope for exactly $50.
Concise: Please enclose a $50 check.

An accurate message includes the correct date, time, figures, and information. Inaccurate messages cause delays and confusion and can lead to poor public relations.

Editing

After you have composed the letter, edit it for both grammatical errors and factual information. Editing is a key step in making your letter a success. Editing entails two steps: proofreading and corrections.

Proofreading. Whenever possible, have a colleague **proofread** (read text and check for accuracy) your letter and provide constructive criticism. Be sure to maintain confidentiality. If you are using a computer, consider printing out a hard copy of your document for proofreading; some individuals find it difficult to proofread a document on the computer screen. Check for the following items:

- Accuracy of all information
- Clarity and conciseness
- Grammar
- Spelling
- Punctuation
- Paragraphs appropriate in length and limited to one subject
- Capitalization
- Logical organization and flow

Use proofreaders marks (Box 3-6) to speed up the editing process. These are standard marks used to indicate corrections. You should become familiar with the basic marks.

Checkpoint Question

4. What is the purpose of proofreading?

Corrections. After making corrections, print a final copy of the letter. As discussed earlier in the chapter, a computer spell check should be used with caution, as it highlights misspelled words but not incorrectly used words.

Types of Business Letters

You will be asked to create and type various letters. Letters that you write will be sent to patients, insurance companies, other health care providers, pharmaceutical companies, and

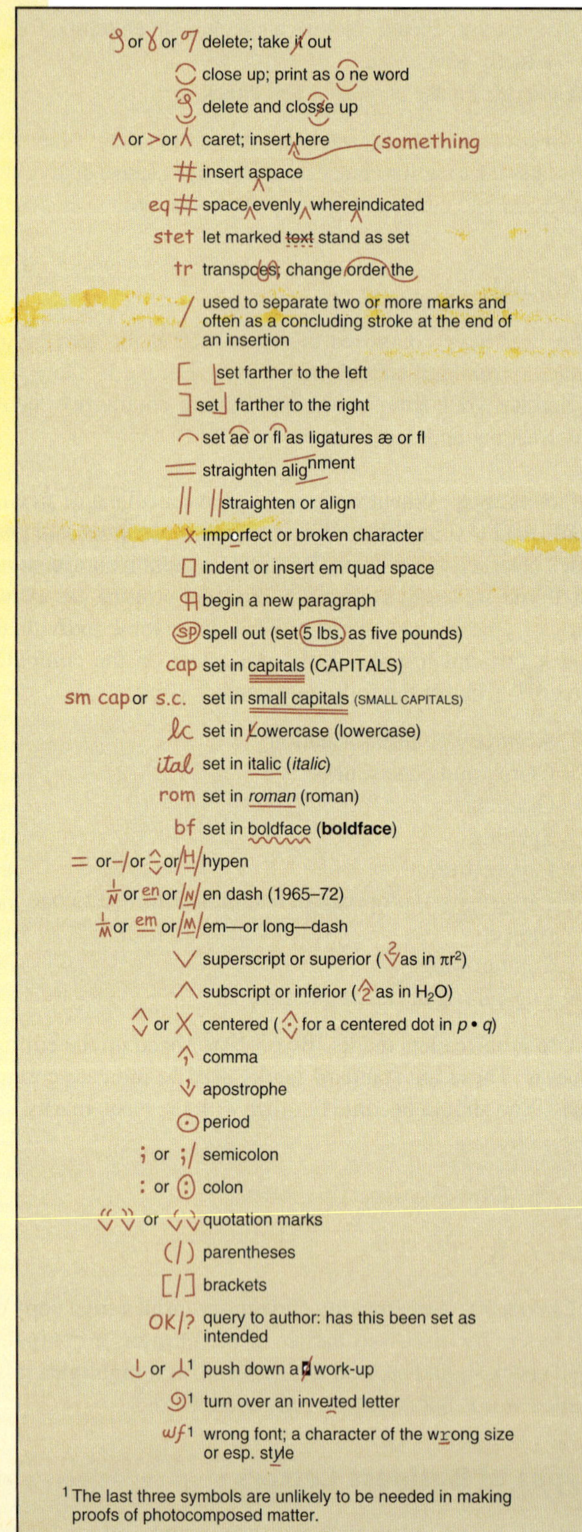

various businesses. Here are some common types of letters that you may write:

- Letters welcoming new patients to the practice
- Letters to patients regarding their test results
- Consultation reports to other health care professionals
- Workers' compensation letters verifying the patient's injury or treatment
- Justification or explanation of treatments to insurance companies
- Cover letters for transferring patients' records to another practice
- Clarification or explanation to patients regarding fees or billing concerns
- Thank you letters to sales representatives
- Physician changes for on-call schedules (generally sent to the hospital and covering physicians)
- Announcements of new services, hours, or office location changes.

MEMORANDUM DEVELOPMENT

A **memorandum** (often called a memo) is for communication within the office or with another department only; it is never sent to patients. It is less formal than a letter and is generally used for brief announcements.

Components of a Memorandum

A memorandum contains the standard elements in the following list. Use these guidelines to complete each element. Figure 3-4 shows a sample memorandum.

1. *Heading.* The word Memorandum is typed across the top of the page.
2. *Date.* Use the same rules for letters when typing the date for memorandums.
3. *To.* List the names of all recipients in either alphabetic or hierarchic order. If the memorandum is going to a particular group (e.g., all department managers, all employees), it can be addressed to the group.
4. *From.* List the name and title of the person sending the memorandum.
5. *Subject.* Insert a brief phrase describing the purpose of the memorandum.
6. *Body.* Write the message of the memorandum here.
7. *Copy (c).* Use the same rules as for letters when sending duplicate copies of memorandums.

Salutations and closings are not used in memorandums. All lines in a memorandum are justified left, and 1-inch margins are used. Writing a memorandum entails the same steps (preparation, composition, editing) as writing a business letter. The memorandum should be read and initialed by the physician before it is distributed. Your computer software will have a memorandum template.

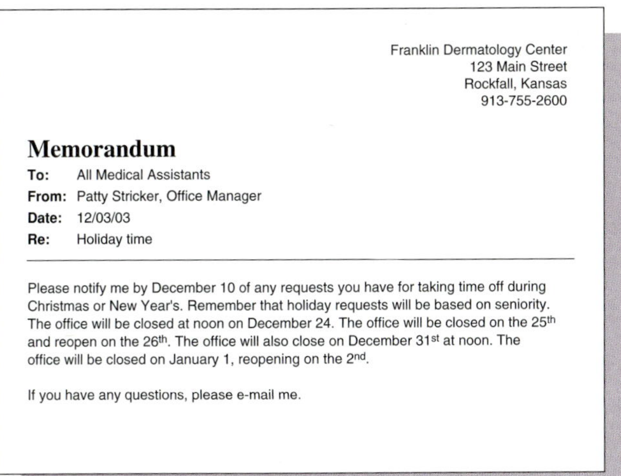

Franklin Dermatology Center
123 Main Street
Rockfall, Kansas
913-755-2600

Memorandum

To: All Medical Assistants
From: Patty Stricker, Office Manager
Date: 12/03/03
Re: Holiday time

Please notify me by December 10 of any requests you have for taking time off during Christmas or New Year's. Remember that holiday requests will be based on seniority. The office will be closed at noon on December 24. The office will be closed on the 25th and reopen on the 26th. The office will also close on December 31st at noon. The office will be closed on January 1, reopening on the 2nd.

If you have any questions, please e-mail me.

FIGURE 3-4. Sample memorandum.

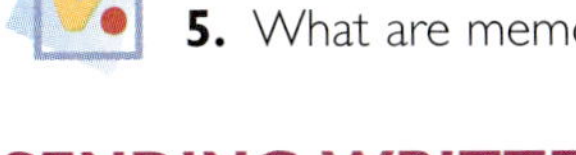

Checkpoint Question

5. What are memorandums used for?

SENDING WRITTEN COMMUNICATION

After the document has been written, proofread, and signed, it is ready for you to send it to its receiver. Fold the letter in thirds and place it in an envelope. Most professional letters are sent through the postal service. Other types of written communications are sent through facsimile machines or by electronic mail. Here are two key steps to remember when sending any type of written communication:

- All attempts must be made to ensure patient confidentiality. The outside of envelopes should be marked confidential when the correspondence contains information about a patient. Send letters only to known or confirmed addresses.
- Return addresses must be used so that mail can be returned if the recipient is no longer at the given address.

Facsimile Machines

Facsimile, or fax, machines allow the medical office to send and receive printed material over a phone line. These machines offer a convenient and cost-effective way to transmit records, orders, prescriptions, test results, and other materials that require quick receipt. Always use a cover sheet (Fig. 3-5) when sending papers through a fax machine. At minimum a cover sheet should have the following information:

- Name, address, telephone, and fax number of the physician's practice
- Name of the intended receiver of the fax
- Number of pages being sent, counting the cover sheet
- Telephone number of the fax machine of the intended recipient
- Date and time the fax was sent
- Confidentiality statement (e.g., "The information in the facsimile message and any accompanying documents is confidential. This information is intended only for use by the individual or entity name above. If you are not the intended recipient of this information you are hereby notified that any disclosure, copying or distribution of this information is strictly prohibited. Please notify the sender immediately by telephone").

When you receive a fax, photocopy it if it is printed on thermal paper (text printed on thermal paper fades quickly), then forward it to the appropriate person. The fax machine should be checked regularly throughout the day, and all items should be sorted quickly.

Sometimes when you fax a given letter, the fax machine may be busy or the number dialed may be busy. If the number is busy, it is not acceptable to leave the fax papers in the machine for redial unless you are sure that no one else will have access to that document. Never leave documents unattended.

Cardiology Associates
Maria Sefferin, MD
897 Bayou Drive
Philadelphia, PA
215-112-9999

facsimile transmittal

To: ______ **Fax:** ______
From: ______ **Date:** ______
Re: ______ **Pages:** ______
CC: ______

☐ Urgent ☐ For Review ☐ Please Comment ☐ Please Reply ☐ Please Recycle

Comments:

CONFIDENTIAL INFORMATION

The information in the facsimile message and any accompanying documents is confidential. This information is intended only for use by the individual or entity name above. If you are not the intended recipient of this information you are hereby notified that any disclosure, copying or distribution of this information is strictly prohibited. Please notify the sender immediately by telephone.

FIGURE 3-5. Sample fax cover sheet.

Electronic Mail

Electronic mail, or e-mail, allows computer-to-computer communication, whether within the same facility or anywhere throughout the world. The communication occurs through a modem. Each computer must be linked to an online service provider. Here are a few things you should remember about sending letters via electronic mail:

- Confidentiality cannot be guaranteed.
- Follow the usual steps of preparation, composition, and editing.
- You can attach letters to an e-mail by clicking on the file attachment icon, locating the letter, and inserting it. It is always a good idea to open the attachment to make sure that you are attaching the correct letter or version.

United States Postal Service

Written communication is commonly sent via the United States Postal Service (USPS). Envelopes must be correctly prepared so that the optical character readers (OCR) used by the USPS can sort the mail quickly and efficiently. The OCR reads the envelope, scanning for information. The OCR scans all envelopes using these margins: 1/2 inch on either side and 5/8 inch from the top or bottom of the envelope. Addresses or notations outside of these margins will not be read.

Addressing Envelopes

The standard business envelope is no. 10. USPS regulations state that the minimal size of an envelope is $3\frac{1}{2} \times 5$ inches. It must be rectangular and no less than 0.007 inch thick. The standard no. 10 business envelope is $4\frac{1}{8} \times 9\frac{1}{2}$ inches.

The return address is placed in the upper left hand corner. It should not exceed five lines. The return address is typed with the same guidelines as for letters and is single spaced. Often, medical offices have the return address preprinted on the envelope.

The recipient's address is typed 12 spaces down from the top and centered on the face of the envelope. All words of the address should begin with a capital letter. Only postal abbreviations for states should be used, and no punctuation is used between the postal abbreviation and the zip code. All addresses must include the five-digit zip code; whenever possible, the four-digit expanded zip code should also be used. The expanded zip code allows the USPS to sort and route the mail faster and more accurately. Envelopes should not be handwritten, as this does not portray a professional image. The entire address should not exceed five lines. Your software may allow you to insert a USPS PostNet bar code. This is generally inserted two to three lines below the address. This bar code accelerates USPS sorting. Always check your software to make sure it is certified by the USPS.

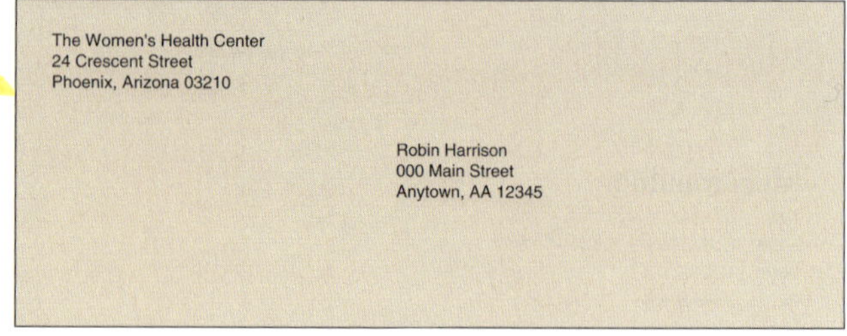

FIGURE 3-6. Properly addressed envelope.

Special notations such as "confidential" or "personal" are placed on the left-hand side of the envelope two lines below the return address. Notations for hand canceling and special delivery are made in the upper right-hand corner of the envelope below the postage. Nothing should be printed in the right lower corner of the envelope, because the USPS uses that space for its bar codes. Figure 3-6 displays a properly addressed envelope.

Here are some additional things to remember regarding envelopes:

- Be sure that graphics or logos do not impede the OCR's ability to read the address.
- Do not use fancy fonts that may impede the OCR's ability to read the address.
- A minimum of eight-point type is recommended by the USPS.
- Do not use dark envelopes.
- White or tan envelope with black type is preferred.
- Do not use the # sign; if it cannot be avoided, leave one space between the # sign and the number (this is a USPS recommendation).
- If you are using an envelope with a window frame, there should be an eighth-inch clearance around the address.

Checkpoint Question

6. What does an optical character reader do?

Affixing Postage

Proper postage must be affixed to the envelope by a stamp, permit imprint, or a postage meter machine. Postal meter machines are in-house machines that are regulated by the USPS. They contain a prepaid amount of postage and can imprint the postage stamp either directly on the envelope or onto an adhesive tape that is applied to the envelope. Some machines weigh, stuff, and seal the envelopes. The date on the postal machine must be changed daily, and the ink roller must be kept full.

The physician may opt to use the USPS permit imprint program. In this case, you take the mail, sealed and ready to be sent, to the post office. The postal clerk passes your letters through the USPS machine, and a permit stamp is placed on the envelope. The postal clerk deducts the postage charges from your prepaid account. The advantages to this

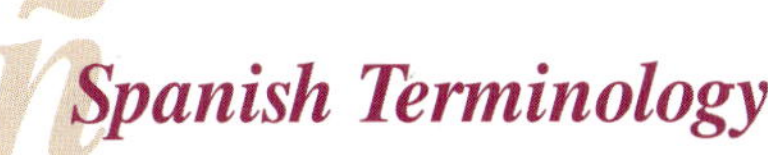

Spanish Terminology

¿Donde está la oficina de correos?	Where is the post office?
Tengo que enviar esta carta.	I need to mail this letter.
¿Cuanto cuesta el franqueo?	How much does the postage cost?

system are that is saves time and does not require the office to care for the postal meter machine.

USPS Mailing Options

Mail can be sent in a variety of ways based on its urgency and value. The following is a brief description of the services offered by the USPS:

- Express mail, the fastest service, ensures delivery of your package by the next day (by noon in most areas). Express mail is delivered 7 days a week. The rate starts at $13.65, and fees increase by weight and destination. Express mail is automatically insured for $500. Additional insurance is available.
- Priority mail, the second fastest service, offers 2-day delivery to most destinations. The maximum weight is 70 pounds, and the maximum size is 108 inches combined length and girth. The rate is based on the weight of the package. You can purchase up to $5,000 of insurance for packages.
- First-class mail is the service used for sending standard mail (letters and postcards) weighing up to 13 ounces. Mail weighing more than 13 ounces will be considered priority mail.
- Standard mail (A) is used by companies to mail books and catalogs. Standard mail (B) is used to mail packages weighing more than 1 pound. The maximum weight is 70 pounds, and the maximum measurement is 130 inches combined length and girth.
- Postal rates, fees, and services are subject to change.

You must stay abreast of the latest information. Use the USPS website for additional information and updates.

USPS Special Services

A certificate of mailing is used to prove that a document was mailed. No record is kept at the post office. It does not provide proof that the letter was received by the addressee.

Certified mail provides a mailing receipt and a record of the mailing at the local post office (Fig. 3-7). This service is available only for first-class and priority mail. Return receipts can be purchased in conjunction with this. Return receipts are used to prove that the recipient received the document (Fig. 3-8).

Registered mail provides the most protection for valuables. It is available only for priority and first-class mail. The maximum insurance that can be obtained is $25,000. This service can be combined with return receipts.

International rates are available from your local post office. Type the address as discussed earlier, and type the name of the country on the last line without abbreviations (Japan, Korea), All physician offices should have a supply of express and priority mail envelopes along with a current fee schedule.

Other Delivery Options

Many other companies specialize in document and package delivery, particularly with next-day or second-day delivery services. Examples of these companies include Airborne

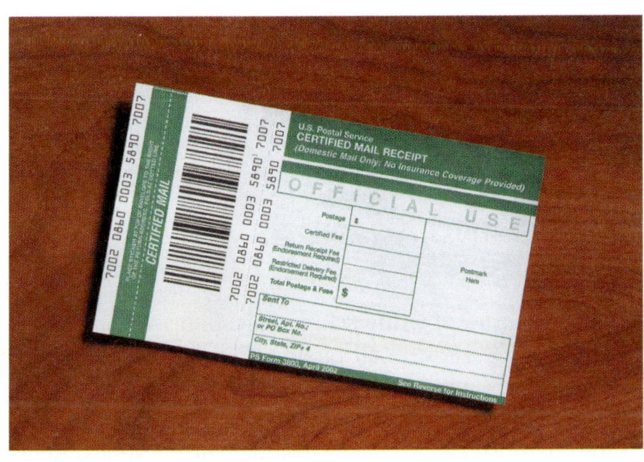

FIGURE 3-7. Certified mail receipt.

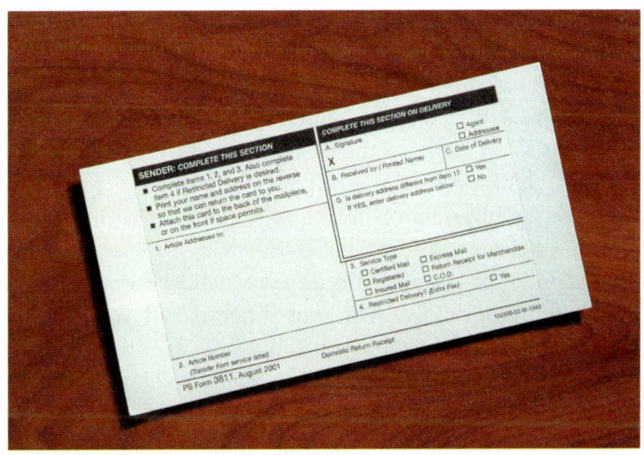

FIGURE 3-8. Return receipt.

Express, Federal Express, and United Parcel Service (UPS). Use the company with which the physician has an account. Fees vary, so you may have to contact each company for prices and available services. These companies offer services such as tracking, pick-up services, money back guarantees, and proof of delivery. The tracking service can be done through their websites.

RECEIVING AND HANDLING INCOMING MAIL

Part of the daily routine for a medical assistant is handling the incoming mail. Sort the mail quickly and promptly to ensure efficient functioning of the office.

Types of Incoming Mail

Many types of mail are received daily in a physician's office:

- Advertisements
- Bills for office services
- Consultation letters
- Hospital communications and newsletters
- Laboratory and radiographic reports
- Office supply magazines
- Patient correspondence
- Payments from insurance companies and patients
- Professional journals
- Literature from professional organizations
- Samples (drugs, laboratory test kits)
- Waiting room magazines

Opening and Sorting Mail

Each physician will have an individual policy on which mail you should open and how you should process it. Any mail marked urgent should be handled first, followed by mail about patient-related issues. Promotional materials should be handled last. Some physicians will have you sort, file, and respond to mail without their review. In some practices, however, all mail is placed in a special file folder and handled only by the physician or office manager. Box 3-7 lists general guidelines for opening and sorting the mail. Most physicians will open and handle their own e-mail. If the physician is on vacation, he or she will apply an auto reply response to his or her e-mail address.

When the physician is away, personal mail is placed on his or her desk and left for the physician to handle. Mail that pertains to patient care issues should be opened and handled appropriately. Ask your supervisor if you are unsure which pieces of mail you should open. If the mail requires an urgent response, the covering physician should be contacted unless otherwise directed. Mail should never be allowed to accumulate in outside mailboxes because patient information is confidential.

Box 3-7

OPENING AND SORTING MAIL

1. Gather the necessary equipment: a letter opener, paper clips, and a date stamp.
2. Open all letters and check for enclosures; paper clip these to the letter. If the letter states that enclosures were sent but they are not in the envelope, contact the sender and request them. Indicate on the letter that the enclosures were missing and the name of the person you contacted.
3. Date-stamp each item.
4. Sort the mail into categories and deal with it appropriately. Generally, you should handle the following types of mail as noted:
   - Use a paper clip to attach test results to the patient's chart; place the chart in a pile for the physician to review.
   - Record promptly all insurance payments and checks and deposit them according to office policy.
   - Account for all drug samples and appropriately log them into the sample book.
   - Dispose of miscellaneous advertisements unless otherwise directed.
5. Distribute the mail to the appropriate staff members. For example, mail can be for the physician, nurse manager, office manager, billing clerk, or other personnel.

Checkpoint Question

7. What mail must be opened first?

Annotation

Some physicians request that letters be annotated. **Annotation** involves reading a document and highlighting the key points. If the letter is very detailed, a summary of the key points should be written in the margins. The summary should be factual and not editorialized.

COMPOSING AGENDAS AND MINUTES

Two other forms of written communication are agendas and minutes. The purpose of an **agenda** (Figure 3-9) is to outline briefly the topics to be discussed at a meeting.

It allows the meeting participants to prepare any necessary reports before the meeting and to anticipate questions. Agendas usually begin with a call to order, followed by a review

Quality Improvement Committee
February 15, 2003
Agenda

I. Call to order
II. Review and acceptance of the minutes from January 10, 2003
III. Old business
   A. Copy machine updates
   B. Insurance updates for overdue accounts
IV. New business
   A. New contract for laboratory supplies
   B. Scheduling guidelines for summer vacations
V. Adjournment

FIGURE 3-9. Agenda.

of previous meeting minutes, old business updates, then new business. Adjournment is the last item on the agenda.

You should type the minutes of a meeting as soon as possible, including the following:

- List of members present
- List of members absent
- Date and time the meeting was called to order
- Statement regarding the acceptance of the previous minutes
- Brief description of discussions
- List of reports that were submitted
- Date and time of the next meeting
- Adjournment time
- Signature of the person who prepared the minutes and the chairperson's signature

Procedure 3-1

Writing a Business Letter

Equipment/Supplies: Paper, writing utensil, computer with word processing software, printer.

Steps

1. Prepare your message by determining who your reader is, what you want them to do, what you want to say, and how you want to organize your message.
2. Select appropriate template or format, margin, and font for the letter.
3. Create a letterhead.
4. Type the date (include month, day, and year) two to four lines below the letterhead.
5. Type the inside address four lines below the date.
6. Type the salutation two lines below the inside address.
7. Type the body of the letter using language that is clear, concise, and accurate.
8. Type the closing two lines below the body of the letter.
9. Leave three lines of space for the signature.
10. Type the name of the person sending the document four lines below the closing.
11. Type the identification line two lines below the typed name.
12. Indicate enclosures, if applicable, two lines below the identification line.
13. Check document for proper grammar, spelling, and punctuation.
14. Check document for accuracy—be sure that all addresses and phone numbers are correct.
15. Check that each paragraph is kept to one topic only.
16. Save document with a proper file name.
17. Print document.

SUMMARY

As a medical assistant, you need excellent written communication skills. Careful attention to detail is essential. Good grammar, punctuation, and spelling are key skills. Be careful when you use your computer spell check. It will not recognize words that are misused. You will use these skills to write letters, memorandums, and other correspondence. These letters will be sent to patients, physicians, and businesses. After writing these documents, you must be able to select the appropriate service for mailing your letters. Your primary goal with all written communication is to get your message across in a clear, concise, and accurate manner.

Critical Thinking Challenges

1. Create a business letter. Include all the components and use the full block format. Print your unedited copy and, using proofreaders marks, indicate your corrections. Make the corrections and reprint a final copy. Ask your instructor to review both copies.
2. Write 10 sentences using terms from Box 3-3. Use some terms correctly and others incorrectly. Exchange your sentences with another student. Correct your peer's sentences.
3. Collect five pieces of mail that you have received at home. What method of affixing postage did they use? Go to your local USPS office. Obtain either a priority mail or express mail envelope. Correctly address the envelope.
4. Suppose the physician told you to read his e-mails while he was on vacation. In doing so, you come across a personal piece of information that you know he would not want you to see. How would you handle it? Would you tell anyone that you saw it? Would you question the physician about it?

Answers to Checkpoint Questions

1. Inaccurate information in a business letter can lead to injuries to the patient and lawsuits and can harm the physician's practice.
2. The inside address is the address of the person to whom the letter is going. The salutation is the greeting. The identification line shows the initials of the person who dictated the letters and the initials of the person who typed the letter.
3. Before you begin to type a letter, select the template, font, and margins that you will use.
4. Proofreading allows you to check the accuracy and content of the letter.
5. Memorandums are used for communication within the office and with other departments.
6. The USPS uses optical character readers to quickly and efficiently sort the mail.
7. Any mail marked urgent must be opened first.

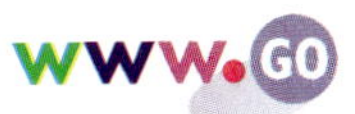

Websites

Here are some Web addresses that may help you:

Airborne Express
www.airborne.com

Medical dictionary
www.medical-dictionary.com

Merriam-Webster's Dictionary
www.m-w.com

United Parcel Service
www.ups.com

United States Postal Service
www.usps.com

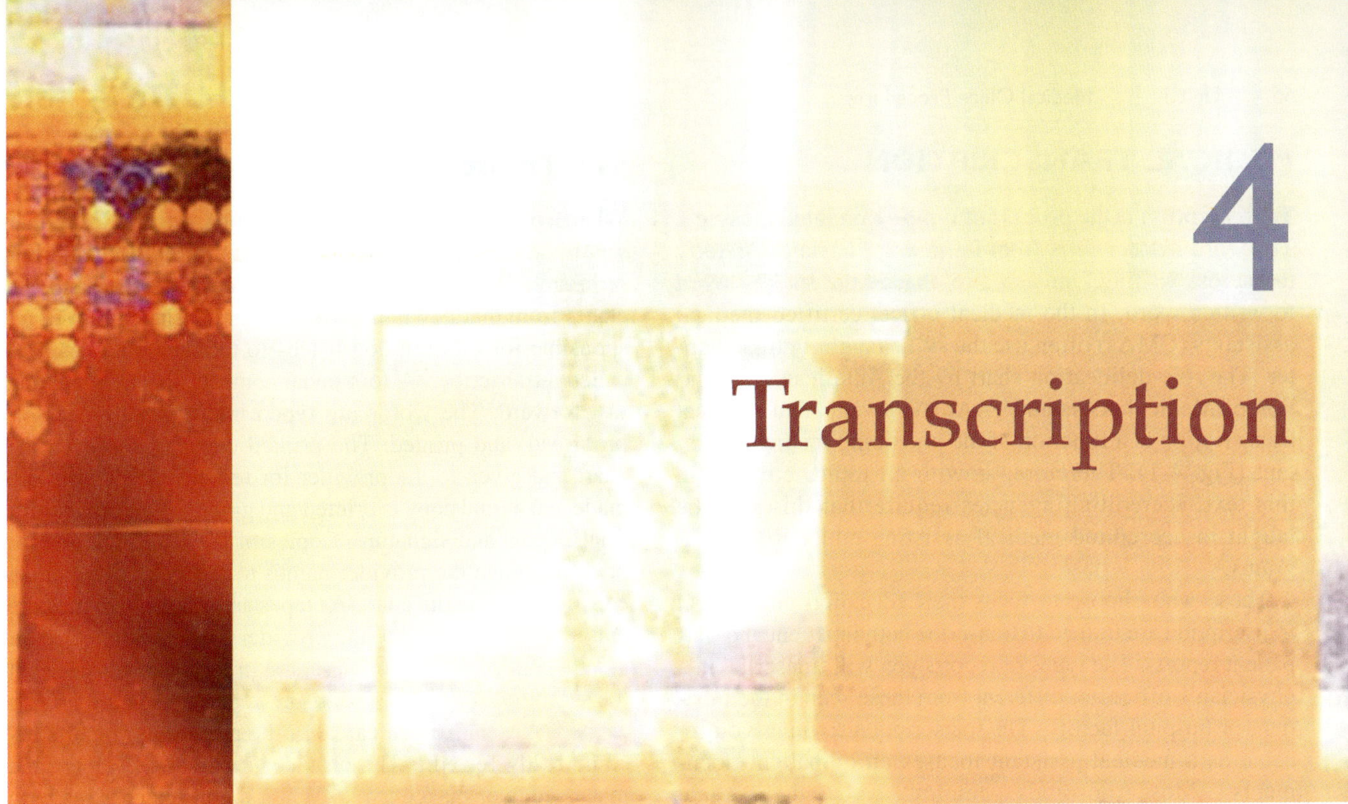

4 Transcription

CHAPTER OBJECTIVES

In this chapter, you'll learn:

1. To explain the role of the medical assistant in performing medical transcription.
2. To explain the roles of the JCAHO and HIPAA on medical transcription.
3. To list the various reports generated in inpatient and outpatient medical facilities.
4. To list the rules of medical transcription as outlined by the AAMT.
5. To discuss the various medical transcription systems.

PERFORMANCE OBJECTIVES

In this chapter, you'll learn:

1. To transcribe various medical reports from taped dictation.
2. To use proper punctuation, grammar, and spelling.

KEY TERMS

analogue
digital
transcription

MEDICAL TRANSCRIPTION

Transcription is the process of typing a dictated message. The word *transcript* is from Latin and translates literally to "across writing," meaning to change the spoken word to written word. In the medical office, certified medical assistants (CMAs) often use the skills taught in this chapter. The role delineation chart by the American Association of Medical Assistants (AAMA) reveals that medical transcription is a function of the practicing medical assistant (Fig. 4-1). Therefore, as with all topics covered in this text, accrediting agencies require that this skill be taught in accredited medical assisting educational programs.

Those who choose to focus their education on medical transcription are trained to transcribe both inpatient and outpatient reports. The types of reports you will transcribe in a physician's office are different from those seen in the inpatient or hospital facility. The transcription training you receive as a medical assistant focuses on outpatient documents. Most hospitals employ certified medical transcriptionists. Some physicians' offices use outside medical transcription companies, and this is another employment opportunity for the trained medical assistant. In today's computerized world, with a modem and sound privacy protection practices, a transcriptionist could conceivably generate and transmit reports from anywhere in the world.

To transcribe well, you must

- Be a fast and accurate typist
- Have a strong vocabulary in medical terminology
- Have a thorough knowledge of grammar, spelling, and punctuation rules
- Have excellent listening skills
- Have good editing skills

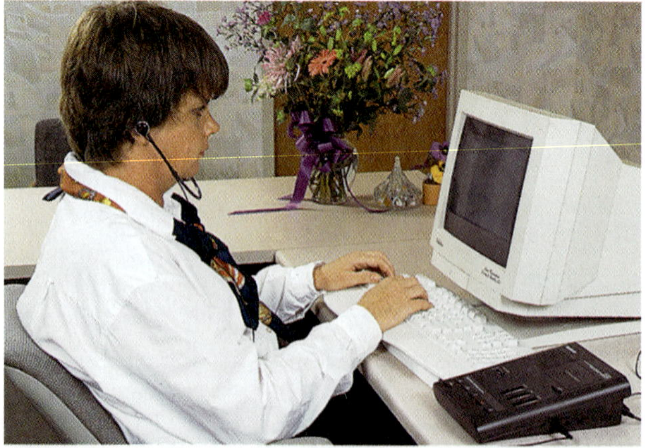

FIGURE 4-1. A transcriptionist must have good communications and computer skills.

The Transcription Process

When a patient visits a physician's office, the provider either writes the findings or dictates a report into a handheld microphone. The provider places the cassette tape and the charts from that day in a designated area. The employee responsible for transcription listens to the tape on a machine called a transcriber. A foot pedal controls play, rewind, and fast forward. The words are typed into a word processor, proofread, and printed. The printed copy is placed on the chart and given to the provider for review. Corrections are made and a final copy is printed and given to the provider for final review and signature. Copies of the report are distributed to anyone the provider names to receive a copy, and a copy is placed in the chart. As tapes are transcribed, they are erased and given back to the provider to use again.

When an office is paperless, the process is the same, but the document is entered into the record instead of being printed. A visual signal can alert the provider as reports become ready for edit. The provider accesses the report and makes edits or marks errors. When the provider is ready to authenticate the report, the stroke of a key "signs" the report. The software allows the provider to check the status of a report at any time.

Off-site Transcription

Many medical offices outsource their transcription through various types of services. Individuals or companies offer services to physicians ranging from picking up tapes and delivering the work on hard copy to transmitting the documents through e-mail.

Several large transcription companies operate solely on the Internet. These websites can be found at the end of the chapter. You can log on, and after passing an online examination, you may begin receiving dictation via modem. The report is transmitted back to the company, which sends it to the provider. Usually, the transcriptionist must buy the necessary equipment. The new regulations of the HIPAA (Health Insurance Portability and Accountability Act) will require changes in practices for transmission of confidential information via modem.

REPORT FORMATTING

There is no set format for each type of medical document. Every facility has its own format and design, but any professional document should be well balanced and attractive, with single spacing, double spacing between headings, and 1-inch margins. Being familiar with the logical sequence and proper sorting of information for each type of document will help you adapt to any prescribed format. Headings and subheadings are used to report the information gathered in the course of a patient encounter. These general headings are seen in the sample reports in Figs. 4-2 to 4-9.

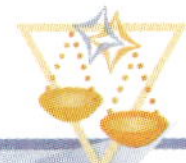

LEGAL TIP

Legal Aspects of Transcription

Health care facilities are expected to adhere to general standards to ensure patient rights and safety. The JCAHO, Joint Commission on Accreditation of Healthcare Organizations, requires that all hospitals and hospital-owned physician practices:

- Use abbreviations from an approved list and provide a key to the reader (if requested.) For a list of accepted abbreviations used in charting.
- Adhere to a specific time frame for review and completion (signing) by physicians.

In addition, HIPAA establishes specific regulations to safeguard the privacy of patient information when using electronic means for medical transcription.

Checkpoint Question

1. List four requirements of any professional document.

TYPES OF MEDICAL REPORTS

Hospital (inpatient) documents and medical office (outpatient) documents are different. The most common documents transcribed in a medical office are history and physical examination (H&P) reports, consultation reports, and progress reports. Practices that offer diagnostic tests are required to generate a report of the findings. For example, a neurologist's practice may perform electroencephalography (EEG) to measure the electrical activity in the brain. The medical assistant transcribes a dictated report of the findings. Other types of documents in outpatient facilities are reports of minor surgical procedures, legal abstracts, and general office correspondence.

Documents that are seen in the hospital setting include H&Ps, consultation reports, radiology and pathology reports, transfer summaries, discharge and death summaries, and autopsies. Many radiologists who work in hospitals also have a private practices and will dictate a report for each radiology procedure done in the office. You need to become familiar with the reports generated in a hospital because they become a part of the office chart and are used for insurance. Figures 4-6 to 4-9 are samples of typical reports generated in a hospital or inpatient setting.

History and Physical Examination Reports

In the inpatient setting, the H&P is a vital part of the quality of patient care. The JCAHO (Joint Commission on Accreditation of Healthcare Organizations) accredits and regulates every aspect of the policies and practices of hospitals and physician offices owned by hospital organizations.

The JCAHO guidelines require hospitals to provide a H&P on a patient's chart within 24 hours of admission in a facility. This report is dictated by the admitting physician and must be signed or authenticated electronically within a specified time. Many times the patient is seen in the office, and the physician makes the decision to admit. The examination takes place in the office, but the report is dictated to the hospital, which is responsible for transcription. Many physicians use the H&P format to record a patient's annual physical examination in the office as well.

The H&P is divided into two sections: the history, which gives an overview of the patient's medical, family, and social history; and the report on the physical examination, which reviews the results of the examination. Figure 4-2 is a sample history and physical examination report.

Checkpoint Question

2. List two requirements of the JCAHO regarding H&Ps.

Consultation Reports

When one provider refers a patient to another, usually a specialist, the consulting physician prepares a consultation

WHAT IF

You are transcribing notes and hear an unfamiliar word or phrase on the tape. What should you do?

You should have a selection of reference materials available at your workstation. Examples of useful reference books include a standard dictionary, a general medical dictionary, a medical dictionary specific to your specialty, a drug reference such as the *Physicians' Desk Reference* (PDR), and a medical textbook on anatomy, physiology, and disease processes. Remember, software that provides a medical dictionary to interact with your word processing spell check is available. If you cannot find the word, leave a blank large enough for the physician to write in the word. The report can be edited before being signed.

CENTRAL MEDICAL GROUP, INC.

Department of Internal Medicine

201 Medical Center Drive • Central City, US 90000-1234 • PHONE: (012) 125-8888 • FAX: (012) 125-3434

PATIENT: COHEN, SARA E. DATE: April 8, 20xx

HISTORY

CHIEF COMPLAINT: Epigastric distress

HISTORY OF PRESENT ILLNESS: This 33-year-old Caucasian female comes in because of excessive burping, epigastric distress and nausea for several weeks. Coffee makes it worse. She complains that it is worse at night when lying down. She gets an acid-like taste in her mouth. She has tried antacids, to no avail.

PAST MEDICAL HISTORY: The patient states that she had the usual childhood diseases. She has had no serious medical illnesses and has been involved in no accidents. Family History: There is some diabetes on her mother's side. Her mother is 52 and has hypertension. Her father, age 56, is living and well. She has a sister who is anemic and a brother who has ulcers. Social History: The patient discontinued smoking ten years ago. Drinks alcohol socially. Allergies: NKDA.
Current Medications: Medications at this time consist of Entex, Guaifed, birth control pills, iron and vitamin supplements.

REVIEW OF SYSTEMS: HEENT: Chronic sinusitis. She sees an ENT specialist and an allergist. Respiratory: Negative. Cardiac: Occasional flutters. Gastrointestinal: As stated above. Genitourinary: Occasional infections. Pap smear is up-to-date and negative. She has had no mammogram at this point. Neuromuscular: Negative.

PHYSICAL EXAMINATION

GENERAL APPEARANCE: Reveals a well-developed, well-nourished female in no acute distress.

VITAL SIGNS: Blood Pressure: 120/80. Pulse: 76 and regular.

HEENT: Head normocephalic. Eyes: Pupils are equal, round, and reactive to light and accommodation. Fundi are benign. Ears, nose and throat are negative. NECK: No thyromegaly. No carotid bruits.

CHEST: Clear to percussion and auscultation. BREASTS: Reveal no masses. HEART: Normal sinus rhythm. No murmurs.

ABDOMEN: Liver, spleen and kidneys could not be felt. Femorals pulsate well, no bruits.

EXTREMITIES: No edema. Pulses are good and equal.

PELVIC & RECTAL EXAMS: Deferred to gynecologist.

NEUROLOGIC EXAM: Physiologic.

IMPRESSION: 1. PROBABLE PEPTIC ULCER DISEASE WITH GASTROESOPHAGEAL REFLUX.
2. POSSIBLE GALLBLADDER DISEASE.

PLAN: Patient started on Pepcid 40 mg, 1 at night. She is given Gaviscon tablets so she can carry them with her. Schedule routine lab work and upper GI series. If negative, schedule ultrasound of the gallbladder.

D. Everley, M.D.

DE:mc
D: 4/8/20xx
T: 4/9/20xx

FIGURE 4-2. Sample history and physical examination report. (Reprinted with permission from Willis MC. *Medical Terminology: The Language of Health Care*, 1st ed. Baltimore: Williams & Wilkins, 1996.)

report to report the findings of the encounter. A consultation report contains a detailed account of the consulting physician's findings and recommendations regarding the patient. These reports are often written in the format of the H&P but are structured as a letter to the physician who referred the patient. Figure 4-3 is a sample consultation report.

Progress Reports

In the outpatient medical facility, the patient's progress is recorded on an ongoing sheet in the chart. When the notes are transcribed, they are printed either directly on this sheet or on special paper with perforations and adhesive backing. The reports are separated and stuck on the progress sheet. Remember, the entries in the medical record must be consecutive. This presents a problem if the transcription is not on the chart when the next entry is made. Entries that are out of order give the appearance of disorganization, improper record keeping, or even an attempt to cover up negligence.

Progress notes are formatted in several ways. The SOAP (subjective, objective, assessment, plan) method of reporting a patient's visit is the most common format used in medical offices. The report is dictated in narrative form using general headings. In the outpatient medical facility, you will transcribe this information. Refer to Figure 4-4 as we examine each part of the report.

SOAP Notes

Subjective. The subjective portion of the report includes information that cannot be detected or measured. This information can only be provided by the patient. Pain and nausea are examples of subjective information. This heading also includes the *chief complaint* (CC), the reason the patient is at the facility. In the subjective section, the provider explains the chief complaint in detail, including how long the symptoms have been present and what remedies the patient has tried, along with their results. This is sometimes called the *history of present illness* (HPI). A subheading titled *Medication* may be included in this section to report medications that the patient is taking.

Objective. The objective information in this section comes from the physical examination, laboratory data, diagnostic test results, and other data that can be measured or observed. The patient's appearance, vital signs, any rash, and results of laboratory tests are examples of objective information. For example, the narrative report might say, "EEG is normal."

Assessment. As discussed earlier, the assessment portion of the report refers to the established or possible diagnosis based on the subjective and objective information provided and gathered. Other subheading titles include *Diagnosis*, *Evaluation*, *Impression*, and *Differential Diagnoses*.

Plan. The plan is the steps the physician intends to take. They are usually typed in a numbered list. Medications prescribed, diagnostic tests ordered, referrals to other physicians, and return appointments are included in this section.

Checkpoint Question

3. Compare subjective and objective information. Give two examples of each.

Hospital Reports

H&Ps, consultation reports, operative reports, pathology reports, radiology reports, discharge summaries, and death summaries are generated primarily in inpatient facilities. Every document generated by a hospital transcription department is "copied to," that is, copied and sent to the physician who dictated it. These documents are kept in the physician's office chart.

Operative Report

Each surgical procedure performed in a hospital is documented. Physicians dictate an operative note immediately after the procedure. It is typed and put on the chart as soon as possible so that others caring for the patient have access to the information. When physicians perform surgery in their outpatient offices, the operative report is transcribed in the physician's office. The terms used in operative reports are often difficult. Many sutures and instruments are named for the person who developed them. A reference book for surgical terms is essential for transcribing. Information included in the operative reports includes the patient's preoperative and postoperative diagnoses, the type of anesthesia used, step-by-step details of the procedure, estimated blood loss, results of sponge and instrument counts, and the condition of the patient at the end of the procedure. The subheadings usually follow that format. Figure 4-5 is a sample operative report.

Pathology Report

Any organ or tissue removed from a patient in the operating room is examined by a pathologist. A pathology report outlines the findings of gross and microscopic examinations performed on organs, lesions, and tissue samples removed in surgery. Figure 4-6 is an example of a typical pathology report on a specimen.

Autopsy Report

Pathologists also dictate autopsy reports. An autopsy report, also called necropsy report or medical examiner report, is generated as the autopsy is performed. Autopsies are done to find the cause of death of a patient or to find or confirm diseases present. The law requires that autopsies be performed in certain situations. The autopsy report includes a preliminary diagnosis, a brief history of the patient, findings from

(text continues on page 63)

CENTRAL MEDICAL GROUP, INC.

Department of Otorhinolaryngology

201 Medical Center Drive • Central City, US 90000-1234 • PHONE: (012) 125-8888 • FAX: (012) 125-3434

Patient: Perron, Carleen DATE: February 17, 20xx

Referring Physician: C. Camarillo, M.D.

CONSULTATION

REASON FOR CONSULTATION: This 28-year-old white female presents with a one week history of upper respiratory infection (URI), sinusitis, and some periorbital headaches in recent weeks. She also has expectorated yellow-green mucus occasionally and has had a history of tonsillitis.

MEDICATIONS: None. ALLERGIES: No known allergies (NKA). SURGERIES: None. HOSPITALIZATIONS: None.

PAST MEDICAL HISTORY/REVIEW OF SYSTEMS: Cardiopulmonary: There is no history of angina, dyspnea, hemoptysis, emphysema, asthma, chronic obstructive pulmonary disease (COPD), hypertension, or heart murmurs. Cardiovascular: There is no history of high blood pressure. Renal: There is no history of dysuria, polyuria, nocturia, hematuria, or cystoliths. Gastrointestinal: There is no history of gallbladder disease, hepatitis, pancreatitis, or colitis. Musculoskeletal: There is no history of arthritis. Endocrine: There is no history of diabetes. Hematologic: There is no history of anemia, blood transfusion, or easy bruising. Gynecological: The patient states her menses are regular, and the start of her last menstrual cycle occurred 15 days ago.

FAMILY HISTORY: The patient states her maternal grandmother has diabetes.

SOCIAL HISTORY: The patient is single and has no children. She denies smoking tobacco. She denies drinking alcoholic beverages. She denies taking drugs.

CHILDHOOD DISEASES: The patient has had the usual childhood diseases.

OTOLARYNGOLOGIC EXAMINATION: Otoscopy: Tympanic membranes (TMs) are dull and slightly congested. Sinuses: There is maxillary fullness. Rhinoscopic examination reveals mild nasoseptal deviation (NSD). Pharynx: There is moderate inflammation; no exudates. Oropharynx: No masses. Nasopharynx: No masses. Larynx: Clear. Neck: Supple. Cervical Adenopathy: There is mild adenopathy.

IMPRESSION:
1. MAXILLARY SINUSITIS.
2. PHARYNGITIS.
3. CHRONIC TONSILLITIS.

DISPOSITION:
1. Warm salt water gargle (WSWG).
2. Ery-Tab 333, #24, 1 t.i.d. p.c.
3. Robitussin.
4. Return to office (RTO) in one week.

P. Rodden MD

PATRICK RODDEN, M.D.

JR:ti
D: 2/17/20xx
T: 2/18/20xx

FIGURE 4-3. Sample consultation report. (Reprinted with permission from Willis MC. *Medical Terminology: The Language of Health Care*, 1st ed. Baltimore: Williams & Wilkins, 1996.)

CENTRAL MEDICAL GROUP, INC.

Department of Otorhinolaryngology

201 Medical Center Drive • Central City, US 90000-1234 • PHONE: (012) 125-8888 • FAX: (012) 125-3434

PROGRESS NOTES

Patient: PERRON, CARLEEN

03/30/20xx

S: The patient presents with a sore throat x 2 weeks.

O: Sinus exam: Maxillary and frontal congestion. Hypopharynx/adenoids: No inflammation.

A: Recurrent pharyngitis/sinusitis x 2 weeks.

P: 1) Ceftin 250 mg, #21, 1 t.i.d. p.o. p.c.

2) Entex LA, #30, 1 b.i.d. p.o.

3) Warm salt water gargle.

P Rodden MD

PATRICK RODDEN, M.D.

05/25/20xx

S: Recurrent sore throat every month.

O: Recurrent tonsillitis, cryptic tonsillitis. Sinus exam: Maxillary and frontal congestion. Neck: Supple; no masses. Hypopharynx/Adenoids: No inflammation. Paranasal Sinus X-ray: Bilateral frontal and maxillary sinusitis.

A: Recurrent tonsillitis, 8-10 times per year. Chronic maxillary and frontal sinusitis.

P: 1) Tonsillectomy discussed with the patient. The risks of general and local anesthesia, as well as the surgical procedure, were discussed with the patient. The consent form was signed.

2) An admitting order was given to the patient for CBC, UA, and BCP-7 to be done one day prior to being admitted.

3) Ceftin 250 mg, #21, 1 t.i.d. p.o. p.c.

4) Entex LA, #30, 1 b.i.d. p.o.

5) Beconase nasal inhaler, 2 sprays each nostril b.i.d.

6) Warm salt water gargle.

P Rodden MD

PATRICK RODDEN, M.D.

FIGURE 4-4. Sample progress report. (Reprinted with permission from Willis MC. *Medical Terminology: The Language of Health Care*, 1st ed. Baltimore: Williams & Wilkins, 1996.)

CENTRAL MEDICAL CENTER

211 Medical Center Drive • Central City, US 90000-1234 • PHONE: (012) 125-6784 • FAX: (012) 125-9999

OPERATIVE REPORT

DATE OF OPERATION: June 3, 20xx

PREOPERATIVE DIAGNOSIS: Chronic tonsillitis.

POSTOPERATIVE DIAGNOSIS: Frequent, recurrent tonsillitis.

SURGEON: Patrick Rodden, M.D.

ASSISTANT SURGEON: None

ANESTHESIOLOGIST: Robert Jung, M.D.

ANESTHESIA: General.

SURGERY PERFORMED: Tonsillectomy.

DESCRIPTION OF OPERATION: After general anesthesia induction, with intubation, the McGivor mouth gag and tongue retractor were utilized for exposure of the oropharynx. Local anesthetic consisting of 6 cc of 0.5% Xylocaine with 1:100,000 epinephrine was utilized. Tonsillectomy was carried out using dissection and air technique. The right tonsillectomy electrocoagulation Bovie suction was utilized for hemostasis. Examination of the nasopharynx was normal.

The patient tolerated the procedure well and went to the recovery room in good condition.

P. Rodden MD

PATRICK RODDEN, M.D.

JR:as
D: 6/3/20xx
T: 6/4/20xx

OPERATIVE REPORT	PT. NAME:	PERRON, CARLEEN
	ID NO:	672894017
	ROOM NO:	312
	ATT. PHYS:	PATRICK RODDEN, M.D.

FIGURE 4-5. Sample operative report. (Reprinted with permission from Willis MC. *Medical Terminology: A Programmed Learning Approach to the Language of Health Care*, 1st ed. Baltimore: Lippincott Williams & Wilkins, 2002.)

CENTRAL MEDICAL CENTER

211 Medical Center Drive • Central City, US 90000-1234 • PHONE: (012) 125-6784 • FAX: (012) 125-9999

PATHOLOGY REPORT

PATIENT: PERRON, CARLEEN
28 Y (FEMALE)

DATE RECEIVED: June 3, 20xx DATE REPORTED: June 4, 20xx

GROSS:

Received are two tonsils each 2.5 cm in greatest diameter.

MICROSCOPIC:

The sections show deep tonsillar crypts associated with follicular lymphoid hyperplasia. No bacterial granules are seen.

DIAGNOSIS:

CHRONIC LYMPHOID HYPERPLASIA OF RIGHT AND LEFT TONSILS.

Mary Needham MD
MARY NEEDHAM, M.D.

MN:gds

D: 6/4/20xx
T: 6/5/20xx

FIGURE 4-6. Sample pathology report. (Reprinted with permission from Willis MC. *Medical Terminology: A Programmed Learning Approach to the Language of Health Care*, 1st ed. Baltimore: Lippincott Williams & Wilkins, 2002.)

the examination of the gross anatomy of the body and its organs, findings of the microscopic examination of the cells, and a determination of cause of death.

Radiology Report

Each radiograph must be interpreted by a radiologist. Even when radiological procedures are performed in an emergency room or walk-in clinic, a radiologist must read the film and dictate a formal report. Radiology reports include the title of the procedure, any contrast medium or nuclear medicine given, and an interpretation of the film (Fig. 4-7).

Discharge Summary

The discharge summary is a chronological account of the patient's hospital stay. If the patient is being transferred to another facility, this report may be titled *Transfer Summary*. It is a concise report of the reason for the patient's admission, tests performed, treatments given, results of those tests and treat-

CENTRAL MEDICAL CENTER

211 Medical Center Drive • Central City, US 90000-1234 • PHONE: (012) 125-6784 • FAX: (012) 125-9999

X-RAY REPORT

LUMBOSACRAL SPINE:
Multiple views reveal no evidence of fracture. There is slight lumbar spondylosis with slight lipping and minimal bridging. The disc spaces appear maintained except for slight narrowing at L4-L5 and L5-S1. There is also a Grade I spondylolisthesis of L5 on S1 and evidence of spondylolysis at L5 on the left. There is also slight dextroscoliosis in the lumbar region and slight increased lordosis in the lumbosacral region. The bony architecture is unremarkable except for eburnation between the articulating facets at L5-S1. The SI joints appear unremarkable. Incidentally noted are slight osteoarthritic changes involving both hips.

CONCLUSION:

1. Slight lumbar spondylosis with hypertrophic lipping and slight narrowing of the L4-L5 and L5-S1 disc spaces, 'rule out discogenic disease. If clinically indicated, CT of the lumbosacral spine may prove helpful in further evaluation.

2. Grade I spondylolisthesis of L5 on S1 with evidence of spondylolysis at L5 on the left.

3. Slight dextroscoliosis in the lumbar region and slight increased lordosis in the lumbosacral region.

M. Volz MD

M. Volz, M.D.

MV:ti

D: 10/19/20xx
T: 10/20/20xx

X-RAY REPORT	PT. NAME:	DORN, JAY F.
	ID NO:	RL-483091
	ATT. PHYS:	T. LIGHT, M.D.

FIGURE 4-7. Sample radiology report. (Reprinted with permission from Willis MC. *Medical Terminology: The Language of Health Care*, 1st ed. Baltimore: Williams & Wilkins, 1996.)

ments, procedures performed, improvements, setbacks, and, finally, the condition of the patient at the time of discharge.

The discharge summary is an excellent tool for members of the health care team involved in the patient's posthospital care. A patient who is recovering from a stroke may receive services from a home health nurse, a physical therapist, and a speech therapist. The discharge summary provides a snapshot of the patient's situation in one document.

Figure 4-8 is a sample discharge summary. Be sure it is in the office chart for the patient's first visit after hospitalization.

CENTRAL MEDICAL CENTER

211 Medical Center Drive • Central City, US 90000-1234 • PHONE: (012) 125-6784 • FAX: (012) 125-9999

DISCHARGE SUMMARY

DATE OF ADMISSION: 10/25/20xx DATE OF DISCHARGE: 10/29/20xx

ADMITTING DIAGNOSIS:
Left ureteropelvic junction obstruction.

DISCHARGE DIAGNOSIS:
Left ureteropelvic junction obstruction.

PROCEDURE PERFORMED:
Left dismembered pyeloplasty and placement of stent.

BRIEF SUMMARY:
The patient is a 19-year-old male who was admitted to the hospital a month ago with left pyelonephritis. He was found to have a left ureteropelvic junction obstruction. The patient was brought to the hospital at this time for repair of the moderately to severely obstructed left kidney. A preoperative urine culture was sterile. The patient underwent the procedure without complication. A double-J stent was placed. The Jackson-Pratt drain was removed on the second postoperative day because of minimal drainage. The patient initially had urinary retention, but this resolved by the third postoperative day. He was doing fine at the time of discharge. His condition on discharge is good.

INSTRUCTIONS TO THE PATIENT:
1) Regular diet. 2) No heavy lifting, straining, or driving an automobile for six weeks from the day of surgery. He should also keep the incision relatively dry this week. 3) Follow up in my office in three weeks. 4) It is anticipated the stent will remain indwelling for six weeks and then will be removed cystoscopically at that time. 5) Discharge medication is Tylenol #3, 1-2 q 4 h p.r.n. pain.

L. Zlatkin, M.D.

LZ:mr

D: 10/29/20xx
T: 10/30/20xx

DISCHARGE SUMMARY	PT. NAME:	MERCIER, CHARLES F.
	ID NO:	IP-392689
	ROOM NO:	444
	ATT. PHYS:	L.ZLATKIN, M.D.

FIGURE 4-8. Sample discharge summary. (Reprinted with permission from Willis MC. *Medical Terminology: A Programmed Learning Approach to the Language of Health Care*, 1st ed. Baltimore: Lippincott Williams & Wilkins, 2002.)

Checkpoint Question

4. List the information found in a discharge or transfer summary.

TRANSCRIPTION RULES

The following section is not intended to be a complete list of rules, but it includes most of the general rules necessary in medical transcription. Different texts give different rules for punctuation, so it is recommended that you follow the guidelines of the American Association of Medical Transcription (AAMT), the source of these rules.

Abbreviations

When you use abbreviations in medical documents, your reader must be able to recognize or translate the abbreviation. Every licensed medical facility is required to keep a list of approved abbreviations, and this list should be updated regularly. Some facilities have local abbreviations that are specific to the facility. Like words in English, many abbreviations have two meanings. The use of capital letters can change the meaning entirely. For example, CC means chief complaint, but cc means cubic centimeters. For this reason, be very cautious in using abbreviations. Some abbreviations have become accepted because they are used more than the long form. BP has come to be easily recognized as blood pressure when used in the vital sign section of the report. In a hospital setting, the use of abbreviations in typed reports is forbidden. For example, you are not allowed to abbreviate the diagnosis on an operative report.

Most doctors' offices use standard abbreviations in the patients' charts, but when you are typing a formal report, it is risky to use abbreviations. If it is the policy of your facility to use abbreviations in letters and formal reports, spell out the words the first time the abbreviation is used, with the abbreviation following in parentheses. In general, "when in doubt, spell it out."

Capitalization

Knowing when to capitalize and when to use lowercase letters is a mark of an excellent transcriptionist. The rules about using capital letters you learned in grammar school still apply, but when you are transcribing medical records, capitals are used in additional situations.

Use capital letters:

1. For headings.
   CHIEF COMPLAINT or Chief Complaint
2. For eponyms (terms formed using the name of a person, usually the name of the researcher or physician who identified a disorder or the inventor of equipment, instruments, supplies, and so on), the second word in the phrase is not capitalized. *Note*: Recent revisions in punctuation guidelines eliminate the possessive apostrophe.
   Down syndrome   Foley catheter   Healy clamp
3. For trade or brand names of drugs and products. Do not capitalize generic names of drugs and products.
   diazepam   Valium
   tissue   Kleenex
4. For the genus of an organism. An example of this classification system of living organisms is *Staphylococcus aureus*. *Staphylococcus* is the genus and *aureus* is the species. A singular genus is capitalized and italicized. If the genus is plural or used as an adjective, it is lower case and not italicized. Use lowercase letters and italics for the species.
   as noun: *Staphylococcus aureus*
   as adjective: staphylococcal infection
5. For a department name when the name is the proper title of a place, but not for department names within a facility.
   The patient was taken to the emergency room.
   The patient was taken to the Forsyth Medical Center Emergency Room.
6. For proper names of languages, races, and religions.
   She is a 23-year-old Hispanic woman.
   Do not capitalize informal designations such as white or black.
7. For acronyms (words formed from initials of words in a phrase).
   NKDA (no known drug allergies)
   CABG (coronary artery bypass graft)
8. To draw attention to vital information, such as allergies.
   ALLERGIES: The patient is allergic to PENICILLIN.

Numbers

Traditional office technology courses teach the rules for using numbers, but many of those rules do not apply to medical documents. When those guidelines have the potential to cause confusion or harm a patient, you must be flexible enough to bend them. The safety of the patient is a goal of the transcriptionist.

Follow these guidelines for using numbers in medical reports:

1. Spell out the numbers one through nine in a narrative report (see guidelines 3 and 6 below). Ten and above are keyed as numerals (e.g., 10, 11) unless they begin a sentence, as in this sentence.
2. If you are using two numbers in one sentence, be consistent. It does not matter whether you choose numerals or words, but they should be consistent.
   Dr. Smith saw 14 patients today; one of them was only 2 days old.

   If using more than one number could cause confusion, spell out the one that is easiest and shortest.
   The patient states that she drinks 12 two-liter sodas per week.

3. Always use numerals with symbols. Do not key a space between the number and the symbol.
   100% oxygen
   $14.27 balance due
   #2 specimen
4. For balance and clarity, add a zero before and after a decimal point. The provider will say, "The specimen measures eight by five and a half by point six."
   Clear: The specimen measures 8.0 × 5.5 × 0.6.
   Unclear: The specimen measures 8 × 5.5 × .6.
5. Key a space between numerals and a unit of measurement, abbreviation, or symbol.
   10 mg%   40 mL   20 mm Hg
6. Use numerals for measurements of vital signs, laboratory values, age, height, weight, and so on.
   BP 110/70   Respirations 20
   Temperature 98.7°F   Wt. 140 lb.
   Pulse 80   Ht. 60 inch.
   FBS (fasting blood sugar) 98
7. Spell out ordinal numbers except in dates.
   She began feeling better the third day after surgery.
   The patient was seen on May 3.
8. Roman numerals are used with cranial nerves, obstetric history, electrocardiographic leads, types and factors, and cancer stages.
   Cranial nerves II through XII are intact.
   Limb leads II through V on the electrocardiogram were not making contact.
   The carcinoma is stage II.

Punctuation

One of the most important skills necessary to be an efficient and productive transcriptionist is the ability to punctuate without direction. Some physicians dictate punctuation, but you should not automatically type these directions unless they follow the AAMT's *Guidelines for Transcription*.

Apostrophes

Use an apostrophe:

1. To show possession
   The patient's appointment is Wednesday.
2. To form contractions
   She's having flu symptoms. (The apostrophe contracts *she* and *is*.)
   Note: "It is" can be shortened to "it's," but there is no apostrophe in the possessive:
   Its length is 4 cm.
3. With units of time and money when they are possessive
   We will give him a week's worth of medication.
   Nine months' gestation is standard.
   He bought 10 dollars' worth of gas.
4. For clarity when using one letter as a word
   The I's were not dotted.
   But not to form plurals
   DRGs
   WBCs
   I've had this dress since the 1970s.
   Unless it is possessive
   The CMA's uniform is neat and clean.

Commas

Use a comma:

1. Between items in a series (the last comma is optional).
   The patient is alert, oriented and talkative.
   Or
   The pain is bilateral, severe, and stabbing.
   Note: Do not use commas between items that modify each other. Even though this seems like a series of adjectives, it is really one unit.
   There is severe, stabbing, bilateral pain in the lower abdominal region.
   The first three adjectives modify *pain* and are separated by commas. "Lower" refers to the abdomen, not the region, so no comma is used.
2. To link two complete sentences that are separated by a conjunction.
   She is a very sick patient, and I will admit her immediately.
   But not when both clauses lack a subject and a predicate
   She is a very sick patient and needs to be admitted.
   "Needs to be admitted" does not contain its own subject. Therefore, no comma is needed.
3. After the conjunctive adverb.
   The medical assistant is in great demand; therefore, most schools have a waiting list.
4. After an introductory phrase or clause with a subject and a verb.
   After she has her chest radiograph, she will come back to the office.
   NO comma is needed when the sentence is reversed.
   She will come back to the office after she has her chest x-ray.
   Lightheaded, she sat down on the floor.
5. To set off clauses within a sentence that provide additional information.
   Electroencephalography, a test that assesses the electrical activity in the brain, is a diagnostic tool used by neurologists.
6. To set off parenthetical expressions.
   The pain, according to the patient, measures 10 on the pain scale.

7. With dates when using the year, place names, and long numbers.
   The patient was seen last on May 2, 2003.
   But: The patient was seen last on May 2 at 2:00 p.m.
   Duke University Medical Center is in Durham, North Carolina.

   Numbers over five figures:
   4500
   567,158,230
8. With quotations.
   The patient said, "I will quit smoking tomorrow."
9. To prevent confusion.
   "The physician came in, in order to see the patient."

Semicolons

Use a semicolon:

1. To separate main clauses that do not have a conjunction such as *and* or *but*
   The patient arrived 10 minutes late; she had car trouble.
2. To separate two main clauses if they are long or you need other commas within the sentence
   She had chest pain, nausea, and headache; and her daughter took her to the emergency room.

Colons

Use a colon:

1. After headings
   FAMILY HISTORY: The patient reports no family history of cancer.
2. To introduce a series after a complete clause but not after a verb
   The physician prescribed the following medications: Keflex, Darvocet-N 100, K Tabs and Prinivil.
   The physician prescribed Keflex, Darvocet-N 100, K-Tabs, and Prinivil.
3. To separate hours from minutes
   Your appointment is scheduled for 10:30 a.m.
4. After a salutation in a business letter
   Dear Dr. Johnsen:

Periods

In addition to ending sentences, periods are used:

1. With lowercase abbreviations
   a.m., p.m. *But:* AM, PM PhD

   Metric measurements do not use periods.
   They had to remove 3 ft. of her colon.
   We removed 15 mL of pleural fluid.
2. After an abbreviation that is a shortened part of a word
   American Association of Medical Assistants, Inc.
3. After a person's initials
   J. T. Weaver, MD

Quotation Marks

Quotation marks enclose:

1. A direct quotation
   The patient stated, "My friend recommended your office to me."
2. Words that are slang or thought to be a quotation.
   The patient stated he was "blown away" by his improved cholesterol reading.
   Jessica thinks her new boyfriend is "Prince Charming."
3. Titles of articles, short stories, subdivisions, and so on
   Please read "Making the Patient Comfortable" in the most recent issue of our professional journal.
   Table 4-1 presents rules for using other punctuation with quotation marks.

Slash Marks

In medical transcription, the slash mark is used:

1. In place of the word *per*. The provider says, "Give the patient one hundred percent oxygen at two liters per minute." You type:
   Give the patient 100% oxygen at 2 liters/minute.

   In some cases, the provider may not say "per," but you insert a slash.
   The student took the class on a pass/fail basis.
2. To separate options and alternatives.
   This is a pass/fail course.

Hyphens

Hyphens are used:

1. In compound words. The general rule is that when two words are used together to form a word, they are joined by a hyphen. Many compound nouns have been used long enough to be consolidated and are now accepted words in their own right. For example, spread-sheet has become spreadsheet.
   mother-in-law figure-of-eight sutures
2. A hyphen can clear up confusion or ambiguity. For example, re-creation is quite different from recreation. Without the hyphen, the reader would misinterpret the meaning.
   We will *re-treat* with a different antibiotic.

   As opposed to
   We went on a weekend *retreat*.

Table 4-1 The Use of Other Punctuation With Quotation Marks

Rule	Example
Place commas and periods inside quotation marks.	"Your bill, explained the patient, "has not come in the mail."
Place colons and semicolons outside quotation marks.	She said, "The doctor told me to come back on Friday"; however, he has no openings.
Place other punctuation inside quotation marks only if they belong in the quotation.	The student asked, "Is that going to be on the test?" *But* Did the patient say, "Yes, I'll come"?
Place commas and periods outside quotation marks when used with single letters or single words.	Even though she made an "A", she felt it was not her best work.

3. When joining the two words would result in two or more identical letters.
   post-traumatic pre-enteric pre-existing
   Note: Otherwise, the hyphen is not used with these prefixes.
   postoperative infection prehistoric
4. When spelling out the compound numbers twenty-one to ninety-nine.
   Fifty-eight percent of our patients are over sixty-five years old.
5. When using compound adjectives before a noun.
   high-frequency hearing loss
   well-developed frame
   22-gauge needle
   6-month-old infant
   Remember, the hyphen is not used when the compound adjective follows the noun it modifies:
   The patient is 6 months old.
6. The hyphen is not used when adverbs modify adjectives.
   very high fever quickly spreading cancer
7. When a compound adjective contains the suffix -free.
   symptom-free
8. When the compound includes an acronym.
   post-CABG care pre-ICU lab results
9. When keying suture sizes.
   2-0 Prolene

Grammar

When a physician dictates a report using incorrect grammar, it is your job to correct the mistake. The physician expects you to produce an error-free report, even though he or she may overlook basic parts of speech and rules of sentence grammar. Although a thorough discussion of the grammar rules in the English language is outside the scope of this text, some basic rules should be mentioned. The most common errors made in medical transcription are those dealing with verb tense.

Always be sure that subjects and verbs agree in number.

One patient: The patient *is* alert.
More than one vital sign: His vital signs *are* normal

Always make sentences within a paragraph agree in tense and subject. Suppose the provider dictates, "The patient was seen in clinic today for pain in the left knee. The examination *is* negative." You will key, "The patient was seen in clinic today for pain in the left knee. The examination *was* negative."

Spelling

When in doubt about the spelling of a word or drug, always use a reference book, dictionary, or spell check to confirm the spelling. Keep in mind that computer spell check will check for spelling only, and a misused word will not be caught if it is spelled correctly. For example, "the patient was late four his appointment" will pass the spell check because "four" is spelled correctly, even though the transcriptionist meant to key "for."

Here are some basic spelling tips:

1. I comes before e except after c or when sounded like a as in neighbor and weigh.
   Examples: achieve, receive (the exceptions are either, neither, weird, leisure, and conscience)
2. For words ending in ie, drop the e and change the i to y before adding ing.
   Examples: die, dying; lie, lying
3. Words ending in o that are preceded by a vowel are made plural by adding s.
   Examples: studio, studios; trio, trios
   Words ending in o that are preceded by a consonant form the plural by adding es.
   Examples: hero, heroes; potato, potatoes
4. Words ending in y preceded by a vowel form the plural by adding s.
   Examples: attorney, attorneys; day, days
   Words ending in y that are preceded by a consonant change the y to i and add es.
   Examples: berry, berries; lady, ladies
5. The final consonant of a one-syllable word is doubled before adding a suffix beginning with a vowel.
   Examples: pin, pinning; run, running
   If the final consonant is preceded by another consonant or by two vowels, do not double the consonant.
   Examples: act, acting; look, looked

6. Words ending in a silent e generally drop the e before adding a suffix beginning with a vowel.
   Examples: ice, icing; judge, judging
   The exceptions are dye, eye, shoe, and toe. The e is not dropped in suffixes beginning with a consonant, however, unless another vowel precedes the final e.
   Examples: argue, argument; pale, paleness
7. For all words ending in c, insert a k before adding a suffix beginning with e, i, or y.
   Examples: picnic, picnicking; traffic, trafficker

You must pay close attention to spelling when transcribing medical documents. Remember, in the medical world a misspelled drug or word can be dangerous.

TRANSCRIPTION SYSTEMS

Vast improvements have been made in dictating and transcribing capabilities and equipment over the past decade. Traditionally, the physician or health care provider uses a dictation machine with a handheld microphone to tape a report of a patient encounter or other correspondence. With the **analogue** or tape system, after the message is taped, the cassette tape will be removed and marked with some form of identification. Cassette tapes range in size from micro to standard.

Traditional Tape Dictation Systems

Each model of transcription machine is slightly different; however, most have the basic parts described next (Fig. 4-9).

- The foot pedal is used to start, stop, fast-forward, and rewind the tape.
- The speed control regulates the speed at which the tape plays. As a beginner, you want to keep the speed slow. As your listening and typing coordination improve, you will be able to increase the speed of the tape. When you become experienced with a particular provider's voice speed, you will be able to set the speed control to match his or her voice speed and your typing speed.
- The tone dial can be adjusted to change the bass or treble of a provider's voice.
- The volume control is used to adjust the sound level.
- The headset is used to eliminate distracting external noises. It is not a good habit to share headset earplugs with fellow colleagues because an ear infection may be transmitted. Ear cushions that attach to the headsets should be used and washed or replaced often.
- The speaker allows the sound to be heard from a speaker in the transcriber instead of the headset. This feature is handy when the transcriptionist needs assistance or clarification in interpreting the dictation.
- Counters are available on most machines for ease in locating certain reports and to judge the length of a document.

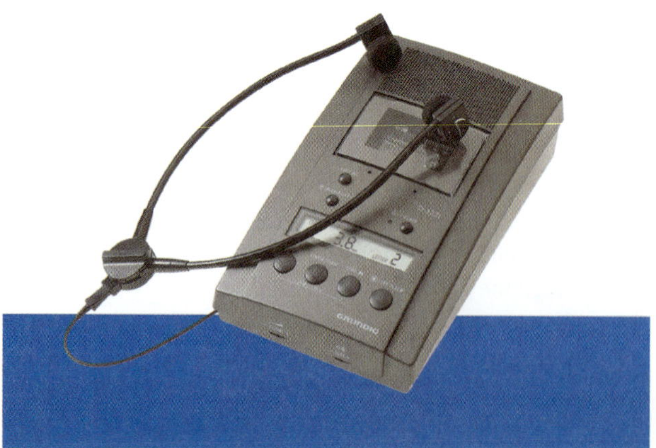

FIGURE 4-9. Transcription machines vary. Speed control is an important function of the machine.

Because every transcription machine is slightly different, you should read the instruction manual before you begin working on a unfamiliar machine. All instruction manuals should be kept in one central location in the office for easy access.

Tapes are usually transcribed in or near the medical records department. Tapes should be erased after the material has been transcribed, reviewed, and signed by the provider. Before discarding a worn-out tape, erase it completely to maintain confidentiality.

Digital Systems

The industry is moving toward a **digital** system, which converts the voice into digits, decodes it, and sends the voice directly to a transcriber through the telephone lines. The system integrates with a computer at the transcriptionist's desk, where a certain code is entered. This code will automatically produce the information and report format on the screen of the computer. In hospitals, most patient care units have dictation phones or ports for digital systems.

Voice Recognition Systems

Voice recognition software and digital voice recording systems have expanded and improved medical transcription. Some people predicted that the invention of voice recognition software would eliminate the need for medical transcriptionists, but the medical community has been slow to respond to the technology. Some limitations are difficult to overcome. For example, if the provider says "there," how does the computer know whether to type "there," "their," or "they're"? Accents, dialects, proper names, and garbled speech are challenges for transcriptionists no matter which system is being used. These same challenges face the inventors of voice recognition software. Even with sophisticated voice recognition systems, there will always be a need for

What If

You are having trouble understanding a particular physician's dictation tapes because of a dialect or foreign accent. How should you handle this situation?

First, rewind the tape and listen again to the phrase. You can try to adjust the speed control to slow the pronunciation of the word. Consider what a word would sound like with the accent on a different syllable or using a short sound instead of a long sound of a vowel. Being familiar with the type of report being dictated will help you anticipate what the provider might be saying. If you are still uncertain about the word or phrase, leave a blank space for that word and continue transcribing. Edit the report to fill in the blank. Never guess! If you have difficulty understanding a provider, discuss the problem with him or her. Open communication will help you both make adjustments. Neither of you wants to take the chance of producing an erroneous report.

transcriptionists or medical language specialists to proofread, punctuate, and edit medical documents.

Transcription With Word Processing Software

When using word processing programs, you may use macros, templates, and other functions that record keystrokes or provide a blank format to speed the process of transcribing reports that contain the same text over and over again. For example, the format for a certain type of report or letterhead and normal dictation for ordinary examinations can be recorded for playback with a quick keystroke. Legal experts warn providers not just to report examination results as "normal." Instead, they should describe the negative findings. For example, when a patient's throat appears normal to the examiner, he or she should report, "The throat appears normal, with no redness or exudate" (pus).

Checkpoint Question

5. Describe the main difference between analogue and digital transcription equipment.

Spanish Terminology

Esto es una máquina de transcripción.	This is a transcription machine.
Yo no lo podría oír con los auriculares.	I couldn't hear you with the headphones on.
¿Qué escucha usted?	What are you listening to?
Escucho y escribo a máquina cartas para el doctor.	I am listening and typing letters for the doctor.

Procedure 4-1

Transcribing a Medical Document

Steps	Purpose
1. Prepare the equipment: transcribing machine, headphones, transcription (dictation) tapes, computer or typewriter, paper, letterhead, and envelopes.	Having everything ready will cut down on interruptions and will help you focus. Concentration is key to being productive.
2. Select a transcription tape with the oldest date, unless there are special requests for priority reports.	Most dictation systems have the capability of *marking* a document for priority status. This alerts you to complete marked dictation first.
3. Turn on the transcriber, and insert and rewind the tape.	Always rewind the tape so that the document starts in the beginning.
4. Put on the headset and position the foot pedal in a comfortable location.	The foot pedal is operated by pressing a certain area for a certain function. In some machines, pressing the left side of the pedal rewinds the tape, pressing the right side fast-forwards it, and pressing the center plays the tape.
5. Play a sample of the tape. Adjust the volume, speed, and tone dials to your comfort.	This promotes efficiency and speed.
6. Select the appropriate format and place proper patient identification on the page.	Proper patient identification is essential for legal and ethical reasons.
7. Play a short segment of the tape by pressing the foot pedal, stop the tape, and type the message.	As your speed and skills progress, you will not need to stop the tape as often.
8. If you come across an unfamiliar term, leave enough blank space for the provider to write it in and continue transcribing. When you have finished the document, contact the physician or colleague or use a reference book to fill in the blank.	A thorough knowledge of medical terminology will minimize time spent looking up words.
9. When you are finished, place the initials of the provider, followed by a slash and your initials, on the bottom of the page. The date that each was done should be added.	The reader must know who dictated the report and who transcribed the document and the dates each was carried out.
10. Spell check the document by using medical spell check software.	The spell checker of standard word processing programs does not recognize most medical terms. Medical spell check software is available to ensure accuracy.
11. Print and proofread the document.	Spell checkers mark only misspelled words, not errors. You need to proofread the hard copy for other errors. After typing a lengthy report, it is common to overlook errors. It is helpful to have a coworker also proofread.
12. Leave the document, along with the tape, in a designated area for review.	After reviewing the document, the provider will sign it, indicating that the report is accurate. If corrections are necessary later, a revised copy must be placed with the original report. The final copy should include a notation to identify it as a revised copy.
13. After the provider has reviewed and approved the document, make a copy of the report for the patient's chart.	Reports can be mailed, faxed, or e-mailed. Be careful to follow the guidelines for protecting patients' privacy.
14. Send the report to the recipient.	This allows the report to be filed.
15. Erase the tape and return it to the dictation area.	Tapes that are not erased cause confusion to the provider when they are recording and may infringe on a patient's right to privacy.

SUMMARY

Medical transcription is a growing industry. The person who possesses the necessary skills transforms vital information about a patient's care and treatment and is an important member of the health care team. Many medical assistants perform this important function in the medical office. The training you receive in your medical assisting education will enable you to perform at entry-level competency, but experience in transcribing will enhance your skills and make you a more desirable employee for medical offices. Medical information is crucial to patient care and must be prepared with proper grammar, punctuation, and spelling. Physicians depend on timely and accurate preparation of their reports to make decisions. This information is confidential and must be handled with great caution and integrity.

Answers to the Checkpoint Questions

1. A professional document should be well balanced and attractive with single spacing, double spacing between headings, and one-inch margins.
2. JCAHO requires that results of the H&P be placed on a patient's chart within 24 hours of admission to a hospital facility. The physician must sign the H&P report within a prescribed amount of time as well.
3. Subjective information is provided by the patient and is information that cannot be seen or measured. Examples are pain and nausea. Objective findings are reported by the examiner and can be observed or detected. Examples are rash and blood pressure.
4. The discharge, transfer, or death summary is a concise report of the reason for the patient's admission, tests performed, treatments given, results of those tests and treatments, procedures performed, improvements, setbacks, and, finally, the condition of the patient at the time of discharge.
5. The analogue system uses cassette tapes to record the voice, and the digital system uses digits that are converted and sent across the telephone lines.

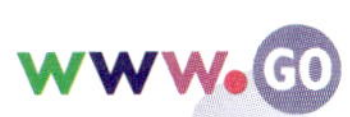

Websites

American Association of Medical Transcription
www.aamt.org
Medical Transcription Jobs
www.mtjobs.com
Medical Transcription Daily
www.mtdaily.com

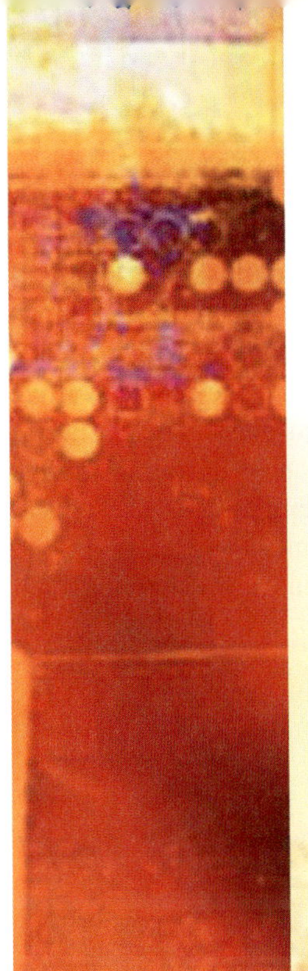

5

Management of the Medical Office Team

CHAPTER OBJECTIVES

In this chapter, you'll learn:

1. To spell and define the key terms.
2. To describe what is meant by organizational structure.
3. To list seven responsibilities of the medical office manager.
4. To explain the five staffing issues that a medical office manager will be responsible for handling.
5. To list the types of policies and procedures that should be included in a medical office's policy and procedures manual.
6. To list five types of promotional materials that a medical office may distribute.
7. To discuss three financial concerns that the medical office manager must be capable of addressing.
8. To discuss four legal issues that affect medical office management.

PERFORMANCE OBJECTIVES

In this chapter, you'll learn:

1. To write a job description.
2. To create policy and procedures manuals.

KEY TERMS

Americans with Disabilities Act
budget
compliance officer
Family and Medical Leave Act
job description
mission statement
organizational chart
policy
procedure

A SUCCESSFUL MEDICAL practice needs an effective medical office management process. This process must be a team effort among the physicians, nurse managers, and the office manager. This chapter provides an overview of medical office management as well as a discussion of a medical office manager's specific responsibilities.

OVERVIEW OF MEDICAL OFFICE MANAGEMENT

Each medical office is organized in a slightly different manner, depending on the size and complexity of the setting.

Organizational Structure

The medical office's organizational structure, or chain of command, is depicted in an **organizational chart**, a flow sheet that allows the manager and employees to identify their team members and to see where they fit into the team. Figure 5-1 displays a sample organizational chart for a physician's office in which there is a partnership between two physicians. In this example, it is assumed that the physicians have an equal partnership in the practice.

Checkpoint Question

1. What is the purpose of an organizational chart?

The Medical Office Manager

The medical office manager must be multiskilled, multitalented, and able to prioritize a variety of issues, juggle responsibilities, and communicate effectively with patients, staff, and physicians. In some settings, the medical office manager may be referred to as the business manager. Managers may be nurses, medical assistants, or administrative support personnel. Although the qualifications and educational requirements for the position vary greatly among health care organizations, a successful medical office manager must be:

- Flexible
- A positive role model for employees
- Honest and fair
- A good communicator
- A resource person for employees
- Supportive of all management decisions
- Well organized
- Able to focus on a given task
- Able to resolve conflicts
- Able to see the big picture

A medical office manager's responsibilities include varied tasks:

- Communicating with patients, physicians, and staff
- Handling staffing issues

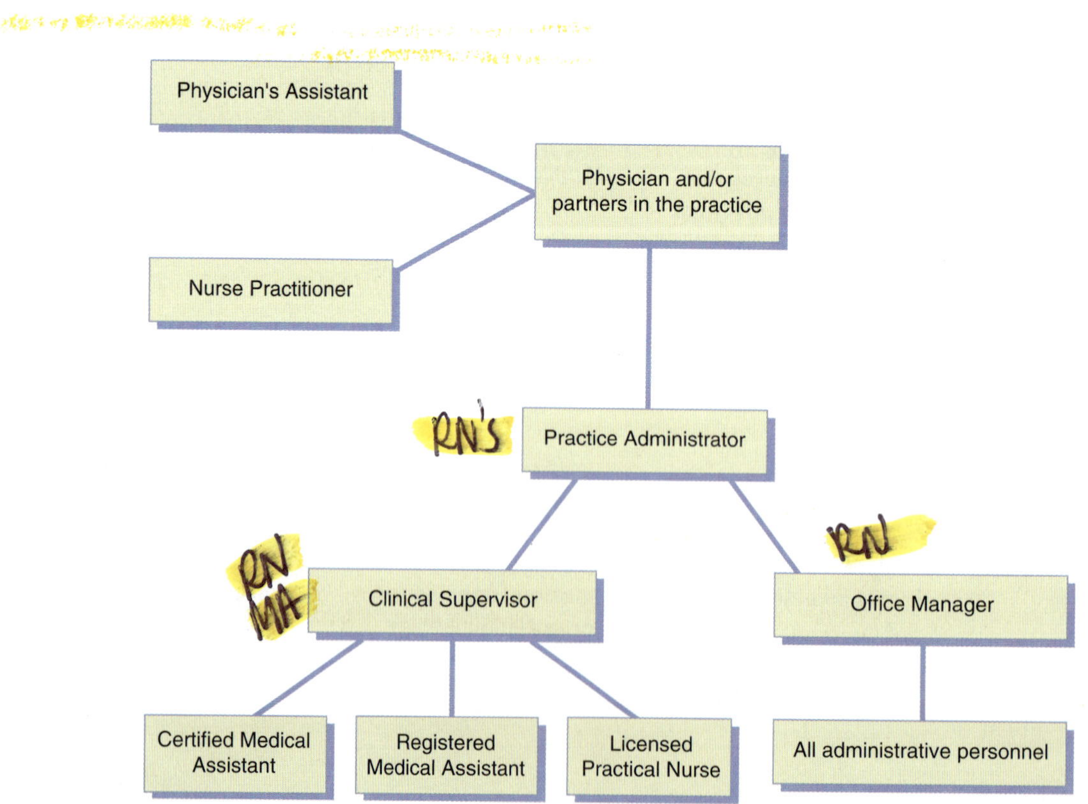

FIGURE 5-1. Sample organizational chart.

- Writing and revising policy and procedures manuals
- Developing promotional materials
- Handling financial concerns
- Handling maintenance and inventory
- Ensuring that the staff receives appropriate education

RESPONSIBILITIES OF THE MEDICAL OFFICE MANAGER

Communication

Perhaps one of the hardest and yet most important aspects of being an effective manager is being able to communicate with fellow employees, colleagues, physicians, and patients. You must be a good listener, have good interpersonal skills, and be aware of your own nonverbal language.

Communicating With Patients

Communication with patients on a management level can often be challenging. Patients come to you with a variety of complaints, such as incorrect billing, poor care, or long waits to see physicians. Of course, you must always be diplomatic. Your goal should be to correct the problem in a timely and professional manner and to alleviate any negative feelings the patient may have.

Communicating With Staff

Communication with staff members can be difficult, depending on the number of employees, number and locations of satellite centers, and the variety of shifts that are in place. There are three ways to promote communication with staff members: staff meetings, bulletin boards, and communication notebooks.

Staff meetings. Staff meetings should be scheduled at a predictable frequency and time to allow the staff to plan (e.g., they might be held the first Monday of every month at 8 A.M.) Meetings should never be canceled except in a true emergency.

Staff meetings must be well organized and should begin and end on time. Agendas should be created prior to the meeting and posted for staff review. The agenda should be followed as closely as possible. Individual staff concerns or complaints should not be handled during a general staff meeting; the meeting should remain focused and constructive and not turn into a battleground for staff disagreements. Minutes should be taken and kept in a notebook for staff to review as needed.

Staff meetings should be conducted in a private area out of patients' sight and hearing (Fig. 5-2). All interruptions except for emergencies should be avoided.

Have the telephone covered by an answering service or a prerecorded message informing callers of the time the staff will be unavailable. Lock the door and place a sign with the time the office will reopen. Of course, you will give clear instructions to callers or visitors who have an emergency. The personnel manual should clearly state the attendance policy for staff meetings. In addition, some offices include attendance as a duty in each employee's job description (statement of work-related responsibilities). To improve attendance at staff meetings, consider serving food or including an educational presentation.

Bulletin boards. Bulletin board postings allow employees to get a quick and easy look at new polices or procedures. To encourage staff members to read the postings, make sure the bulletin boards are attractive, well organized, and updated regularly. It is a good idea to have employees initial all messages on the bulletin board after reading them.

Communication notebooks. A simple notebook can serve as a two-way communication tool: You can write messages to employees, and they can write back to you. Such a notebook is usually kept in the staff lounge. Again, staff members should initial any important messages after reading them. If the message is directed to you, be sure to respond as soon as possible.

Emails

Communicating Electronically

E-mail has become popular and is an easy and time-saving way to communicate with staff. Messages can be printed and kept in a binder for easy reference. E-mail messages eliminate the need for memos that must be posted or circulated. Your e-mail system will provide you with an address book that can be customized to include groups such as all employees, all clinical employees, employees and physicians, and so on.

Sometimes, the stress of daily duties prevents managers from communicating with staff members on a personal level. To be an effective manager, you should communicate not

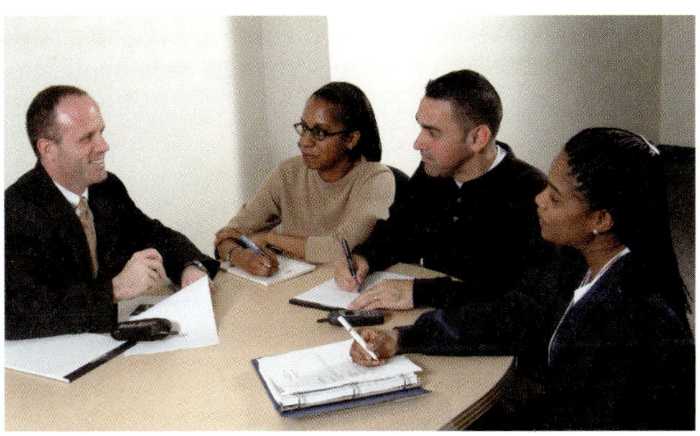

FIGURE 5-2. Staff meeting being conducted in a private area.

only bad news but also positive messages to your employees. You can communicate positive messages through birthday and holiday cards and employee recognition awards.

Checkpoint Question

2. What are three ways to promote communication with staff members?

Staffing Issues

Staffing issues will occupy most of your time as an office manager. These concerns include writing job descriptions, hiring new employees, evaluating present employees, taking disciplinary actions, handling terminations, and scheduling.

Writing Job Descriptions

Each job must have a description. The purpose of a **job description** is to inform the employee about the duties and expectations for a given position. Job descriptions also help you in interviewing applicants and evaluating existing employees.

Each employee should receive a copy of his or her job description at the time of hiring and after any revisions to the description are made. Some medical offices have a policy requiring the employee to read and sign the job description at the time of hiring.

Formats for writing job descriptions vary among offices. In general, the following elements are included: job title, supervisor, position summary, hours, location, employment requirements, physical requirements, duties, and the evaluation process (Fig. 5-3). The description should also include the date it was written and date of any revisions.

If possible, involve staff members in writing and revising their job descriptions. Employee participation leads to greater cooperation.

Hiring and Interviewing Employees

Only after creating or reviewing an existing job description can you begin the process of interviewing and hiring a new employee. Finding applicants for most medical office positions is usually not a problem. You can seek applicants through advertising in local newspaper classified sections,

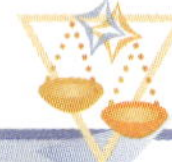

Legal Tip

Verify the credentials of an applicant by calling the appropriate state licensing board or certification registry. Is the applicant's license or certification current? Unfortunately, some people are dishonest and unethical. A person who is not misrepresenting himself or herself will not mind you checking. A CMA's status can be obtained by calling 1-800-ACT-AAMA. Many state medical assisting societies also have certification registries. Try going to the particular profession's website.

placement personnel at local schools that offer medical assisting programs, networking, and employment agencies.

All applicants should complete an application. State laws vary regarding the types of questions that can be asked on applications. In general, you must avoid any questions pertaining to an applicant's age, sex, race, religion, and physical or mental disabilities. If your medical facility requires a criminal background check and drug testing, the form should include this information with a place for the applicant to give necessary permission with a signature. Any employee application form should be reviewed by legal counsel prior to its use. It is always a good idea to request that the applicant bring a résumé to the interview.

Before interviewing an applicant, prepare a list of questions. Again, use caution; under law you are not permitted to ask about some topics. During the interview, assess the applicant's ability to do the following:

- Perform technical skills
- Treat patients in a caring manner
- Fit into your organization
- Communicate in a professional yet friendly manner
- Remain flexible

Evaluating Employees

All employees must be evaluated annually. The evaluation should be a positive experience for the employee. Employee evaluations must be fair, accurate, and objective. Some type

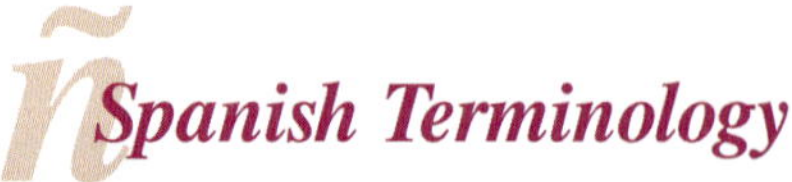

Busco un trabajo.	*I am looking for a job.*
¿Tiene usted cualquier abîerto?	*Do you have any openings?*
¿Dónde estan las aplicaciones?	*Where are the applications?*
Soy el director.	*I am the manager.*

Job Description

Title: Medical Assistant

Supervisor(s): Clinical Supervisor

Office Manager for Administrative Duties

Position summary: This is a 40-hour position that will require the employee to perform various duties including administrative, clinical, and laboratory procedures. Scheduling will be variable to meet the needs of the office.

Hours: Hours will vary to meet the needs of the office. Hours will rotate from 8:00 AM–4:30 PM and 10:00 AM–6:30 PM. You will be expected to work one Saturday per month.

Location: Our main office is located at 129 South Main Street. The satellite office is located at 56 West Road, Suite 102. This position will primarily require you to work at our main office. However, occasional days may be assigned at the satellite office.

Employment Requirements: The employee must have graduated from a medical assisting program. CMA or RMA is preferred. The employee must have a current CPR and First Aid card. One year of experience or completion of an externship is preferred.

• *Language skills:* The employee must be able to read and interpret documents and respond appropriately (verbally and/or in writing). Must be able to document in a professional manner.

• *Mathematical skills:* The employee must be able to add, subtract, multiply, and divide whole numbers and fractions.

Physical requirements: The following are physical requirements for this job: Standing: 6–8 hours/day; Sitting: 6–8 hours/day; Lifting: 50 pounds; Twisting and rotating: 45 degrees; Squatting: As needed to assist patients or to perform office tasks.

Duties: You will be expected to perform the following duties after completing the orientation process. This is a partial list; and other duties can be added as necessary.

Administrative:

Scheduling appointments	Processing mail
Transcribing documents	Operating the telephone
Filing	Providing patient education
Completing insurance forms	

Clinical/Laboratory:

Operating centrifuge	Obtaining vital signs
Performing phlebotomy	Administering vaccines and other medications as ordered
Performing HCT/HGB/CBC	Providing patient education
Performing pregnancy and monospot tests	Assisting the physician as directed
Obtaining visual acuities	

Evaluation process: Three evaluations will be conducted in the first year. Thirty days from start date, ninety days from start date, and then at the one-year anniversary date. Following the first year of employment, annual evaluations will be done.

I have read my job description, and I understand what is expected of me. I am able to physically perform all the required duties.

Signature of employee: ______________________ Date: __________

Signature of supervisor: ______________________ Date: __________

Signature of supervisor: ______________________ Date: __________

Dates: original JD - 1977, revised March 1998.

FIGURE 5-3. Sample job description.

of written evaluation should be given to the employee to read, sign, and comment on. Most forms ask employees to list their objectives and goals for the coming year. Figure 5-4 displays a sample evaluation form. Some organizations call evaluations performance appraisals.

New employees should be evaluated 1 month after their start date, again in 90 days, and then at their 1-year anniversary date. This process helps new employees gain confidence and improve weaknesses.

Taking Disciplinary Action

Most offices have policies regarding documentation of disciplinary action. Disciplinary actions can be verbal or

Employee Evaluation Form

Employee: ______________________________

Evaluation Date: ______________________________

Job Title: ______________________________

Ratings:

Traits	Score
Appearance	
Communication Skills	
Attendance	
Quality of work	
Reliability	
Initiative	
Other:	
Total Score:	

Rating scale:
5—excellent
4—above average
3—meets job expectations
2—below job expectations
1—does not meet job expectations

Supervisor comments:

____

____

Employee goals for the next year (to be completed by employee):

____

____

____

Employee Comments:

____

____

____

Supervisor signature: ______________________ Date: ________

Employee signature: ______________________ Date: ________

FIGURE 5-4. Sample employee evaluation form.

written. Verbal warnings are generally done for a first-time minor occurrence (e.g., not showing up for work and not calling in). A note should go into the employee's file stating that a verbal warning was given, the date, any actions that were taken, and any comments that the employee made.

Written notices are used for more serious problems (e.g., breaching patient confidentiality, substance abuse) or recurrent minor ones. Employees should sign any written warning notices. These documents can be used as evidence in the event that the person is fired and brings a lawsuit for wrongful discharge. Figure 5-5 shows a sample written disciplinary action form. Determine whether the employee's credentialing agency should be notified of serious infractions.

Terminating Employees

Having to terminate (fire) an employee is never an easy or pleasant task. It is essential that policies regarding termination be followed precisely. All disciplinary actions must be clearly and objectively stated. Terminating employees for unlawful reasons or failing to follow the organization's termination policy can result in lawsuits against you and the office. Some reasons for termination:

- Excessive tardiness or absenteeism
- Inappropriate dress or behavior
- Alcohol or drug use
- Endangering patients

- Lying or stealing
- Falsifying medical records or time sheets
- Breaching patient confidentiality

Scheduling

The primary goal of scheduling is to meet the needs of the office. The secondary goal is to meet the requests of your employees. You must be fair in scheduling and always follow your organization's policies for weekend and holiday or personal day requests. If possible, employees should be given time off with pay when attending seminars and meetings of their professional organization. This practice will keep morale high and encourage employees to stay current with their skills. Depending on the number of employees that you have to schedule and the complexity of the hours or shifts, you can either schedule by hand or use a computer program. If your organization is small and cohesive, you may want to assign a senior staff member to do the scheduling, or you might allow the employees to self-schedule. No matter what scheduling format is used, you are ultimately responsible for ensuring that the appropriate number and type of employees needed are scheduled.

Requests for time off should be put in writing. Depending on the size of the organization, such requests may have to be received by a given date or time. For example, the policy may read, "A request for a day off in May may have to be submitted by April 15. Any requests for time off filed after the cutoff date will be approved whenever possible." This eliminates repeated adjustment of the staffing schedule.

Checkpoint Question

3. What is the medical office manager's primary goal in scheduling?

Policy and Procedures Manuals

Every business needs written rules and regulations to ensure that its practices are within legal and ethical boundaries. Employees need written procedures to ensure consistency in the practices of the business. In the outpatient medical facility, these written policies and procedures are *required* by regulatory and accrediting agencies.

It is the office manager's responsibility to coordinate the orientation and training of any new employee. A personnel

Discipline Record

Employee Name: ______________ #: ________ Date of Warning: ________

Warning

Date of Violation: ________ Time: ______ Place: ______________

Description of Violation:

____

____

____

____

____

____

________ Verbal Warning

________ Written Warning

________ Probation ________ Days

________ Suspension ________ Days

________ Termination

Action To Be Taken:

____

____

____

____

____

____
Supervisor's Signature

____
Date

Employee's Remarks

Do you agree with the details above: Yes: ______ No: ______

Comments: ____

____

____

Employee's Signature: ______________________ Date: ______________

FIGURE 5-5. Sample disciplinary action form.

What If...

You receive a call requesting a reference for an employee who was fired. What should you say?

Be careful! This situation can turn into a legal nightmare if not handled appropriately. If you give a wonderful report to the potential employer and say, "She was great; never had any problems," you and the office may be sued by the former employee for wrongful discharge. In court, you would be asked: "If she was so wonderful, why did you fire her?" On the other hand, if you say, "She was a terrible employee, and we fired her," you can be sued for defamation of character. Because of the legal concerns in providing employment references, most organizations have a policy stating that the only information to be released is verification of employment dates and job titles. When in doubt, give no information. Ask for the caller's name and phone number; discuss the issue with the physician in charge, and then return the phone call.

manual that includes the organization's policies and outlines step-by-step procedures for each task performed in the facility becomes the new employee's information source. Even veteran employees may have to refer to the proper procedure for a task. As new procedures become available or existing procedures are changed, this is added to the procedures manual.

Most organizations create a policy and procedures manual that is written, maintained, and regarded as one document. A **policy** is a statement regarding the organization's rules on a given topic. A **procedure** is a series of steps required to perform a given task. Policies and procedures must be written in a clear, concise, and understandable format. Each policy or procedure is signed by the employees, indicating they have read, understand, and will adhere to the policy or procedure. Policies regarding medical office management are signed by the physician and supervisory staff.

Tips for Writing Personnel Manuals

- Form a personnel committee. If staff members help develop the policies and procedures, they are more likely to follow them.
- Determine the rules and regulations of the office with the physician and managers.
- Contact local organizations, medical offices, or ambulatory care centers and ask for copies of their personnel manuals including policies and procedures.
- Research state and federal laws that regulate the medical office.
- Ensure compliance by appointing a **compliance officer**.
- Personnel manuals must be kept in a central location and be available to each employee for review.
- Review all policies and procedures annually to assess for currentness and accuracy.

Types of policies and procedures. There are many types of policies and procedures. In general, the following areas are included in a policy and procedures manual:

1. Mission statement
2. Organizational structure
3. Human resources, or personnel
4. Quality improvement and risk management
5. Clinical procedures
6. Administrative procedures
7. Infection control

Section 1: mission statement. A **mission statement** describes the goals of the practice and whom it serves. Often a mission statement provides a philosophical look at an organization. It is generally one to two paragraphs long (Fig. 5-6).

The mission statement should not only be included in the policy and procedures manual; it should also be available to patients. Often it is framed and placed in the waiting room or printed in the practice brochure.

Section 2: organizational structure. The organizational chart is included in this section along with policies regarding the following:

Box 5-1

TYPES OF HUMAN RESOURCES POLICIES

- Absentee policies
- Cafeteria plans
- Confidentiality policy
- Continuing education requirements
- Disciplinary action procedures
- Emergency procedures
- Employee benefits (health and dental insurance)
- Evaluation and performance appraisals
- Grievance procedures
- Grooming, uniforms, appearance
- Holiday coverage and compensation for holidays
- Jury duty
- Office hours
- Orientation
- Overtime reports
- Parking
- Payroll
- Personal phone calls
- Resignations
- Sexual harassment
- Sick leave and family leave
- Staff meetings
- Tardiness
- Termination process
- Time recording
- Vacation days

North Shore Family Practice is a group practice dedicated to providing quality care through compassion, innovation, performance and education. It is our goal to provide medical care to the community of Rochester, New York. The physicians, nurse practitioners, and all staff members are committed to working together as a team to provide the patient with the best care possible.

FIGURE 5-6. Sample mission statement.

- Chain of command
- How and when to contact various members of the team
- Coverage for managers
- Physician on-call policies

Section 3: human resources, or personnel. This section consists of policies relating to staff responsibilities, benefits, and rules and regulations for employees. Box 5-1 lists the kinds of policies found in this section of the manual. A sample human resources policy is displayed in Fig. 5-7.

Section 4: quality improvement and risk management. This section includes policies outlining who is in charge of quality improvement, the steps for developing a quality improvement plan, and explanations of incident reporting.

Section 5: clinical procedures. Any task that requires intervention with a patient should be listed in this section. (Some offices separate laboratory procedures into a different section for convenience.) In addition, clinical procedures should include specific infection control guidelines for the particular procedure, patient education guidelines, and instructions for documentation. Sample documentation forms should be included in this section. It is a good idea to complete the sample form correctly so that it can serve as a model. In the medical office, these procedures may vary slightly to meet the needs of the office, physicians' requests, or manufacturers' guidelines.

Section 6: administrative procedures. This section includes procedures on all tasks that the administrative office staff must perform. Sample forms should also be included and updated as necessary. Examples of administrative tasks follow:

- Accounting and bookkeeping
- Appointment scheduling
- Collections
- Computer care and operations
- Insurance filings
- Medical records management
- Mail and postal machines operations

Section 7: infection control. Depending on the length of this section, some offices opt for a separate manual dedicated to

Benjamin William, MD
2295 Matthews Drive
Boca Raton, Florida 33432
POLICY AND PROCEDURE MANUAL

Policy title: Human Resources, Call offs
Purpose: The purpose of this policy is to advise all employees of the policy for call offs and to prewarn employees regarding the disciplinary steps that will be taken as a result of not complying with this policy.
Equipment/Forms necessary: No equipment or forms are required.
Explanation:

- If you are going to call in sick, you must call in two hours prior to your assigned time. Messages should be left with the answering service if the office is not open.
- If you have personal days accrued, you can use them for compensation.
- If you are going to be out sick for more than three consecutive working days, you will need to obtain a physician's note to document the illness.
- Employees are allowed six (6) call offs per year without disciplinary action. Seven (7) call offs will result in a verbal warning regarding attendance. Eight (8) call offs will result in a written warning. Nine (9) call offs will result in termination. Exceptions to disciplinary action will be reviewed on an individual basis and are at the joint discretion of the office manager and physician.

Susan Rogers, RMA
Office Manager

Benjamin William, MD

date: original policy - 06/96, revised 07/98
HR: 14

FIGURE 5-7. Sample human resources policy.

infection control and prevention. Examples of these policies are:

- Types of personal protection equipment available
- Biohazardous waste disposal
- Handling of various disease identities
- Handling of employee exposures and needlesticks
- Documentation required by the Occupational Safety and Health Administration (OSHA)
- Employee education for infection control

Checkpoint Question

4. Which seven elements must be included when writing a policy or procedure?

Developing Promotional Materials

The medical office manager is often responsible for developing and distributing promotional literature for the practice. Depending on the budget, promotional materials can be created and produced at commercial printing shops or done in the office with desktop publishing programs. Examples of promotional materials follow:

- Education pamphlets and booklets for patients
- Practice brochure
- Newsletters
- Holiday cards
- Birthday cards (usually used by pediatricians)
- Newspaper articles
- Yellow pages
- Direct mail
- Business cards

Follow these guidelines when creating promotional materials:

- Double-check all spelling and grammar.
- Ensure accuracy.
- Use clear and specific language.
- Avoid abbreviations and complex medical terms.
- Use brightly colored materials.

If you are using a commercial printer, be sure to review the proofs carefully before the final printing.

Financial Concerns

Budgets

A **budget** is a financial planning tool that helps an organization estimate its anticipated expenditures and revenues. Budgeting has many purposes for an organization:

- Forcing the manager and physician to plan
- Causing managers and staff to become cost conscious
- Promoting communication among staff and managers
- Helping the organization achieve a financial goal

The medical office generally has both an operating and a capital budget. Operating budgets consist of all costs to run the office. These include but are not limited to payroll, office and medical supplies, education, promotional materials, and electricity and telephone services. Capital budgets consist of large outlays of money. These usually include large purchases (usually over $500), building maintenance, property management, and equipment.

Developing and writing a budget takes practice and instructions from the financial officer or physician. In general, the previous year's expense report is reviewed, revenues are projected for the following year, and figures are assigned to ensure that income balances with the outgoing expenses.

Checkpoint Question

5. What are the two basic types of budgets?

Payroll

Another financial concern for the manager is payroll. All employees expect to receive the correct amount of pay on time, and those expectations must be met. Payroll is a complex task that must satisfy state and federal laws regarding deductions for Social Security and other taxes. Because of this and because payroll is so time-consuming, some offices outsource this service.

Petty Cash

Most offices keep a small amount of cash in the office. Petty cash is used to purchase small items (e.g., postage, emergency office supplies) or to reimburse employees for small items. It is essential that the office manager keep close tallies on the petty cash fund. Most offices have some form of a petty cash receipt. Petty cash must be kept in a separate drawer from the change box.

Maintenance and Inventory of Supplies

One of the medical office manager's key responsibilities is to keep the office neat, clean, and well organized. Most offices have an outside cleaning agency to maintain the lobby, examination rooms, and offices. Special attention to waiting room toys is necessary because they can pose a safety threat to children. Staff should be encouraged to check the lobby periodically for neatness and to assist in routine cleaning and straightening.

Service Contracts

The medical office manager is responsible for keeping track of all service contracts. A service contract is an agreement between the medical organization and a service company in which the company agrees to perform regular inspections of and care for a specific piece of equipment. Service contracts are usually obtained for copiers, computers, fax machines, and other large and expensive pieces of equipment.

Inventory

Extensive amounts of supplies are needed to run a medical office. As a medical office manager, you must develop a logical system to keep track of them. There should be a policy outlining who is responsible for ordering supplies and the procedure for ordering. There also must be some process to check that deliveries of supplies are complete and accurate.

Education

Staff Education

The medical office manager must keep the staff up to date on medical procedures, drugs and vaccines, insurance coding and billing regulations, and any other topics that promote good patient care. In addition to these topics, annual education is usually conducted on cardiopulmonary resuscitation (CPR), infection control, and fire and electrical safety. Most allied health professionals are required to accumulate continuing education units (CEUs). CMAs must receive 60 CEUs every 5 years to retain the CMA credential. The office manager may choose to keep a file for each employee with the necessary documentation. This will assist the staff in the recertification process.

As the medical office manager, you should select an educational topic for each month. In some offices, the educational topic is covered during the monthly staff meetings, whereas other offices have separate educational programs. After choosing the monthly topic, select an appropriate presenter. Suggestions for presenters include colleagues, physicians, sales representatives, local hospital staff development coordinators, and specialists. Presenters for CPR classes must be CPR instructors who are approved by a national organization. To promote attendance, create informative flyers and distribute them to all staff members. Keep attendance records for all classes given.

In addition to formal educational programs, there are other ways to keep your staff up to date. For instance, educational videos can be rented or purchased for staff viewing; consider developing a posttest to assess for comprehension. Also, many professional magazines have continuing education articles on various topics, usually accompanied by a posttest. Finally, staff members should be sent to one or two seminars a year. Outside seminars help increase employee productivity, self-esteem, and retention.

Patient Education

All members of the health care team must constantly contribute to educating patients. As a manager, you may not provide patient education directly, but you are responsible for assisting the staff in performing this task. You can help the staff with patient education by creating booklets, developing posters, and by teaching your staff how, when, and what to teach patients and families.

Patient education brochures should be colorful and easy to read. Close attention to spelling, grammar, punctuation, and accuracy is essential. All brochures should be reviewed by a physician. Depending on your office's clientele, the brochures should be printed in various languages.

Manager Education

Managers should attend workshops and conferences and read appropriate printed materials to enhance their knowledge and skills in managing a medical office. All new managers can benefit from courses on time management, stress management, solving personnel conflicts, and budget preparation. Memberships in professional organizations can also assist the new office manager. Two such organizations are:

Medical Office Management Association
1355 South Colorado Boulevard, Suite 900
Denver, CO 80222-3331

Professional Association of Health Care—Office Managers
Suite 102
2929 Langley Avenue
Pensacola, FL 32504-7355

LEGAL ISSUES REGARDING OFFICE MANAGEMENT

Americans with Disabilities Act

Formerly called the Rehabilitation Act, the **Americans with Disabilities Act** (ADA) was expanded in 1994. All companies with more than 15 employees must comply with regulations designed to meet the needs of people with

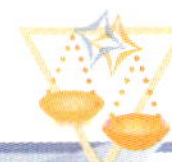

LEGAL TIP

Many acts and regulations affect health care organizations and their operations. As a medical office manager, you must keep current on all legal updates. Most states publish a monthly bulletin that reports new legislation. Every state has a website that will link you to legislative action. Read these regularly. Each office should have legal counsel who can assist in interpreting legal issues. It is important for a new manager to meet with the medical office's attorney to discuss legal concerns for the practice.

physical and mental disabilities. This act requires that all buildings be accessible to physically challenged people. Following is a partial list of ways the medical office can comply with this act:

- Entrance ramps
- Widened rest rooms and doors to be wheelchair accessible
- Elevated toilet bowls for easier transferring from wheelchairs
- Easy-to-reach elevator buttons
- Braille signs
- Access to special telephone services to communicate with hearing-impaired patients

Sexual Harassment

Sexual harassment of any employee or patient is illegal. Sexual harassment comes in many forms. As a medical office manager, it is your responsibility to be alert for signs of harassment and to have in place a policy for handling complaints regarding this.

Family and Medical Leave Act

The **Family and Medical Leave Act**, approved in 1993, allows an employee to leave his or her job for up to 12 weeks (unpaid) to meet family needs (e.g., the birth or adoption of a child; serious illness of a child, parent, spouse, or self). Employers must hold the employee's job position or offer the employee a position of similar nature on return.

Other Legal Considerations

The Clinical Laboratory Improvement Amendments (CLIA) of 1988 contain specific rules and regulations regarding laboratory safety.

OSHA is a federal agency that sets standards for employee safety.

The Joint Commission on Accreditation of Healthcare Organizations (JCAHO) is a private organization that sets standards for health care administration.

Each state also has specific laws regarding patient care, insurance billing, payroll management, and so forth that a medical office manager must understand.

Checkpoint Question

6. What are some legal issues of concern to the medical office manager?

Procedure 5-1

Creating a Procedures Manual

Equipment/Supplies

- Word processor
- 3-ring binder
- Paper

Steps	Reason
1. Gather product information; consult government agencies, as needed. If the procedure is for using new equipment, ask the sales representative for educational pamphlets. Some companies offer printed sample procedures.	This ensures that you are using products and equipment according to the manufacturer's suggestions and that you are practicing within legal and ethical boundaries.
2. Title the procedure, e.g., Infection Control Procedure for Handwashing.	A logical, easily identifiable format will allow easy retrieval.
3. Number the procedure, e.g., "HR 14" means human resource section, policy 14.	All policies and procedures should be numbered to allow for easy access and identification.
4. Define the overall purpose of the policy. This should be a sentence or two at most explaining the intent of the procedure.	Provides the staff with a rationale for the policy.
5. List any necessary equipment or forms. Include everything needed to complete the task. Also indicate so if no special equipment or forms are necessary.	The employee will be prepared before beginning the procedure if he or she has everything needed at hand.
6. List each step with its rationale. The steps must be complete and in order. Never assume the reader knows how or when to perform a given step, such as handwashing. The employee will be able to follow specific steps, ensuring patient safety.	Listing the steps in order promotes compliance and accuracy for policy completion.
7. Provide spaces for signatures. Administrative procedures are signed by the physician and office manager. Clinical procedures usually are signed by the clinical manager and a physician. Employees must have a space to sign.	The employee's signature will verify that he or she has read and understands the policy.
8. Record the date the policy was written. If changes are needed, the procedure is rewritten, signed, and dated again. The previous dates also are generally listed.	By recording the date, you ensure that you are reading the most current revision. It will also help you know when a new revision should be considered.

Procedure 5-2

Performing an Inventory of Supplies and Equipment

Equipment/Supplies: Computer with spreadsheet software, list of supplies, printer, paper.

Steps

1. Turn on the computer, monitor, and printer.
2. Open the spreadsheet software program.
3. Create a file called Supply Inventory.
4. Type the title of the spreadsheet (e.g., Medical Office Supplies for Inventory) in the appropriate cell.
5. Create a row for each type of supply, and columns to indicate the number of each supply available, the amount of each supply on hand during each month of the year (January through December), and how many supplies must be reordered each month.
6. Create formulas in the appropriate cell that will allow automatic calculations for the amount on hand each month. Also create formulas to automatically calculate how many supplies will need to be ordered each month.
7. Create a "total" amount column at the end of the spreadsheet and create a formula to automatically calculate the yearly total amount reordered.
8. Save all work.
9. Print the finished spreadsheet.

SUMMARY

Effective management of the medical office is essential for a health care organization to succeed in the competitive marketplace. A good manager must be able to perform a variety of tasks in an organized and efficient manner. These tasks include communicating with patients and staff, handling staffing issues, developing policy and procedures manuals, creating promotional materials, preparing budgets, and overseeing educational programs. In addition, the medical office manager must keep current on legal requirements related to office operations.

Critical Thinking Challenges

1. Review the list of qualities that a manager should have. Which ones do you have? How would you acquire the others? Should any other qualities be listed?
2. Review the types of sections that are often included in policy and procedures manuals. Now assume that you are to help a physician set up a practice. How would you organize your policy and procedures manual? Create one sample sheet for each section of your manual. Be sure to include all necessary elements when you write your policies and procedures.
3. Write a description of your ideal job. How would you go about finding this position?

Answers to Checkpoint Questions

1. An organizational chart is a flow sheet that allows the manager and employees to identify their team members and to see where they fit into the team.
2. Three ways to communicate with staff members are through bulletin boards, staff meetings, and communication notebooks.
3. The primary goal of scheduling is to ensure that the needs of the office are met.
4. The elements that must be in a policy or procedure are document name, purpose, equipment or forms needed, steps or explanations, signatures, numbering system, and dates.
5. The two basic types of budgets are operating and capital.
6. Some of the legal issues are the Americans with Disabilities Act, sexual harassment laws, Family and Medical Leave Act, CLIA, and OSHA.

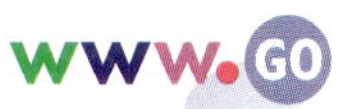

Websites

Medical Group Management Association
www.mgma.org
Physician Practice Group
www.physicianspractice.com
Family Leave Act/Department of Labor
www.dol.gov
Americans with Disabilities Act/U. S. Department of Justice
www.ada.gov
www.usaoj.gov

Unit 2

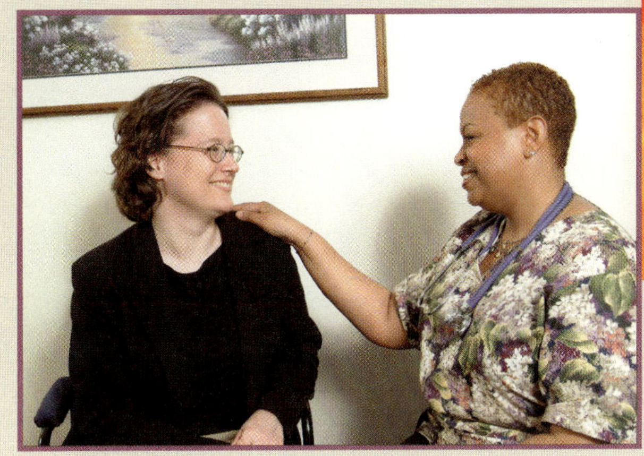

Medical Accounting Procedures

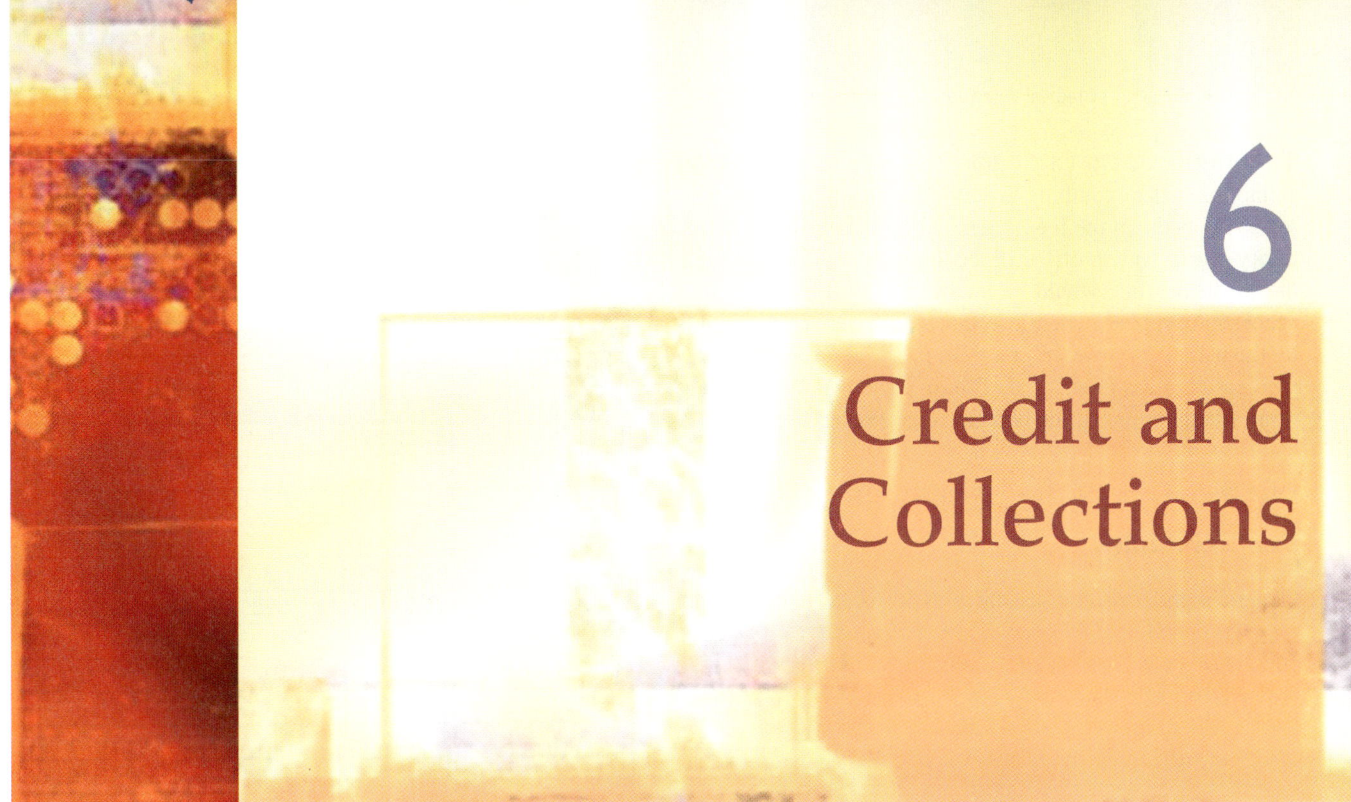

6 Credit and Collections

CHAPTER OBJECTIVES

In this chapter, you'll learn:

1. To spell and define the key terms.
2. To explain the physician fee schedule.
3. To discuss forms of payment.
4. To explain the legal considerations in extending credit.
5. To discuss the legal implications of credit collection.
6. To describe three methods of debt collection.

PERFORMANCE OBJECTIVES

In this chapter, you'll learn:

1. To use an aging schedule.
2. To write a collection letter.

KEY TERMS

adjustment
aging schedule
collections
credit
installment
participating providers
patient co-payment
professional courtesy
write-off

THE MEDICAL PRACTICE MUST operate in a financially sound manner to continue to serve the patient's needs. The office depends on the fees generated by patient visits, laboratory work, and in-office procedures. Without these fees, the medical office would be unable to pay for staff, office space, and supplies. Therefore, collecting fees, whether paid by the patient, an insurer, or a third party, is essential for the medical practice to succeed. Box 6-1 shows how to determine whether your office is collecting fees satisfactorily.

FEES

Fee Schedules

Generally, the physician sets the fees for office visits, laboratory work, and in-office procedures based on the UCR concept: (1) U (usual) fair value of the service; (2) C (customary) competitive rates charged by other physicians; and (3) R (reasonable), that which meets the other two criteria. Fee setting also considers the resource-based relative value scale (RBRVS), by which fees are based on the relative value of a particular service and adjusted for geographical differences. A physician's fee schedule also takes into consideration the costs of operating the office, such as rent, utilities, malpractice insurance, salaries, and so on. A list of the services and procedures offered in an office along with descriptions, procedure codes, and prices must be available to patients. Federal regulations require that a sign to this effect be posted in the office.

Code	Key	Mod	Par Fee	Non Par Fee	Limiting Charge
50010			$690.30	$655.79	$754.16
50010			$690.30	$655.79	$754.16
50020			$1,112.72	$1,057.08	$1,215.64
50021			$522.30	$496.19	$570.62
50040			$1,009.84	$959.35	$1,103.25
50045			$921.52	$875.44	$1,006.76
50060			$1,116.74	$1,060.90	$1,220.04
50065			$1,128.28	$1,071.87	$1,232.65
50070			$1,172.52	$1,113.89	$1,280.97
50075			$1,451.88	$1,379.29	$1,586.18
50080			$976.28	$927.47	$1,066.59
50081			$1,336.92	$1,270.07	$1,460.58
50100			$1,033.66	$981.98	$1,129.28
50120			$945.54	$898.26	$1,033.00
50125			$980.30	$931.29	$1,070.98
50130			$1,010.09	$959.59	$1,103.53
50135			$1,110.42	$1,054.90	$1,213.14
50200			$138.72	$131.78	$151.55
50205			$696.55	$661.72	$760.98
50220			$1,015.02	$964.27	$1,108.91
50225			$1,168.36	$1,109.94	$1,276.43

FIGURE 6-1. Sample Medicare fee schedule.

There may be several fee schedules based on the reimbursement schedules of different insurance companies. **Participating providers** are those who agree to participate with managed care contracts and other third-party payers in exchange for building a solid patient base. Patients covered under participating plans will have a different fee schedule from patients who are private pay (paying with no money from insurance). Each managed care plan, workers' compensation company, Medicaid carrier, and Medicare has a different fee schedule.

A Medicare fee schedule has three columns. A participating fee is the amount paid to physicians who participate or agree to accept a certain fee. A nonparticipating fee is the amount paid to physicians who do not have agreements with Medicare. A limiting charge is the amount a physician can charge a Medicare patient. Figure 6-1 is a sample Medicare fee schedule.

Discussing Fees in Advance

It is always a good policy to discuss fees with patients in advance. This ensures that patients are aware of the charges. Patients will need to know in advance whether the medical office is a participating provider with their insurance carrier. Managed care companies usually require that the patient pay

Box 6-1

DETERMINING A PRACTICE'S COLLECTION PERCENTAGE

Medical practices should evaluate their method of collections periodically to determine the effectiveness of their practices. A collection analysis lets you identify the strengths and weaknesses of the system.

To do a collection analysis, determine the monthly production from the first day of each month to the last day. This will be the total charges posted to all patients' accounts. Next determine the revenues the practice received. Computer systems will automatically total payments received during a specified time. Divide revenue by production to determine the collection percentage. Analysis of the collection percentage should reveal the percentage of the collection of all outstanding debts to the practice.

Collection percentage =
monthly production ÷ monthly revenue received

Most medical practices average 8 to 20% loss yearly. Experts consider a collection percentage above 80% to be reasonable. Performing a 2-year collection percentage comparison analysis will help you evaluate past collection effectiveness.

a certain share of the bill, known as the **patient co-payment, or co-pay.** A good and easy way to initiate a discussion of fees is by providing an office brochure that lists not only the office's address, telephone number, and hours but also office policies regarding fees and collections, third-party payments, and how they are handled. Patients should understand that co-pays are to be paid at the time of service. Such information should be included in the office brochure. Many offices post a sign in the waiting area stating this.

Always collect the entire amount due from a new patient on the first visit. Most problems associated with collection (acquiring funds that are due) come from patients who go from one practice to another. Be sure you get a picture identification, such as a driver's license, on a patient's first visit.

Forms of Payment

Depending on the medical office's policies, the patient can usually pay for services in one of two ways: with cash or by personal check. If a new patient is paying by check, get two forms of identification. Many larger practices accept credit and debit cards (Visa, MasterCard, Discover) also. By agreeing to accept a credit card payment, the medical office also agrees to pay the credit card company a percentage (usually 1.8%) of the total charge. Although this may seem costly, it is sometimes more cost effective to receive payment by credit card than to receive it in installments—or not at all—from the patient.

Payment by Insurance Companies

By far the largest proportions of fees are paid by insurance companies. Therefore, it is imperative that patients' insurance information be kept current. Most medical practices require that a patient submit a medical insurance card for each visit; this way, changes in insurance can quickly and easily be noted. Always make a copy of both sides of the patient's insurance card and staple it to the appropriate section of the chart for billing reference.

Adjusting Fees

Sometimes, **adjustments** (changes in a posted account) must be made to a standard fee, as when the medical office accepts a set insurance rate for a service that is lower than the practice's rate. You must charge the patient the normal fee for the service; when the insurance carrier sends payment, however, the explanation of benefits (EOB) will show how much you may collect for the service. The difference between the physician's normal fee and the insurance carrier's allowed fee will be adjusted in the credit adjustment column on the patient's account.

Other fee adjustments include **professional courtesy** fees, in which other health care professionals are charged a reduced rate. The physician may choose not to charge a fee at all; this too is considered a professional courtesy and should not be confused with writing off a fee. (A **write-off** is cancellation of an unpaid debt; these generally can be claimed on the practice's federal taxes.) Again, you charge the normal fee and then adjust the designated amount in the adjustment column with "professional courtesy" in the description column.

Checkpoint Question

1. To avoid collection problems, what should you get from a new patient on the first visit?

CREDIT

Extending Credit

It is not always possible for patients to pay the entire bill when such costs are incurred. Depending on the medical office's policy, **credit** may be extended to patients on an installment plan. Collection experts have estimated that billing one patient costs the practice about $8 per month. This total includes the time it takes to prepare the statements, the supplies needed, and so on. Extension of credit to a patient is a decision that is often made solely by the physician.

Legal Considerations

When a medical practice extends credit to a patient, it may charge interest on the patient's unpaid balance. If this is the case, the medical office is legally required to disclose this information to the patient, along with any other fees or charges incurred by the patient's acceptance of credit. This legal documentation, called a truth-in-lending statement, must be filed in the patient's medical chart.

Different states have different laws concerning the extension of credit. Generally, credit cannot be denied based on age, gender, race, marital status, religion, national origin, or source of income (e.g., if a patient receives public assistance). If your facility has given credit to one patient, you typically may not refuse the same arrangement to another patient. Some states have laws limiting the amount of interest that can be charged. The practice's accountant should be able to provide the information required by the state and municipality.

Checkpoint Question

2. On what grounds should credit *not* be denied?

COLLECTIONS

When a patient has an unpaid bill or has not paid an installment per a credit agreement, those funds must be collected. Collecting an unpaid debt is costly to any business. Collecting fees can also be time consuming, and collecting practices are regulated by a variety of consumer protection laws. Many medical practices outsource their billing to companies specializing in billing and debt collection.

Box 6-2

RULES FOR TELEPHONE DEBT COLLECTION

When attempting to collect a debt by telephone, a debt collector may not:

1. Contact the patient at his or her place of employment if the employer objects
2. Tell anyone other than the patient or responsible party about a debt without court authorization
3. Contact the patient before 8:00 A.M. or after 9:00 P.M.
4. Contact the patient at all if the patient has filed for bankruptcy
5. Harass or intimidate the patient; that is, use abusive language, provide false or misleading information, or pose as someone other than a debt collector

Box 6-3

COLLECTING DEBTS FROM A PATIENT'S ESTATE

When a patient dies, the family needs time to grieve and accept the death. Collecting debts from an estate requires professionalism and tact. Never contact the family regarding a debt immediately after a patient's death. Most offices have a policy stating that family members of deceased patients will not be contacted until a week after the funeral. At the appropriate time, call the next of kin listed in the patient's chart. Offer your sympathy and ask for the name of the patient's executor, the individual responsible for handling the patient's affairs after death. The executor may be an attorney, spouse, friend, or other relative. Call the executor and introduce yourself. Obtain the executor's address and send a final bill. It is important that all claims on a patient's estate be made promptly. In case the estate does not have enough funds to meet all of its debts, the probate court will decide the priority list for debt collection.

Legal Considerations

Certain procedures should be followed in attempts to collect a debt. A debt collector—in this case, the administrative medical assistant or billing clerk—must exercise reasonable restraint when contacting a patient about a bill. Box 6-2 displays guidelines for collection attempts by phone.

Attempting to collect a debt from a patient's estate requires particular diplomacy. Box 6-3 offers some guidelines to follow in such a situation.

Collecting a Debt

Monthly Billings

The easiest way to collect a debt or an installment is by monthly billing. Once a month, the medical office sends bills to its patients who have unpaid balances. Larger offices set up a billing cycle and divide the alphabet, sending statements once a week to each selected group. For example, patients with names beginning with the letters A to G might be billed on the 1st of the month, H to N on the 8th, O to S on the 15th, and T to Z on the 22nd. If your facility changes a billing cycle, you are legally required to notify patients of the change 3 months before the change takes effect.

The uncomputerized office normally just copies the ledger cards of the patients who owe balances. It is important to make each entry on the ledger card with consistency and provide a key for office codes or abbreviations. The patient should be able to understand each entry. When a practice is computerized, the staff can easily send statements. Medical office software usually gives the option of printing a separate message at the bottom. For instance, you may add "Happy Holidays" to every patient's December statement or "Time for your flu shot" in the September statements.

If the account is on an **installment** plan, the patient receives a bill that lists the amount due for that month, any third-party payments or adjustments applied to the account, the total amount due, and the amount the patient owes. This

Spanish Terminology

Necesito recoger el total en su cuenta.	I need to collect the balance on your account.
¿Puede pagar usted algunos de su deuda?	Can you pay some of your balance?
Esto es una carta de la colección.	This is a collection letter.
Usted debe este dinero a esta oficina.	You owe this office money.

way, the patient has the option of paying more than is due for that particular month (and thereby reducing the amount of any interest charged) and is aware of the current balance.

Aging Accounts

Unpaid accounts must be monitored to determine how far overdue or in arrears they are. Aging of an account is calculated from the first date of billing, not by the procedure date. For example, a patient has an office visit on January 5 and the first statement is sent on February 1. The account will not be past due until March 1.

For this purpose, the medical office keeps an **aging schedule** that lists the patient's name, balance, any payments, and comments, such as reminders or second notices sent. Such a schedule can be kept on a large sheet of paper or by a comprehensive computer billing program. Figure 6-2 is a sample of a manual report. Figure 6-3 shows a computer screen that automatically places the amounts charged under the proper heading based on the age of the account. This account shows that $132 of the charges are current, or less than 30 days old. The $95 represents charges that were incurred and posted at least 120 days ago.

Aging of accounts is a measure of the practice's ability to collect its fees. Nearly all fees (80%) should be collected within 30 days. If the aging shows a high percentage (50%) of fees being collected 30 days or more after billing, the practice's billing and collection procedures should be reviewed.

Collecting Overdue Accounts

The three most common ways of collecting an overdue account are sending an overdue notice to the patient, telephoning the patient to let him or her know the account is overdue, and informing the patient at the next office visit.

Overdue notices. With a manual system, overdue notices are fairly simple to prepare. Often, they consist of a copy of the patient's monthly billing with the words "overdue" or "second notice" stamped in red. Alternatively, a form letter with spaces for the patient's particulars may be sent. Figure 6-4 is a sample collection letter. If a computer billing program is used, the computer often can automatically generate overdue notices.

Telephoning the patient. If written notices bring no response, you may have to telephone the patient to inquire about an overdue account. Always ask when payment may be forthcoming and document the reply on the patient's account. If payment is not received as promised, contact the patient again.

Aging of Accounts Receivable Report: April 30, 2003

Patient Name	Account Number	Due Date	Amount
Accounts 30 Days Past Due:			
Doe, John C.	000-00-0000	3/6/03	625.00
Graham, Paula R.	000-00-0000	3/29/03	450.00
O'Toole, William Q.	000-00-0000	3/13/03	25.00
Parker, Mary W.	000-00-0000	3/25/03	299.00
Reeves, Chris A.	000-00-0000	3/11/03	58.00
South, Cheryl C.	000-00-0000	3/8/03	385.00
Yarkony, Ralph M.	000-00-0000	3/11/03	108.00
Accounts 60 Days Past Due:			
Forest, Patricia L.	000-00-0000	2/19/03	476.00
Heany, Beverly O.	000-00-0000	2/13/03	57.00
Thomas, Walter T.	000-00-0000	2/27/03	185.00
Accounts 90 Days Past Due:			
Glick, Rhonda K	000-00-0000	1/4/03	28.00
Payne, Robert A.	000-00-0000	1/25/03	456.00
Accounts 120 Days or More Past Due:			
Baird, Jane C.	000-00-0000	10/3/02	45.00
Wallace, Michael S.	000-00-0000	12/15/02	349.00
Total Overdue Accounts Receivable			**$3,546.00**

FIGURE 6-2. Sample aging of accounts receivable report.

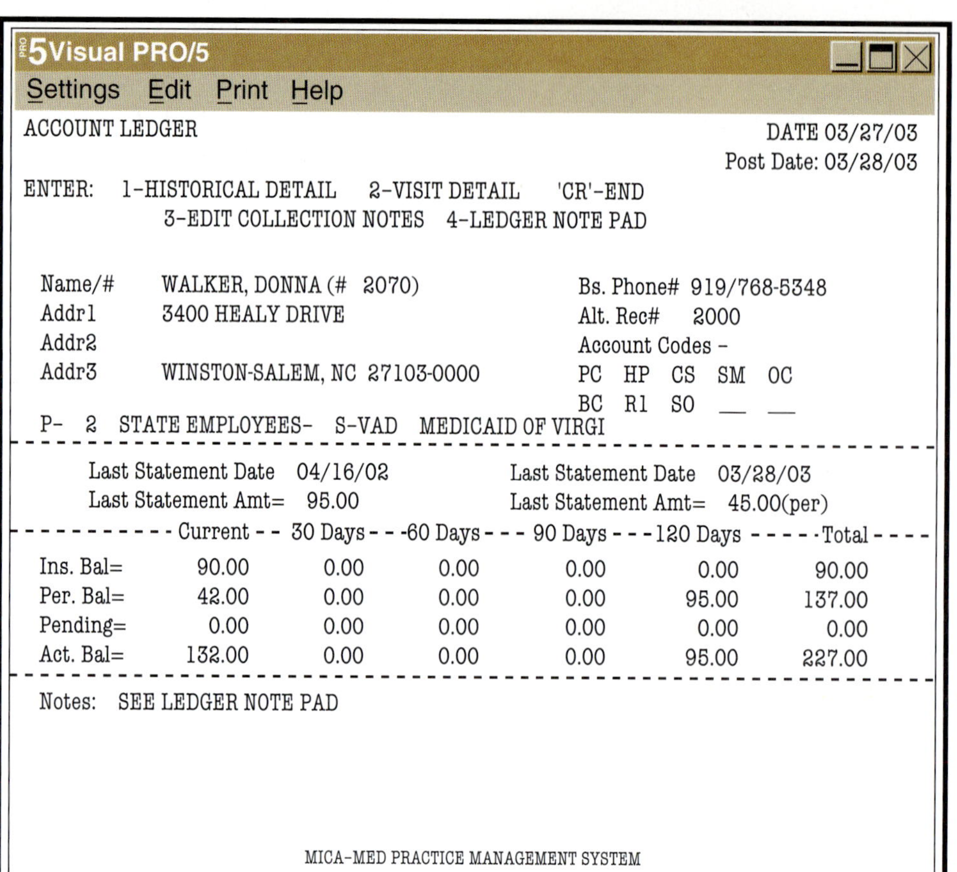

5Visual PRO/5

Settings Edit Print Help

ACCOUNT LEDGER — DATE 03/27/03
Post Date: 03/28/03

ENTER: 1-HISTORICAL DETAIL 2-VISIT DETAIL 'CR'-END
3-EDIT COLLECTION NOTES 4-LEDGER NOTE PAD

Name/# WALKER, DONNA (# 2070) — Bs. Phone# 919/768-5348
Addr1 3400 HEALY DRIVE — Alt. Rec# 2000
Addr2 — Account Codes -
Addr3 WINSTON-SALEM, NC 27103-0000 — PC HP CS SM OC
BC R1 SO __ __
P- 2 STATE EMPLOYEES- S-VAD MEDICAID OF VIRGI

Last Statement Date 04/16/02 — Last Statement Date 03/28/03
Last Statement Amt= 95.00 — Last Statement Amt= 45.00(per)

	Current	30 Days	60 Days	90 Days	120 Days	Total
Ins. Bal=	90.00	0.00	0.00	0.00	0.00	90.00
Per. Bal=	42.00	0.00	0.00	0.00	95.00	137.00
Pending=	0.00	0.00	0.00	0.00	0.00	0.00
Act. Bal=	132.00	0.00	0.00	0.00	95.00	227.00

Notes: SEE LEDGER NOTE PAD

MICA-MED PRACTICE MANAGEMENT SYSTEM

FIGURE 6-3.
Sample computer screen.

Family Practice Associates
2345 Oak Street
Forest, OR 77777
(234) 567-8900

June 23, 2003

Mary W. Parker
300 Red Bird Lane
Lake, OR 77771

Dear Ms. Parker:

It has recently come to our attention that your account with our office is slightly overdue. Your balance of $299.00 is over 30 days past due. Please pay this amount as soon as possible. If you are having trouble paying this amount, please call our office and make arrangements to pay your balance.

If you have recently paid this amount and your payment is on the way to us in the mail, please disregard this letter. If you have any questions or concerns, feel free to contact me at the phone number above.

Sincerely,

Kathy Porter
Accounting Manager

FIGURE 6-4.
Sample collection letter.

WHAT IF

A patient who has an overdue account wants to schedule an appointment. What should you do?

As a medical assistant, you are not responsible for deciding whether a patient who has an outstanding balance gets to be seen by the physician. Schedule the appointment, then discuss the issue privately with the physician. Ethically, the physician may opt to care for the patient until the disorder is resolved. Legally, the physician is obligated to care for this patient until the physician–patient relationship is terminated.

In-Office Reminders. A patient can be reminded of an overdue balance when he or she comes to the office to see the physician. To handle this situation discreetly, simply give the patient a copy of the most recent overdue notice. Once again, ask when payment may be forthcoming and follow through. Computer systems may offer the option of a flashing computer screen when the patient's overdue account is retrieved. This alerts anyone working with the patient either to discuss payment or to refer the patient to someone in the office who will explain that payment is expected.

Collection Alternatives

Sometimes, it is more cost effective for **collections** to be handled outside the medical office. Three common options include collection agencies, small claims court, and credit bureaus. Collection agencies specialize in collecting debts. For either a fee or a percentage of the debt, the collection agency attempts to collect the monies due by the methods listed earlier. In addition, the collection agency can represent the medical practice in small claims court and can have the bad debt listed with credit-reporting agencies.

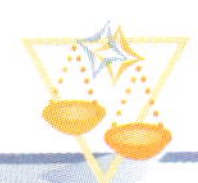

LEGAL TIP

The Fair Debt Collection Act

The Fair Debt Collection Act is a federal law that states how and when a collector can attempt to collect a debt. It is a violation of the law to threaten to send a patient to a collection agency if you do not intend to do so. Unlawful threats can result in a lawsuit for harassment against the caller. Box 6-2 shows the guidelines for telephoning patients to attempt to collect a debt.

The medical practice can, of course, sue patients in small claims court or list patients with credit bureaus itself, but it is often more time and cost effective to hire an outside agency.

Checkpoint Question

3. What are three ways of collecting overdue accounts?

SUMMARY

The financial status of a medical office is based on the ability of the staff to collect the physician's fees. This must be done in a professional manner and in accordance with state and federal laws. Technology affords the medical office the ability to streamline procedures, and collection practices are more efficient with computer systems. Aging accounts and communicating with patients in a fair and professional manner ensures a constant cash flow and success in managing the finances of the outpatient medical practice.

Critical Thinking Challenges

1. Under what circumstances might a patient need credit? To what local resources could you refer this patient?
2. A patient has an overdue account balance. What steps would you take to collect the debt?
3. Create a collection letter for a patient account that is 60 days' overdue. Create a collection letter that you would send to a patient's executor or patient's estate.

Answers to Checkpoint Questions

1. On a new patient's first visit, collect the entire amount due and get a picture identification.
2. Credit cannot be denied based on age, gender, race, marital status, religion, national origin, or source of income.
3. Overdue accounts can be collected by sending overdue notices, telephoning patients, and informing patients at the next office visit.

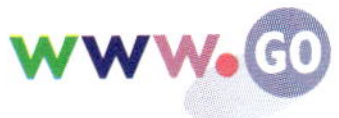

Websites

Credit and Collections World
www.collectionsworld.com

Fair Debt Collection Practice/Federal Trade Commission Statutes
www.ftc.gov

National Credit Systems
www.nationalcredit.com

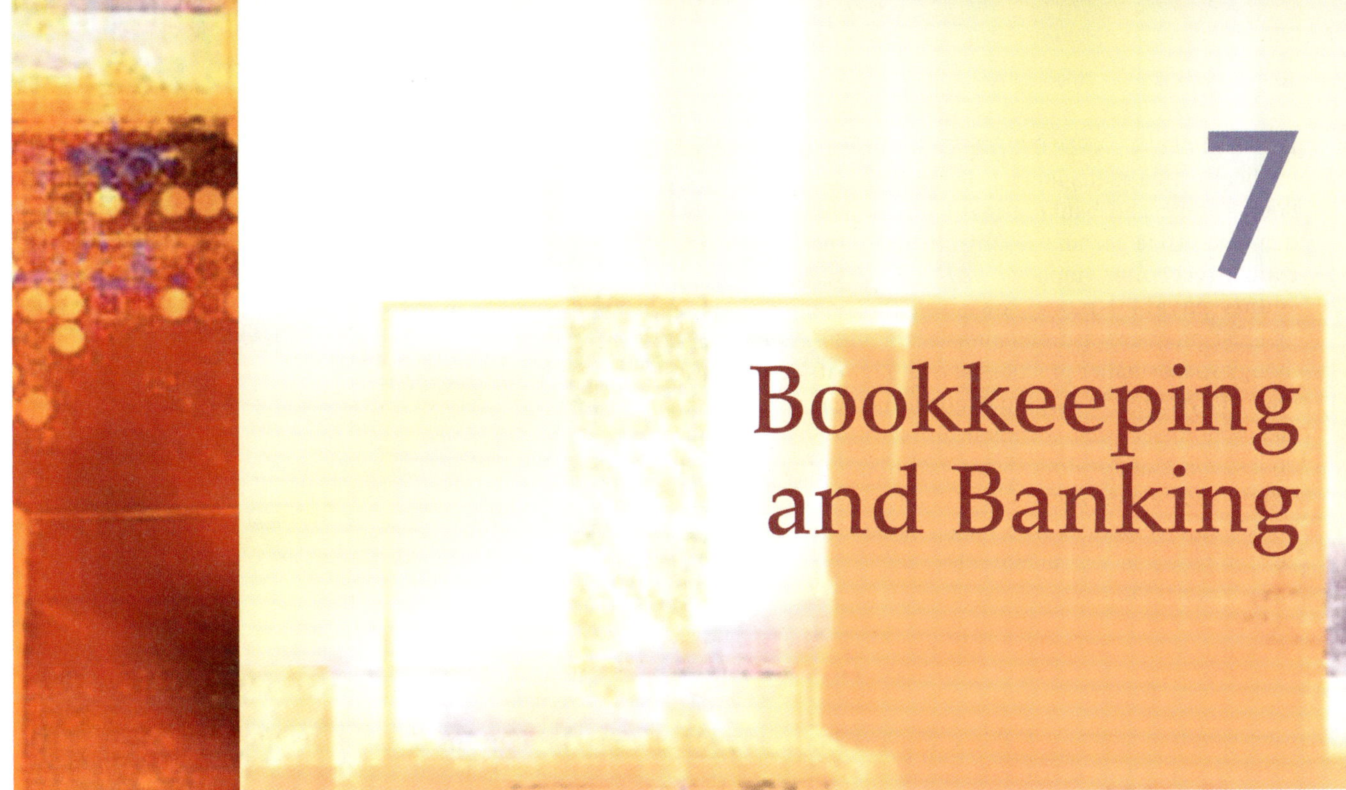

7 Bookkeeping and Banking

CHAPTER OBJECTIVES

In this chapter, you'll learn:

1. To spell and define the key terms.
2. To explain the concept of the pegboard bookkeeping system.
3. To describe the components of the pegboard system.
4. To identify and discuss the special features of the pegboard day sheet.
5. To describe the functions of a computer accounting system.
6. To list the uses and components of computer accounting reports.
7. To explain the services and procedures of the bank.

PERFORMANCE OBJECTIVES

In this chapter, you'll learn:

1. To record financial transactions, such as charges, payments, credits, and adjustments to patient ledger cards.
2. To balance a day sheet.
3. To complete a bank deposit slip and make a deposit.
4. To reconcile a bank statement.
5. To write a check.
6. To maintain a petty cash account.

KEY TERMS

accounts payable
accounts receivable
adjustment
balance
bookkeeping
charge slip
credit
day sheet
debit
encounter form
ledger card
posting
returned check fee
service charge

BOOKKEEPING AND BANKING are important facets of medical office management. In most medical practices, bookkeeping and banking involve maintaining both patient and office account records, including petty cash, **accounts receivable** (money owed to the practice), and **accounts payable** (money owed by the practice). Most medical practices use computer accounting systems, although some smaller practices and satellite offices still use manual systems. In large outpatient medical conglomerates with many sites, a central billing office may handle bookkeeping and billing. Some practices outsource their billing and related accounting functions. Although daily bookkeeping practices are handled in the office, the office also employs an accountant who receives reports of the daily financial functions.

DAILY BOOKKEEPING

Bookkeeping is defined as an organized and accurate record-keeping system of financial transactions for a business. The daily financial transactions of a medical office include patient payments that arrive through the mail, patient payments from patients seen in the office, and patient charges that are added to the accounts receivable. Most medical practices use the single-entry bookkeeping system.

The foundation of accounting is this equation:

$$\text{Assets} = \text{liabilities} + \text{equity}$$

Assets are all things of value owned by or relating to the practice. Liabilities are monies owed. Equity refers to the amount of capital the physician has invested in the practice. Because the two sides of the accounting equation must always **balance** (be equal), each transaction requires a **debit** (charge) on one side of the equation and a **credit** (payment) on the other side of the equation; the amount of the debit and credit must be equal. Double-entry systems are usually used by accounting firms and corporations.

Most medical facilities use the *cash basis* type of accounting, which means that income is considered as income only when money is collected and that payables (money owed) are considered expenses only when money is paid.

The most popular formats for daily bookkeeping are the manual pegboard system and computer systems.

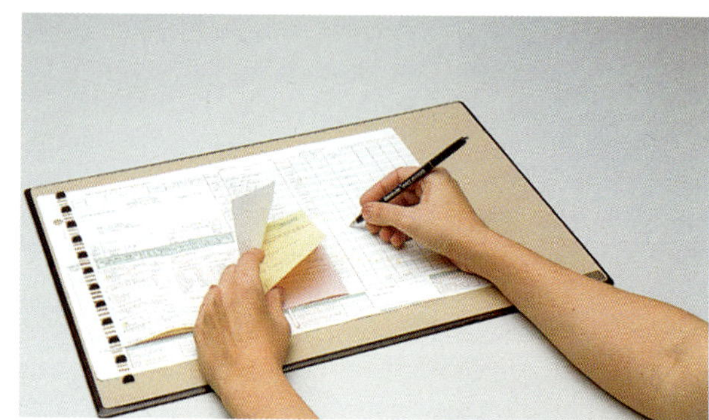

FIGURE 7-1. Sample day sheet with ledger card and charge slip. (Courtesy of Control-o-fax, Waterloo, IA.)

MANUAL ACCOUNTING

Pegboard Bookkeeping System

The pegboard, or write-it-once, bookkeeping system uses a board with pegs running down the left side. The pegs hold a **day sheet**, or daily journal, in place on the board. All transactions for the day are recorded on this day sheet. Each patient has a ledger card (record of the patient's financial activities). When a patient transaction occurs, the bookkeeper places the ledger card over the day sheet and the **charge slip** (preprinted patient bill) over the ledger card on the next available entry line and makes the appropriate entry on the ledger card. Figure 7-1 is a sample day sheet.

Day sheets come with a sheet of carbon paper; thus, the entry recorded on the ledger card, even when a charge slip is not used, is also recorded on the day sheet. When a payment received in the mail is posted, for example, no charge slip is needed. As the day progresses, each patient's ledger card is placed on the next available line on the day sheet, so that the day's entries appear consecutively. At the end of the day, all of the transactions are added.

The various components used in a pegboard system and the specific steps for recording patient transactions are discussed in greater detail next.

Day Sheet

The day sheet keeps track of daily patient transactions, such as charges for services to patients, payments received from

Spanish Terminology

Esto es su total.	This is your balance.
Esto es su crédito.	This is your credit.
No pague esta cuenta.	Do not pay this bill.
Su cheque se volvió para fondos de insuficiente.	Your check was returned for insufficient funds.
Su cuenta ha sido mandada a una agencia de la colección.	Your account has been sent to a collection agency.

patients and insurance carriers, and adjustments to patient accounts. A day sheet should be kept for each day that the physician sees patients; on busy days or for practices with more than one physician, more than one day sheet may be required.

The day sheet has several sections: a deposit slip, distribution columns, a section for payments, a section for adjustments, and a section for **posting** proofs (listing financial transactions in a ledger).

The deposit slip is a detachable portion of the day sheet. All payments received are noted on the deposit slip, and at the end of the day it is separated from the day sheet and deposited with that day's payments.

The distribution columns are used to assign charges for various services. How these columns are used depends on the needs of the individual practice. In a group practice, each practitioner has his or her own column. Some practices may assign columns to the various insurance plans they accept. Finally, these columns can be used to provide information on quality improvement issues. The distribution columns, regardless of how they are assigned, provide the physician with important information about how the practice earns its income.

An **adjustment** is an entry to change an account. The adjustments section allows for reductions in office fees, as with professional courtesy discounts and insurance disallowances. The adjustments section also allows for crediting an account for uncollectible monies without using the payment column. It can also be used to return charges to an account if the patient's payment has been returned by the bank for insufficient funds.

The posting proofs section is where the day's totals are entered and the day sheet is balanced, much as one would balance a checkbook. Once the day sheet is complete, each column or section is totaled individually. It is best to total each column twice to make sure that no errors have been made. After all the columns have been totaled, the posting proofs section is filled out.

If the posting proofs do not balance, an error has been made on the day sheet. To locate the error, go over each transaction one by one. Add the previous balance to the fee or subtract the payment from the previous balance to check whether the new balance listed is correct. If the posted charges are correct, total each column again. Do not erase or white-out errors, but draw a line through the erroneous entry and enter the transaction on a new line. When you reenter a transaction on the day sheet, use the ledger card again. Box 7-1 outlines some basic bookkeeping tips.

WHAT IF

You cannot balance the day sheet. What do you do?

First, take a short break. Then return to the day sheet and double-check each entry and your arithmetic (a common error is transposing numbers, such as entering 69 instead of 96). If you are still unable to find the error, ask a colleague to check the day sheet. After all attempts to balance the sheet have been exhausted, notify the physician or office manager.

Box 7-1

BASIC BOOKKEEPING TIPS

- Always use black ink; do not use pencil.
- Write legibly.
- *Never* erase or white-out errors. Draw a single line through the incorrect entry, record the correct information, and initial the change.
- Always double-check each entry.

The day sheet is important because it keeps track of accounts receivable. The accounts receivable total changes every time a charge, payment, or adjustment is made to an account. You should perform a trial balance at the end of each month. Add the totals of each ledger card with an outstanding balance. The total should match the running total kept on the day sheet. This practice ensures the accuracy of your financial records.

Completed day sheets are filed chronologically in a ledger (a book of accounts) with the most recent day sheet on top. Completed day sheets are important legal documents and must be kept for at least 7 years for tax purposes. They should be stored in a safe, dark area to avoid loss or fading.

Checkpoint Question

1. What are five sections of a pegboard day sheet?

Ledger Cards

The **ledger card** is a financial record for each patient. Most ledger cards include areas for the responsible person's name, address, telephone number, and insurance information. Fig. 7-2 is a sample ledger card. Other information, such as employment information and primary and secondary insurance information, may appear on the ledger card. Patient information appears on the top of the ledger card; the bottom portion is used to record the patient's financial activities.

Many practices use photocopies of an individual's ledger card as a bill, mailing the photocopy to the patient each time payment is required. If you use a copy of the ledger card for billing, make sure that no information other than the billing name and address is visible through the window

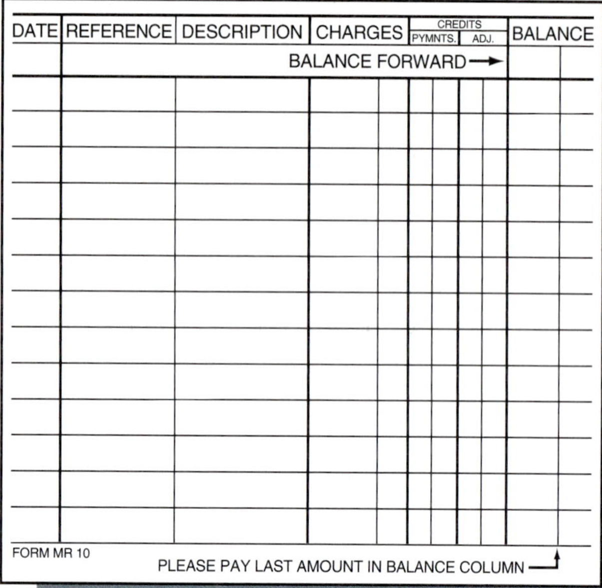

DATE	REFERENCE	DESCRIPTION	CHARGES	CREDITS PYMNTS.	CREDITS ADJ.	BALANCE
	BALANCE FORWARD →					

FORM MR 10

PLEASE PAY LAST AMOUNT IN BALANCE COLUMN

FIGURE 7-2. Sample ledger card.

of the envelope. Allowing other information to be visible is a breach of privacy.

The ledger card is a legal document and should be kept for the same length of time as the patient's medical record. Ledger cards are filed alphabetically in a ledger tray. A medical practice may require more than one ledger tray. Ledger cards with outstanding balances are kept separate from paid ledger cards; this makes it easier to photocopy the monthly bills or find a ledger card when a patient calls about an outstanding bill. If the office uses only one ledger tray, the ledger cards with outstanding balances are filed alphabetically in the front of the ledger tray, with the paid ledger cards filed alphabetically in the back.

Encounter Forms and Charge Slips

The **encounter form** and the **charge slip** are preprinted patient statements that list codes for basic office charges and have sections for the patient's current balance and next appointment. Most encounter forms and charge slips have three-part copies:

1. The first copy is kept by the facility for auditing purposes (all are numbered).
2. The second copy is given to the patient for insurance filing (if the patient files the insurance claims).
3. The third copy, which has a carbon line at the top to match your ledgers and day sheets, is given to the patient as a receipt of services.

Charge slips are smaller versions of an encounter form and are designed to be used in conjunction with ledger cards. They often have different-colored no-carbon-required (NCR) copies. Figure 7-3 shows a computer-generated encounter form and a charge slip used in a manual system.

Checkpoint Question

2. How do ledger cards and encounter forms differ?

Posting a Charge

The charge column of the day sheet is for original charges incurred for services received by the patient from the physician or staff on a specific date. Examples include office visits, electrocardiogram, blood work, hospital visits, consultations, and fees for returned checks. Charges in a medical office are based on a fee schedule or list of charges determined by the usual, customary, and reasonable charges of similar providers in similar localities who practice under similar circumstances. Procedure 7-2 outlines the steps for posting a charge.

Posting a Payment

Payments received by the practice may include insurance checks received in the mail, money orders, credit card payments, or cash received from patients. Procedure 7-3 outlines the steps for posting payments and adjustments.

Posting a Credit

Sometimes an account is overpaid, either by the patient or the insurance company. Such an overpayment is termed a credit (money owed to the patient or insurance carrier). This will show on the patient's ledger card as the last balance, with brackets (e.g., [25]) indicating a credit. Brackets are used to show the opposite of the column's normal meaning. For example, the balance column normally shows patients' debits, or amounts patients owe to the doctor. Brackets around an amount indicate the opposite, namely, that the doctor owes the patient money.

Credits are handled in one of two ways: (1) the credit stays on the account and is subtracted from the charges on the patient's next visit, or (2) the patient is mailed a refund for the amount of the overpayment. How an overpayment is handled depends on office policy and the amount of the overpayment. Generally, overpayments under $5 are left on account as a credit, whereas overpayments over $5 are refunded.

Posting a Credit Adjustment

The adjustments section is used to indicate nonstandard office fees and to credit an account for uncollectible monies. Below are three specific situations that require a credit adjustment.

Patient Name: ______________________ | Encounter #: ______________________

Patient ID #: __________ DOB: __________ Sex: __________ | Service Provider: ______________________

PCP: ______________________ | Appt. Status: ☐ Scheduled ☐ Same Day ☐ Walk-in

SSN: __________ Financial Class: __________ | Check-in Time: __________ Check-out Time: __________

Escorted to Exam Room: __________ Time Patient Seen: __________

Phone: __________ (home) __________ (work) | Appointment Time: __________

Medical Record #: __________ Date of Service: __________

Is Patient Being Seen in Relation to:
☐ Motor Vehicle Accident ☐ Workman's Compensation

Benefit Pkg: __________ Copay $ __________

Appointment Failure Reason:
☐ Patient Cancel ☐ No Show ☐ Walk Out ☐ PHA Cancel

TYPE OF VISIT

✓	CODE	DESCRIPTION	FEE	✓	CODE	DESCRIPTION	FEE	✓	CODE	DESCRIPTION	FEE	✓	CODE	DESCRIPTION	FEE
		OFFICE VISITS-EST.				**OFFICE VISITS-NEW CONT.**				**PREVENTATIVE, NEW**				**COUNSELING**	
	99211	Minimal			99204	Compreh.			99385	E&M 18-39			99401	15 Min.	
	99212	Focused			99205	Comp. & Complex			99386	E&M 40-64			99402	30 Min.	
	99213	Expanded				**NURSE VISIT**			99387	E&M 65 & over			99403	45 Min.	
	99214	Detailed			99211	Minimal				**CONSULTATION**			99404	60 Min.	
	99215	Compreh.				**PREVENTATIVE, EST.**			99241	Focused					
		OFFICE VISITS-NEW			99395	E&M 18-39			99242	Pre-Op Consult					
	99201	Focused			99396	E&M 40-64			99244	2nd Opinion					
	99202	Expanded			99397	E&M 65 & over									
	99203	Detailed													

PROCEDURES

✓	CODE	DESCRIPTION	FEE	✓	CODE	DESCRIPTION	FEE	✓	CODE	DESCRIPTION	FEE	✓	CODE	DESCRIPTION	FEE
	88170	Aspiration - Cyst			11200	Skin Tag Removal				**IMMUNIZATIONS/INJECTIONS**				**IMMUNIZATIONS/INJECTIONS CONT**	
	20600	Aspiration - Joint (Small)			20550	Trigger point/Tendon Inj.			G0009	Administration Fee - Pneumovax			J2203	Triamcinolone Inj.	
	20605	Aspiration - Joint (Interm.)							G0010	Administration Fee - Hepatitis B			J3420	Vitamin B_{12}	
	20610	Aspiration - Joint (Large)				**SPECIALTY SERVICES**			95115	Allergy Injection Single				**IN-HOUSE LABORATORY**	
	16020	Burn Dressing			99070	Ace Bandage			95117	Allergy Injection Multiple			89050	Cell Count, except blood	
	69210	Ear Irrigation			E0110	Crutches			90788	Antibiotic IM			89060	Crystalanalysis	
	10120	Foreign Body Removal, Skin			29130	Finger Splint			J2910	Aurothioglucose			82948	Glucose	
	10060	I&D Abscess, simple			29125	Wrist Splint			G0008	Flu Vaccine			85013	HCT	
	90780	IV Infusion Therapy			99080	Form Completion			J1600	Gold Injection			85018	Hemoglobin Screen	
	12001	Laceration Repair, Simple				**TESTING/SCREENING**			90731	Hepatitis B			81025	Pregnancy	
	13160	Laceration Repair, Extens.			95004	Allergy - Skin Test			90741	Immune Globulin			81002	Urinalysis, Dipstick	
	64450	Medial Nerve Infiltration			92557	Audiometry			90724	Influenza			81000	Urinalysis, Full	
	17110	Molluscum/Wart Rmvl			93000	EKG			J9217	Lupron 3.75 mg			G0001	Venipuncture	
	94640	Nebulizer			92506	Hearing Screen			J9217	Lupron 7.5 mg				**OTHER PROCEDURES**	
	82270	Stool for Blood (Hemocult)			86580	PPD			J9250	Methotrexate 2-5 mg					
	12001	Suturing, Superficial			94010	Pulmonary Function			90732	Pneumovax					
	13100	Suturing, Complex			94760	Pulse Oximetry, Single			90718	Td					
	11050	Skin Les./Wart Cautery			45330	Sigmoidoscopy, Flexible			90782	Therapeutic SQ or IM					

P = PRIMARY S = SECONDARY S1-S9 = NUMBERED SECONDARY

DIAGNOSIS

✓	CODE	DESCRIPTION	✓	CODE	DESCRIPTION	✓	CODE	DESCRIPTION
	789.0	Abdominal Pain		780.6	Fever		462	Pharyngitis (sore throat)
	879.8	Abrasion/Laceration		704.8	Folliculitis		486	Pneumonia
	995.3	Allergic Reaction		535.5	Gastritis		V70.3	Pre-Marital Testing
	477.9	Allergic Rhinitis		558.9	Gastroenteritis		V72.81	Pre-op Cardiac Exam
	285.9	Anemia		274.9	Gout		V72.83	Pre-op Exam, Other
	413.9	Angina		V72.3	Gyn Exam		601.0	Prostatitis
	300.00	Anxiety		784.0	Headache		600	Prostatism
	716.90	Arthritis		389.9	Hearing Loss		782.1	Rash
	427.9	Arrhythmia		536.8	Heartburn/Indigestion		569.3	Rectal Bleeding
	493.90	Asthma		573.3	Hepatitis		530.81	Reflux
	611.72	Breast Lump		455.6	Hemorrhoids		V81.2	Screening for Cardiac Condition
	490	Bronchitis		553.9	Hernia		780.3	Seizure Disorder
	727.3	Bursitis		401.9	Hypertension (NOS)		473.9	Sinusitis
	354.0	Carpal Tunnel Syndrome		272.4	Hyperlipidemia		848.9	Strain/Sprain
	682.9	Cellulitis		242.00	Hyperthyroidism		438	Stroke
	786.50	Chest Pain		251.2	Hypoglycemia		305.90	Substance Abuse
	575.1	Cholecystitis		380.4	Impacted Cerumen		099.9	STD
	372.3	Conjunctivitis		780.52	Insomnia		727.00	Tenosynovitis, Tendonitis
	496	COPD		564.1	Irritable Bowel Syndrome		451.9	Thrombophlebitis
	414.9	Coronary Artery Disease		719.40	Joint Pain		246.9	Thyroid Disease
	290.9	Dementia		592.0	Kidney Stones		435.9	TIA
	311	Depression		464.0	Laryngitis		463	Tonsillitis
	692.9	Dermatitis		724.2	Low Back Pain		011.90	Tuberculosis
	250.01	Diabetes, IDDM		710.0	Lupus		465.9	Upper Respiratory Infection
	250.00	Diabetes, NIDDM		V70.0	Medical Exam/Physical		599.0	Urinary Tract Infection
	558.9	Diarrhea		346.9	Migraine		V04.8	Vaccination, Flu
	562.10	Diverticular Disease		278.0	Obesity		V03.9	Vaccination, Pneumovax
	780.4	Dizziness		382.9	Otitis Media		616.10	Vaginitis
	995.2	Drug Reaction		614.9	Pelvic Inflammatory Disease		424.9	Valvular Heart Disease
	782.3	Edema		533.9	Peptic Ulcer Disease		079.9	Viral Syndrome
	780.7	Fatigue/Tiredness/Malaise		443.9	Perpheral Vascular Disease			

Comments:

PREVIOUS BALANCE	$
TODAY'S CHARGES	$
PAYMENT	$
BALANCE	$

RETURN APPOINTMENT:
____ Days ____ Weeks ____ Months

APPT. LENGTH: PROVIDER:

APPT. REASON:

PROVIDER SIGNATURE:

Adult

Philadelphia
Health Associates
Tax ID #23-2350500
PHA Group # PH75923

❑ 3550 Market Street
Philadelphia, PA 191(
(215) 823-8660

❑ The Bourse Building
111 S. Independence
East • 7th Floor
Philadelphia, PA 191(
(215) 625-9100

OTHER DIAGNOSIS

✓	CODE	DESCRIPTION	✓	CODE	DESCRIPTION

FIGURE 7-3. Sample encounter form and charge slip.

Example 1. The physician wishes to give a registered nurse a 25% professional discount on charges incurred for an office visit. You enter the fee from the fee schedule in the charge column, show in the description column an office visit with a professional discount of 25%, and put the 25% in the adjustment column. Assume an office visit is $40. You put $40 in the charge column and $10 (25% of $40) in the adjustment column. The patient owes your facility $30 for this visit.

Example 2. Most medical offices participate with certain insurance groups, which means the physician has signed an agreement with the insurance carrier to accept the fee for services set by that carrier instead of the physician's normal fee. Again, you must charge the same fee for the same procedure. When payment is received, however, the explanation of benefits from that carrier will show the agreed-on amount for that procedure. You will post the payment in the normal way, but you must write off the difference between the physician's standard fee for this procedure and the agreed-on amount. Assume the doctor charged $40 for an office visit and the insurance carrier's agreed-on amount was $35. You would post $40 in the payment column and $5 in the adjustment column to arrive at the agreed-on amount.

Example 3. Most facilities request that you write off the balance of an account when you turn it over to a collection agency to keep better control of the accounts receivable. Therefore, if the patient's balance is $1200, you would show "collection agency" in the description column of the ledger and put the $1200 in the adjustment column, which would bring the balance to 0. Procedure 7-4 lists the steps for posting an adjustment.

Checkpoint Question

3. What do brackets around an amount listed in a column indicate?

Posting a Debit Adjustment

Generally, a credit adjustment reduces the patient's account balance, whereas a debit adjustment adds to the patient's account balance. Below are three specific situations that require a debit adjustment.

Example 1. You receive an insufficient funds (NSF) check from the bank today from a payment made earlier by a patient and posted as such to his account. The previous payment is no longer valid. Therefore, you must eliminate that payment because the patient now owes it again. Because this is not an original charge, you may not use the charge column for this entry. To post this debit adjustment to the patient's account, you will show NSF in the description column and the amount of the NSF check in the adjustment column with brackets.

Example 2. Assume that you have turned over an account to a collection agency and the patient comes in later to pay the amount owed. You must first put the money back on the account, or you will create a credit balance. Place the ledger card on the day sheet and in the description column write "reverse collection." Again, this is not an original or new charge, so you do not use the charge column. Show the amount in the adjustment column in brackets because you are adding the amount to the patient's balance. You may now show the payment in the payment column.

Example 3. Your office requires that you refund all money over $5 to the patient or insurance carrier. You must also post this to eliminate the credit balance on the account. Place the ledger card on the day sheet and in the description column write "refund to patient" (or insurance carrier). To eliminate a credit balance, you must debit the account. You put the amount of the refund in the adjustment column in brackets, indicating that it is a debit, not a credit adjustment.

Checkpoint Question

4. How does a credit adjustment differ from a debit adjustment?

Posting to Cash-Paid-Out Section of Day Sheet

Sometimes, the physician may take cash from the day's receipts. When this happens, your bank deposit for that day will be short by the amount taken out. The best way to account for this is to have the physician sign in the cash-paid-out section of the day sheet for the amount. This documents the transaction and prevents anybody else from being able to do this.

Some insurance carriers adjust for money overpaid to your facility by holding that amount out of money they are paying your facility for other patients. Although you are posting the correct amounts in the payment column for each patient, the check amount from the insurance carrier is short the refund or kept-out money. You write this in the cash-paid-out section of the day sheet, explaining, "insurance refund on account of [patient's name]." It is also a good idea to make a copy of the explanation of benefits and staple it to the back of your day sheet for future reference.

COMPUTER ACCOUNTING

Most medical office accounting software available today is easy to use and requires a minimum of computer skills. Computer programs fulfill many of the same functions as a pegboard system but do so much faster. Instead of recording entries on a day sheet, you key entries into a computer. You can print out invoices and receipts for patients and insurance companies. Since most practices have computer stations in several locations, the patient's account can be quickly and easily retrieved in all areas of the office, enabling everyone

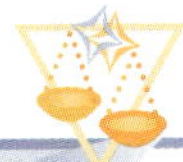

LEGAL TIP

Overpayment of an account is more common than you might realize, especially when multiple insurance companies are billed along with the patient. If your office receives an overpayment by an insurance company, notify the company and send the overpayment back. Be sure to discuss this with the physician first. Legally and ethically, it is wrong to keep overpayments.

involved in the patient's care to access information about third-party coverage, co-payments required, and so on.

Computer bookkeeping programs have a variety of advantages over pegboard bookkeeping. Computer programs work as expanded calculators and perform the arithmetic functions, such as balancing individual accounts and the day's totals. Many bookkeeping programs also can write checks. Some programs manage electronic banking between the office and bank. The office may have computerized many functions, including bookkeeping, making appointments, and generating other office reports, such as forms for insurance reimbursement. It is essential that data stored on computer be backed up in a reliable way in case the computer crashes.

Posting to Computer Accounts

If you understand the fundamentals of accounting and how to post entries manually, you will be able to use a computer system with ease. To post payments, first retrieve the patient's account. The software will take you through the process. You enter the source and amount of the payment, the allowed amount for the service, and any necessary adjustments. As in a manual system, this information is provided on the insurance carrier's explanation of benefits (EOB). Calculations are automatic and error free.

When you post charges into the computer database, in most systems you use a local code to indicate a certain procedure or service. For example, you may enter 211 to post a level 2 office visit for a new patient. When the information prints on the claim form, the CPT (current procedural terminology) code 99212 will appear.

Computer Accounting Reports

Depending on the software package, you can easily generate daily, monthly, and yearly reports or reports on transactions of an individual physician in a group practice. Daily and weekly reports provide the same information found on the bottom of a day sheet in a manual accounting system. At any given time, you can request a report that displays the practice's period-to-date and year-to-date financial status.

Computer systems record the daily activities described earlier for the manual system, and bookkeeping software enables you to create a closing report that prints a list of the day's financial activities. You may run a trial daily report or a final daily report. In a trial report, the information keyed in that day is printed for review. You correct any errors before running a final report. As on the day sheet, you categorize receipts as cash, check, and so on. A check register report can print the amount of the daily deposit and a list of checks for the day.

BANKING

Banks and Their Services

Besides physical location, several factors are important when choosing a bank for the office business account. These factors include the monthly service fees, overdraft protection programs (protection against bouncing checks), interest-bearing accounts, and returned check fees.

Checking Accounts

A checking account allows you to write checks for funds that are deposited in the account. Each day you will deposit to a checking account the money collected in the office. At the time a new checking account is opened, checks are ordered with a check order form. The administrative medical assistant must maintain the checkbook and ensure that checks are reordered as needed.

Banks offer a variety of options for checking accounts. Variables include monthly service charges, maximum amounts of checks written, minimum balance requirements, and so on. Interest-bearing checking accounts pay interest if the balance is kept above a certain amount. Most banks set the minimum checking account balance at $500 to $2500. The bank pays this interest in exchange for the use of your money for loans and other transactions. If you drop below the minimum balance, however, you will not earn interest. Most banks also charge a monthly service fee and a fee for each check written for the period the balance was below the limit. Some banks waive the monthly service fee if the office agrees to maintain a minimum balance in another account, such as a savings account.

Savings Accounts

The medical practice may use a savings account for money that is put aside for long-term plans or money that is not needed for writing checks. A savings account pays interest at a higher percentage rate than a checking account, allowing the money to grow. Funds can be transferred to the checking account as needed.

Money Market Accounts

Money market accounts are a combination of a savings account and an interest-bearing checking account. The minimum balance is usually much higher than that of a checking account (as much as $2500), but the interest rate also is much higher. These accounts offer limited check-writing privileges, including an initial deposit of $2000 and minimum balance of $500 per check.

Bank Fees

Banks charge fees for services. In an effort to get new business, banks offer special services and plans for small business, including the medical office.

Monthly Service Fees

Bank policies concerning monthly fees or service charges vary widely. A **service charge** is a fee charged monthly for using an account. The charge can be a fixed amount or may be an individual charge for each check written on the account. As discussed, some banks do not levy a service charge if a specific minimum balance is maintained for the account.

Overdraft Protection

Overdraft protection guarantees that checks written against the account will be paid even when there is not enough money in the account at the time. Usually, the bank pays the checks and retrieves the money owed to it when the account balance is restored. Many banks offer overdraft protection only up to a certain dollar amount.

Returned Check Fee

Some banks charge a **returned check fee**, which is a fee charged for any check that is deposited into the checking account but that is later returned to the bank because the account it was issued from had insufficient funds with which to pay the check. Such a check is often referred to as a bounced check. Most facilities charge this amount to the patient. Because this is an original charge, the bad check fee is listed in the charge column of the patient ledger and day sheet, with the amount of the check being recorded as a debit adjustment.

Types of Checks

Most medical offices use the standard business check, but when certain circumstances require, there are other types available:

- Certified checks are stamped and signed by the bank to verify that the amount of the check is being held in the account for payment. The check is written from the customer's account.
- Cashier's checks are sold to a customer for cash or a personal check. The check is written by the bank, giving the recipient the added guarantee that the check is good.
- Traveler's checks are a convenient and safe way to carry cash when traveling. They are available in denominations of $10, $20, and $50, and if lost, they can be replaced. Traveler's checks are signed when bought and are countersigned (signed again) in the presence of the payee.
- Money orders, although not checks, can be purchased with cash from a bank or the U.S. Postal Service. Money orders, which guarantee payment to the recipient, are often used for mailing payments, since it is not safe to mail cash.

Box 7-2 highlights other terms used in the language of banking.

Box 7-2

DO YOU SPEAK "BANKING?"

ABA number: A number originated by the American Bankers Association to identify the bank on which the check is written. It is written in the form of a fraction and is usually found above or below the check number. The top number of the fraction indicates the geographic location, and the bottom number identifies the bank.

ATM: Automated teller machines have made 24-hour banking possible. With the use of a card you insert in a slot and a personal identification number (PIN), you can make deposits, withdrawals, and transfers at an ATM. If your bank owns the ATM, this convenience is usually free. If you use any other ATM, a service fee of up to $3.50 is charged. The ATM screen gives you the opportunity to cancel the transaction if you are not willing to pay the service fee.

Debit card: A card with a magnetic strip that is presented for payment directly from your checking account. When a transaction occurs, you record it in your check registry.

Online banking: Electronic or online banking gives you the opportunity to view your account at any time. Withdrawals and deposits are listed and can be printed, and transfers can be made.

Stale check: A check that has not been cashed within a certain time, usually 6 months. Some checks must be cashed within a shorter time, but that requirement must be printed on the check.

Checkpoint Question

5. List three types of checks available through banks.

Writing Checks for Accounts Payable

Another financial duty of the medical assistant may be to handle accounts payable, or pay the bills. The accounts payable in a medical office usually include rent, utilities, taxes, salaries, vendors of supplies and services, patient refunds, and petty cash reimbursement. The accounts are usually paid by check. Banks require signature cards for each person authorized to sign checks. In most cases, this is limited to the physician or physicians. Some medical offices require two signatures, especially if the check is over a certain amount. Computer systems allow you to enter information in the proper field and print checks. Software systems also keep track of every transaction using a check. When using a manual system, type or write legibly. Use the current date and write the amount of the payment in both figures and words and the name of the payee. Complete the memo line for reference. Record the date, check number, amount of the check, and payee on the check registry. Post this transaction to the appropriate account in the general ledger or apply it to the proper category in a computer system by entering the type of payment on the proper screen. Recording transactions in the proper account or category is important when preparing the office taxes. Subtract each amount from the check register balance.

Receiving Checks and Making Deposits

When checks are received in the office, they are first endorsed. To endorse a check requires writing (or rubber stamping) on the back of the check the name and number of the account into which it will be deposited (Fig. 7-4). This way, if the payments are lost or stolen, no one else can cash them. It also ensures that the bank deposits the payments to the correct account. An endorsement stamp can be purchased from your bank or a stationery store.

After all payments are posted, total all of the checks and all cash received that day. This total should match the totals of the payments column on your day sheet. Detach the deposit sheet from the day sheet and stamp the back with the endorsement check stamp. If a computer program is used, print out a deposit slip. Wrap the deposit slip around the checks and complete a bank deposit slip for the account to which the deposit is made. The deposit can be hand-delivered or mailed to the bank.

A hand-delivered deposit may be taken to a teller, who will issue a deposit receipt, or dropped in a depository. If the deposit is mailed, make sure sufficient postage has been affixed to the envelope. Never include cash payments in a deposit that is mailed or placed in a depository. Cash deposits should always be hand-delivered, and a teller's receipt should always be obtained.

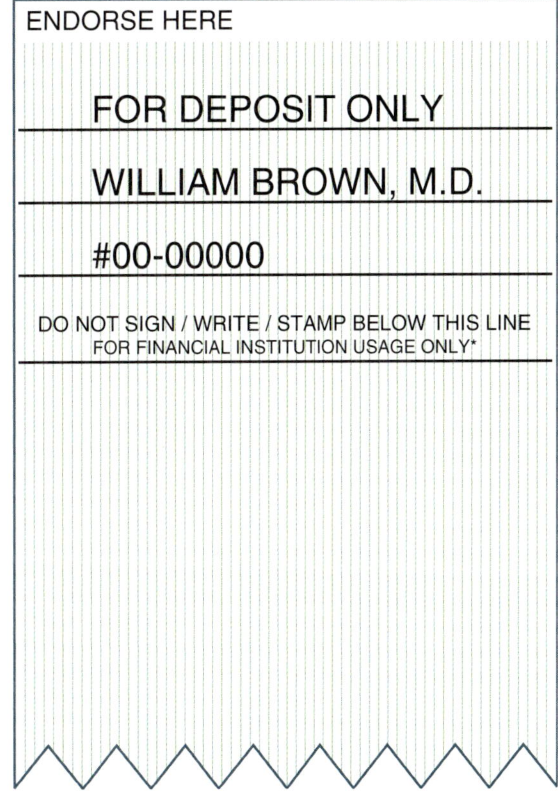

FIGURE 7-4. An endorsed check.

Reconciling Bank Statements

All banks mail monthly statements to account holders on which are listed all transactions since the last closing date. This bank statement must be reconciled, or compared for accuracy, with your records each month.

The statement consists of a list of all checks written and their amounts, all deposits made and their amounts, any electronic transactions, and any service charges. Verify that all checks and deposits are listed correctly. Make a check mark on the checkbook stub of each check that has been paid by the bank. On the back of the statement is a worksheet that explains how to balance the account (Fig. 7-5). Following the steps listed on the worksheet makes balancing the account fairly easy. The steps for reconciling a bank statement are listed in Procedure 7-5.

Checkpoint Question

6. What information is found on a bank statement?

1. Subtract any fees or charges that appear on this statement from your checkbook balance.
2. Add any interest paid on your checking account to your checkbook balance.
3. List the checks you have written that have not been paid (these checks did not yet appear on your bank statement). You can also include in this list any withdrawals you have made since the ending date of the banking statement that do not appear on the statement.

Check Number	Amount
________	________
________	________
________	________
________	________
Total	________

4. If you have entered deposits or other additions to your checkbook that do not appear on the statement, list them there:

Date	Amount
________	________
________	________
Total	________

5. Enter the ending balance from your statement here: ________
   Add the total deposits from Step 4: + ________
   Subtract the total from Step 3: − ________
   Total (this should equal your checkbook balance): ________

If these balances do not equal your checkbook balance:

- Check the addition and subtraction in your checkbook
- Check the amount of each transaction in your checkbook with the amount shown on your statement
- Check to see that all transactions from your previous statement have been accounted for
- Call your bank manager for assistance

FIGURE 7-5. Bank statement reconciling worksheet.

PETTY CASH RECEIPT

__________ 20 ____

To Office Manager:
Please furnish for________________

Supplies:		
Postage:		
Travel Expenses:		
Other:		
Approved	TOTAL	

Received Above Amount

____

FIGURE 7-6. Petty cash voucher.

PETTY CASH

A petty cash account is a cash fund kept in the office specifically for small purchases, such as buying postage stamps or office supplies. The value of the petty cash account should always remain the same. A petty cash fund is always a designated sum of money. When money is taken from the fund, a voucher (Fig. 7-6) or receipt is placed in the fund to verify the purchase. The remaining cash and the sum of the vouchers should always equal the designated sum; for example, a petty cash fund of $40 with $13 in actual cash should have receipts that amount to $27.

Petty cash funds should be kept separate from patient cash payments. All cash should be kept in a securely locked area. One person should be designated to maintain the petty cash fund and issue vouchers. A voucher with an attached receipt should always be placed in the petty cash box, both to provide proof of the purchase and to keep the account balanced. The petty cash fund normally is replenished once a month. To replenish the fund, cash a check in the amount of the total of the vouchers. The money is placed in the fund, and the vouchers are removed and filed.

Some offices keep a petty cash expense record. This record is similar to a checkbook that keeps track of the account balance as checks are written, such as personal checkbook. This expense record also categorizes purchases so that they can be included with the monthly office expenses. Purchases such as stamps and office and medical supplies can be deducted as office expenses and added to the accounts payable expense record.

Checkpoint Question

7. List six guidelines for managing petty cash.

Procedure 7-1

Balancing the Day Sheet

Equipment/Supplies

- Calculator
- Current day sheet with yesterday's previous balance total
- Carbon
- All ledger cards with transactions on the day sheet
- Pencil
- Pen

Steps	Reason
1. Determine if all entries are complete.	If all charge slips listed on the day sheet are not returned to you, the day sheet will not balance. Make sure you have finished the transaction on each account.
2. Add each column with a calculator and place the total in pencil in the appropriate column.	Day sheets include a portion for performing a daily proof (verifying the accuracy of the entries). Using pencil will enable changes if needed.
3. Add the totals from today to the totals from the previous day sheet.	A running total is kept by placing the ending figure for each day under the column for the beginning figure on the next day's sheet. This gives you a total accounts receivable amount at any time.
4. To verify the accuracy of the entries: • Add the total of the previous balance column to the total of the current balance column • From this total, subtract the totals of the payment and adjustment columns • This amount equals the current balance	This allows for double verification of current totals.
5. When the totals are verified, go back over them in pen.	Day sheets are legal documents that are retained. They must be written in ink.

Procedure 7-2

Posting Charges to the Patient's Account

Equipment/Supplies

- Day sheet
- Carbon paper
- Pegboard
- Ledger card
- Charge slip and/or encounter form
- Calculator
- Form
- Pen

Steps	Purpose
1. Take the charge slip from the patient and check to be sure it is complete, signed by the provider, and belongs to the patient whose ledger card or account is in hand.	It is difficult to undo entries to the wrong account. It's best to be accurate the first time. Just as in the clinical area, identify your patient.
2. If using a ledger card, post the total amount of today's charges in the charge column on the ledger card. Each service can be listed in the description column by using abbreviations such as OV, INJ, LAB for office visit, injection, and laboratory services, respectively.	Since the manual billing system uses a copy of the ledger card for a statement, it is important that patients be able to understand your abbreviations. Provide a key at the bottom of the ledger card.
3. If using a computer, post each charge separately on the charge screen. Most programs require a local code for a particular service. When you enable this code or the CPT code, the computer will automatically post the appropriate charge in the proper field.	Proper computer entry allows for accurate financial records to be maintained.

Procedure 7-3

Posting Payments to a Patient's Account

Equipment/Supplies

- Day sheet
- Carbon paper
- Pegboard
- Ledger card
- Charge slip and/or encounter form
- Calculator
- Form
- Pen

Steps

1. Align the patient's ledger card on the day sheet. If the patient is paying for services received by the physician today, the charge slip that shows today's charges should also be in place on the day sheet.
2. Enter the patient's name and previous balance in the appropriate columns. If using a charge slip, make sure you place the charge slip number in the receipt number column. Enter the posting date in the date column.
3. Enter the type of payment being made in the description column, whether personal check (pers. ck.), money order (m. o.), credit card (MC, VISA), or insurance check (ins. ck.). Enter the amount of payment in the payment column and on the deposit section of the day sheet in the cash or checks column.
4. Subtract the payment amount from the previous balance and record the new balance. If only a payment is being posted, no entry is made in the fee area. If an entry has been made in the fee area, you will start with the previous balance, add the charges, subtract the payment, and record the new balance.

Procedure 7-4

Posting a Credit Adjustment

Equipment/Supplies

- Day sheet
- Carbon
- Pegboard
- Ledger card
- Calculator

Steps	Reason
1. Align the patient's ledger card on the day sheet.	Proper alignment is needed for accurate record keeping.
2. Record the patient's name, previous balance, and the date in the appropriate columns.	Payments and adjustments can be posted at the same time. The payment is recorded in the payment column, and the adjustment is entered in the adjustment column. Both are subtracted from the previous balance, and the new balance is recorded in the new balance column.
3. Record [in brackets][a] the amount of the adjustment in the adjustment column of the ledger card. Enter a description of the adjustment in the professional service column, that is, insurance adjustment or correction adjustment.	A description of the adjustment is needed for proper financial record keeping and quality assurance.
4. Subtract the amount of the adjustment from the previous balance and record the new balance in the balance column.	Knowing the balance of an account is essential for the financial stability and growth of a business.

[a]Brackets indicate that the amount is subtracted.

Procedure 7-5

Reconciling a Bank Statement

Equipment/Supplies

- Monthly bank statement
- Check register
- Calculator
- Pen

Steps	Reason
1. Determine which portion of the checkbook is covered on this bank statement.	You must know where your last bank statement ended and where the current one begins.
2. Find the ending balance and the list of checks and deposits on the bank statement.	
3. Check your checkbook register or record of disbursements against the bank statement and place a check mark against each check and deposit on your record that has been recorded on the bank statement.	To balance the account, you must identify which checks or deposits are recorded by the bank and which ones are outstanding.
4. Total all checks not listed on the bank statement. Place this total in the space provided on the back of the bank statement (outstanding checks).	Since there is no standard form, each bank's worksheet may be different, but there will be a space reserved for the total of all outstanding checks and withdrawals.
5. Total all deposits that do no appear on the bank statement and place this total in the space provided on the worksheet (outstanding deposits).	Outstanding deposits must be accounted for to balance the bank statement.
6. Note any additional charges, such as for services, ATM use, or returned checks.	Miscellaneous charges must be taken into account when balancing the checkbook
7. Calculate the correct balance by starting with the ending balance from the bank. Then, add the outstanding deposits to that balance (from Step # 5). Then, subtract the outstanding withdrawals (from Step # 4).	Outstanding deposits and withdrawals must be accounted for to reconcile the bank statement.
8. Verify that the correct balance (from Step # 7) matches with your checking account amount.	This allows verification that, as of today, your checking account balance agrees with your bank statement.
9. If the figure is not the same, recheck your work. If the two numbers still do not match, contact the bank to check for possible bank errors.	This allows you to verify your records with the bank's record. It is easy to transpose numbers or misread figures when using a calculator. You should add the columns again. It is helpful to have a coworker add the columns also.

Procedure 7-6

Preparing a Bank Deposit

Equipment/Supplies: Calculator with tape, currency, coins, checks for deposit, deposit slip, endorsement stamp, deposit envelope.

Steps

1. Organize currency by arranging bills face up and sorting with the largest denomination on top.
2. Count currency and coins and record the total in the cash block on the deposit slip.
3. Endorse the back of each check with pre-printed stamp, "For Deposit Only."
4. Record the amount of each check beside an identifying number on the deposit slip.
5. Total the amount of checks and record in the total of checks line on the deposit slip.
6. Total the amount of cash and the amount of checks and record in the total deposit line on the deposit slip.
7. Record the total amount of the deposit in the office checkbook register.
8. Make a copy of both sides of the deposit slip for office records.
9. Place the cash, checks, and the completed deposit slip in a envelope or bank bag for transporting to the bank for deposit.

Procedure 7-7

Posting Payments Using a Pegboard System

Equipment/Supplies: Pen, pegboard, calculator, day sheet, encounter forms, ledger cards, previous day's balance, list of patients and charges, fee schedule.

Steps

1. Place a new day sheet on the pegboard and record the totals from the previous day sheet.
2. Align the patient's ledger card with the first available line on the daysheet.
3. Place receipt to align with the appropriate line on the ledger card.
4. Record the number of the receipt in the appropriate column.
5. Write the patient's name on the receipt.
6. Record any existing balance the patient owes in the previous balance column of the daysheet.
7. Record the source and type of the payment in the description line (e.g., BlueCross/Blue Shield (BC/BS) check for date of service (DOS) 5/28/05).
8. Determine any discounts or adjustments and record in the adjustment column.
   a. Check the explanation of benefits (EOB) for any disallowed amounts from participating third-party payers. Record the difference in the charge and the allowed amount in the adjustment column.
   b. Record professional discounts, discounts for cash, etc. in the adjustment column.
9. Record the total payment in the payment column on the receipt, pressing down firmly so that the writing will transfer to the ledger card and the day sheet.
10. Subtract the payment and adjustments from the outstanding or previous balance, and record the current balance.
11. Return the patient's ledger card to its storage area.

Procedure 7-8

Processing a Credit Balance

Equipment/Supplies: Pen, pegboard, calculator, day sheet, ledger card.

Steps

1. Determine the reason for the credit balance.
2. Place brackets [ ] around the balance indicating that it is a negative number.
3. Write a refund check following the steps in Procedure 7-9: Processing a Refund.

Procedure 7-9

Processing a Refund

Equipment/Supplies: Pen, pegboard, calculator, day sheet, ledger card, checkbook, check register, word processor letterhead, envelope, postage,copy machine, patient's chart, refund file.

Steps

1. Determine who gets the refund, the patient or the insurance company.
2. Pull patient's ledger card and place on current day sheet aligned with the first available line.
3. Write the amount of the refund in the adjustment column [in brackets] indicating it is a debit, not a credit, adjustment.
4. Write "Refund to Patient" or "Refund to _______" (name of insurance company) in the description column.
5. Write a check for the credit amount made out to the appropriate party.
6. Record the amount and name of payee in the check register.
7. Mail the check with letter of explanation to the patient or insurance company.
8. Place a copy of the check and the letter in the patient's record or in the refund file.
9. Return the patient's ledger card to its storage area.

Procedure 7-10

Posting an NSF Check

Equipment/Supplies: Pen, pegboard, calculator, day sheet, ledger card.

Steps

1. Pull patient's ledger card and place on current day sheet aligned with the first available line.
2. Write the amount of the check in the payment column [in brackets] indicating it is a debit, not a credit, adjustment.
3. Write "Check Returned For Nonsufficient Funds" in the description column.
4. If your facility assesses a fee for returned checks, post that amount in the charge column.
5. Write "Bank Fee for Returned Check" in the description column.
6. Call the patient to advise them of the returned check and the fee.
7. Write a letter of explanation and mail it to the patient with a copy of the ledger card.
8. Place a copy of the letter and the check in the patient's file.
9. Make arrangements for the patient to pay in cash.
10. Flag the patient's account as a credit risk for future transactions.
11. Return the patient's ledger card to its storage area.

Procedure 7-11

Posting Collection Agency Payments

Equipment/Supplies: Pen, pegboard, calculator, day sheet, ledger card.

Steps

1. Review check stub or report from the collection agency explaining the amounts to be applied to the accounts.
2. Retrieve the account records by pulling the patients' ledger cards or pulling the patient's account up in the computer system.
3. Post the amount to be applied in the payment column for each patient.
4. Write off the amount representing the percentage of the payment charged by the collection agency.
5. Return the patients' ledger cards to the appropriate storage area.

SUMMARY

Whether a medical practice uses a manual bookkeeping system, such as the pegboard system, or a computer system, you may be responsible for keeping records of accounts payable, accounts receivable, and petty cash. You may also be responsible for banking functions, such as receiving checks, making deposits, and reconciling monthly bank statements. To carry out these responsibilities effectively, you must record all transactions accurately and promptly. Computers have made the daily bookkeeping practices much easier, but you must understand the principles of accounting applied in the manual system if you are to use the computer system. Using the appropriate banking services will allow the day-to-day financial operations to be efficient, accurate, and secure.

Critical Thinking Challenges

1. Your day sheet deposit slip and your posting proofs do not agree. How do you find the error?
2. An employee is prosecuted for stealing money for more than a year from her physician employer's funds. Investigation reveals that she was stealing any cash payments given to her. How could she do this for so long without being caught? What necessary monthly action would make this crime impossible?
3. Your office is considering going from a pegboard system to a computer bookkeeping system. What features should you look for in the software?

Answers to Checkpoint Questions

1. Five sections of a pegboard day sheet include the distribution columns, adjustment column, deposit slip, payments section, and posting proofs section.
2. Ledger cards provide an overall financial record of a patient; encounter forms provide documentation of today's financial activity.
3. Brackets indicate the opposite of the normal meaning of that column.
4. Generally, a credit adjustment reduces the patient's account balance, whereas a debit adjustment increases the patient's account balance.
5. Three types of checks offered by banks include cashier's checks, certified checks, and traveler's checks.
6. The statement consists of one or more pages that lists all checks written and their amounts, all deposits made and their amounts, any electronic transactions, and any service charges.
7. These are the six guidelines for managing petty cash:
   - Keep petty cash separate from patient cash payments.
   - Keep in a secure, locked area.
   - Designate one person to maintain the petty cash fund and issue vouchers.
   - Place a voucher with an attached receipt in the petty cash fund.
   - Replenish the petty cash fund once a month.
   - Remove and file all vouchers.

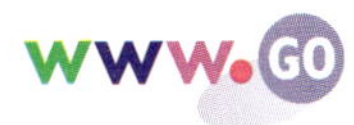

Websites

Superbill Forms and Creations
www.physicianshelp.com

Comptroller of Currency Administrator of National Banks
www.occ.treas.gov

Maximum Returned Check Fees allowed by state
www.checkagain.com/statefees.asp

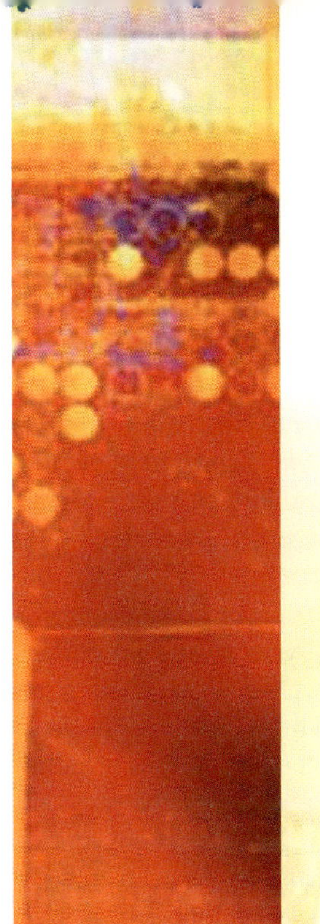

8

Accounts Payable and Payroll

CHAPTER OBJECTIVES

In this chapter, you'll learn:

1. To spell and define the key terms.
2. To describe the accounting cycle.
3. To describe the components of a record-keeping system.
4. To explain the process of ordering supplies and paying invoices.
5. To discuss the types of payroll records.
6. To explain which taxes are withheld from paychecks.

PERFORMANCE OBJECTIVES

In this chapter, you'll learn:

1. To issue a payroll check, using the pegboard system.
2. To calculate the amount of an employee's payroll check for a given pay period.

KEY TERMS

accounting cycle
audit
check register
check stub
FICA
federal unemployment tax
gross income
Internal Revenue Service (IRS)
invoice
liabilities
net pay
packing slip
payroll
payroll journal
profit-and-loss statement
purchase order
summation report
withholding

ACCOUNTING IS THE compilation of a business's financial records. It is necessary for assessment of the practice's financial history and current financial stakes, which serves as the basis for sound financial management. The medical office, like other businesses, requires strict adherence to sound record-keeping practices. Records must be maintained in an orderly fashion so you can retrieve financial information at any time and present an organized picture of the business's finances. A system of checks and balances is an integral part of record management. Generally, the check-and-balance status of accounts is examined monthly by comparing the total of all accounts with outstanding balances against the running total taken from the daily logs of all financial transactions. The practice's accountant will also closely scrutinize these records at scheduled intervals for tax-reporting purposes.

Although manual accounting systems are still used widely, computer accounting is available as part of most medical software packages, and the many advantages include efficient tracking and analysis of critical information, improved productivity, and smarter business decisions. General ledger, payables, receivables, inventory, purchasing, cash flow, bank reconciliation, collections, fixed assets, and many other applications integrate with each other so you can manage the office's core processes efficiently and effectively.

ACCOUNTING CYCLE

The finances of medical practices operate in one of two 12-month intervals or durations. The office **accounting cycle** follows either a fiscal year (a consecutive 12-month period starting with a specified date) or a calendar year (January through December). The yearly interval used depends on the way the practice's accountant has structured the business. For example, the medical practice can exist as a sole proprietorship or as a professional corporation.

The federal **Internal Revenue Service (IRS)** examines a business's income statements for the amount of profit and owed tax four times a year by quarterly estimated tax returns. The practice's annual tax return is a summary of the quarterly returns and reports the final year-end profit or loss (income minus expenses equals profit or loss) for the fiscal or calendar reporting period. If financial records are scrupulously maintained all year, preparation of the annual income tax return should merely be a summation of existing accounting facts. Well-maintained office records not only facilitate IRS returns but also provide data that define the practice's business picture.

There are many reasons for a physician along with an accountant to review financial data on a regular basis. Financial records reflect growing expenditures and growth in the business. Conclusions drawn from financial data can affect future financial decisions. For example, analysis of the practice's accounts receivable can predict the amount of salary increases. Tax records must be available in case of an IRS inquiry or **audit** (review of accounts). Records such as receipts should be retained for 7 years, but records such as bank statements, canceled checks, and IRS tax returns should be kept for the duration of the business.

RECORD-KEEPING COMPONENTS

The practice's financial records should include a running record of income, accounts receivable, and total expenditures, including **payroll** (employee salaries), cash on hand, and **liabilities** (amounts the practice owes). Expenditures can be broken down into categories (Box 8-1). This is important because it enables the record keeper to track the practice's expenses and provide the physician and accountant with a cohesive picture of the practice's expenses at tax time.

Categories can be accommodated by several types of bookkeeping systems; a simple business checkbook does not allow this. Pegboard systems allow the bookkeeper to write the check once over the **check register** (a place to record checks) or the ledger sheet and then have multiple pages with columns to distribute an expense into categories, including a back sheet for payroll. These columns are totaled and balanced at the completion of each check register sheet and can be subtotaled monthly, quarterly, and annually (discussed later in the chapter). Keeping a monthly accounts payable disbursement sheet lets the administrative medical assistant easily compare past years' expenses for the same part of the year.

Box 8-1

CATEGORIES OF EXPENDITURES

- Office supplies: items used by the facility's employees, such as paper, pencils, day sheets, ledger cards
- Medical supplies: items used for patients, such as examination gowns, electrocardiograph paper, syringes, tongue depressors
- Drugs: drug purchases, such as injectables; some facilities keep a separate column for these purchases and others put this amount in the medical supplies category
- Payroll: gross amount paid to employees
- Taxes: taxes paid, such as FICA, Medicare, federal withholding, state withholding, listed separately
- Rent: amount paid to rent the facility
- Utilities: gas, electric, telephone
- Maintenance: routine care of the facility, such as cleaning personnel
- Travel: physician's car lease payment, gas mileage if paid to employees, and so on
- Personal: any money used personally by the physician

Legal Tip

It is unethical and illegal to falsify any financial documents. Accurate record keeping is essential. The IRS will examine the practice's financial records. You may be held liable for errors or omissions to these documents. If you are not comfortable posting a payment, calculating payroll deductions, always ask your supervisor for clarification. If the employee's W-4 form is illegible, ask the person to complete a new form. W-4 forms should not have any eraser marks or cross-outs. If any do, obtain a new form from that employee.

Software packages offer the most sophisticated way to maintain financial records, not just for the categorization of expenses but also for the rapid formation of financial reports. Automating accounts payable does, however, require a personal computer (PC), software, and the training to use it.

There are advantages and disadvantages to both computer systems and paper records. Each practice should make this decision based on its particular volume and needs. Either system (pegboard or computer) can provide the practice and its accountant with the ability to pay and track expenses and to furnish the financial data necessary to create reports.

Multiple **summation reports**, such as the payroll report, itemized category report, account balances, and the **profit-and-loss statement**, must be prepared for the practice's accountant. If financial data are entered diligently into the bookkeeping system, preparing monthly, quarterly, or yearly reports should not be a daunting task. Income tax accounting cycles are divided into quarters: January through March, April through June, July through September, and October through December. Payroll reports show the amount of taxes being withheld and made monthly, quarterly, or annually. Normally, the practice's accountant will send you necessary reports and have you mail the checks.

ACCOUNTS PAYABLE

Ordering Goods and Services

There are many economical ways to purchase office supplies or equipment. For instance, purchasing cooperatives (co-ops) offer bulk rate discounts by allowing physicians to order in a pool with other purchasers. Vendors may offer discounts for buying in volume or for paying promptly. Large warehouse-type merchandisers and companies with discount catalogs also offer competitive prices. Researching and cost-comparing office products and medical supplies can be time consuming, but it is worth the effort, especially for items used frequently. Compare past invoices with prices in new catalogs.

Besides cost, other considerations come to bear when purchasing office supplies. For example, office supply companies often provide free delivery, but office warehouse chains may charge a fee or require a minimum order for free delivery. Quality also plays a role. Supplies should be of standard quality as well as economical. It is common to use several office supply vendors according to quality or pricing of specific goods.

Office supplies or equipment can be ordered in a number of ways. Once an account is set up, offices can place orders by telephone, fax, mail, or e-mail. These orders can be paid monthly by check or by credit card. It is preferable to pay for supplies by check or credit card rather than by cash, but when cash purchases are necessary, retain a detailed receipt for tax purposes. Credit card purchases can be made over the telephone or by mail, but for security reasons, credit card account numbers should not be faxed.

When placing orders for supplies, give the office's account number to the vendor or write it on the order form. It is a good idea to use a **purchase order** that lists the supplies ordered and their order numbers, so that order numbers for frequently ordered items can be pulled from the previous purchase order; this saves time with subsequent orders. Be sure to record the charges for your order and verify them against the bill later. It is also handy to keep a list of all vendors, telephone numbers, and account numbers.

Checkpoint Question

1. When purchasing office supplies, what factors besides price should you consider?

Receiving Supplies

When goods are delivered to the office, a receipt or **packing slip** listing the enclosed items should always accompany the order. The office staff member who receives the supplies must check the packing slip against the actual contents to ensure that all supplies are in the shipment. The person should initial the packing slip, which shows that all goods were received. When it is time to issue checks for payables, the assistant can then pay the **invoice** or bill. These receipts or packing slips should be placed in a bills pending file, so that they may be compared to the bill when it arrives. If the bill has already been paid by check or credit card, the invoice should be placed in the appropriate accounts paid file; there should be such a file for each fiscal or calendar year.

Paying Invoices

Invoices for supplies and other types of bills payable by the practice should be kept together in a bills pending file to avoid loss or misplacement of a bill. Bills can be paid daily, weekly, biweekly, or monthly.

Manual Payment

Manual payment of bills requires a checkbook and checks. The practice's accountant may recommend use of a log or record book into which is entered information about each check, such as payroll taxes or the breakdown of expenses for a monthly credit card bill. The large checks and checkbooks available from banks and business printers offer more space for writing memos or itemizing a check. Each check, once written, is detached from a **check stub**, which remains in the checkbook. If you make a mistake while writing a check, void the check and stub and staple the voided check to the stub. Never make corrections on the facility's checks. Check stubs should be filed with other fiscal or calendar year records and kept for the life of the practice.

The information recorded on the check stub includes the check number, the date the check was issued, the payee (the party to whom the check was written), and the full amount of the check. Notes should be written on both the memo section of the check and on the check stub. For example, when entering the purchase of a new beeper, the note might read, "payee: Office Communications" or "new beeper for Dr. Smith." The check is then attached to the bill or invoice and signed by an authorized individual.

Memos or notations on check stubs can be referenced later if a question arises concerning payment by a particular check. A log or record book enables the bookkeeper to make entries for each expense, categorize expenses, and maintain detailed payroll records. Unlike one-write (pegboard) or computer systems, multiple entries must be made by hand to track office bill paying. This can seem laborious when compared to other bookkeeping systems, but it may be ideal for smaller practices.

Pegboard Payment

The same pegboard system that is used for accounts receivable may be used for bill paying; it has several advantages over the ordinary manual method of paying bills. Instead of using a day sheet, a **check register** page is used to record the checks that have been written. The check is then aligned on the pegboard over the register page and is filled out as with any other check (Fig. 8-1). Pegboard checks have a carbon or transfer strip, and on this strip is written the date, the payee, the check number, and the amount. The information written on the strip is recorded automatically on the check register. These check-writing systems are referred to as one-write systems for this reason. The check can be addressed directly beneath the payee line and mailed in a window envelope, which saves the time it would take to address an envelope.

The pegboard check register has approximately 20 columns that can be used to categorize expenses, such as rent, insurance, office supplies, utilities, service contracts, postage, and any other applicable categories. All entries on the check register are totaled when the register is completed; these totals are carried forward to the new register page. Each fiscal or calendar year begins with a new first page (page 1), and the last check register page will have totals for the entire year. The check register provides a system of checks and balances even before the bank statement arrives because the check register must be balanced, as with a bank statement.

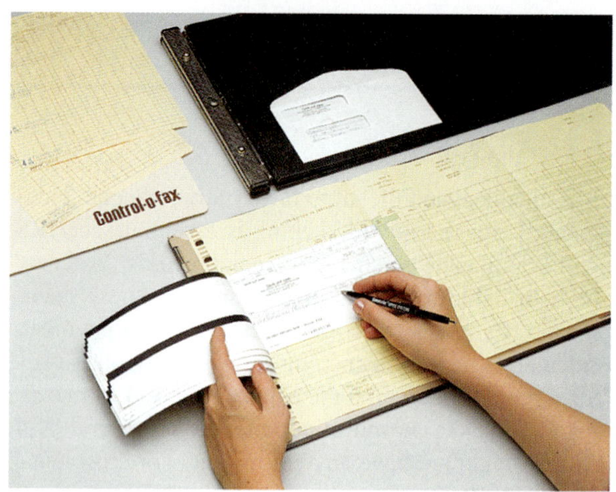

FIGURE 8-1. Sample pegboard check and check register. (Courtesy of Control-o-fax, Waterloo, IA.)

The check register also allows entries for bank deposits, and the back page of the register is used for payroll record keeping. As with pegboard accounts receivable, completed pegboard check registers are filed in a separate binder in chronological order, with the most recent register on top.

Computer Payment

A computer accounts payable system has all the advantages that a pegboard system offers: access at a glance to check registers, itemized categories and their totals, payroll records, and entries for bank deposits. To use such a system, you must have a PC, accounts payable program software, printer, and bank checks that are compatible with the software and printer. The initial expense with a computer system is much higher than that of manual or pegboard systems. Office personnel will need computer training to use the program. Also, since it runs on electricity, a computer may not work during power failures. A good computer accounting program will, however, provide functions for both accounts receivable and accounts payable. Financial data should be recorded in three forms: on the computer's hard drive, on a magnetic tape or floppy disk, and in printout form (hard copy).

Although entering data in the computer at first may be time consuming, this becomes less of a concern with practice. Furthermore, financial reports can be compiled and printed in a fraction of the time required with manual or pegboard systems. The computer program can also perform the record-keeping arithmetic; as a result, mathematical errors are practically nonexistent.

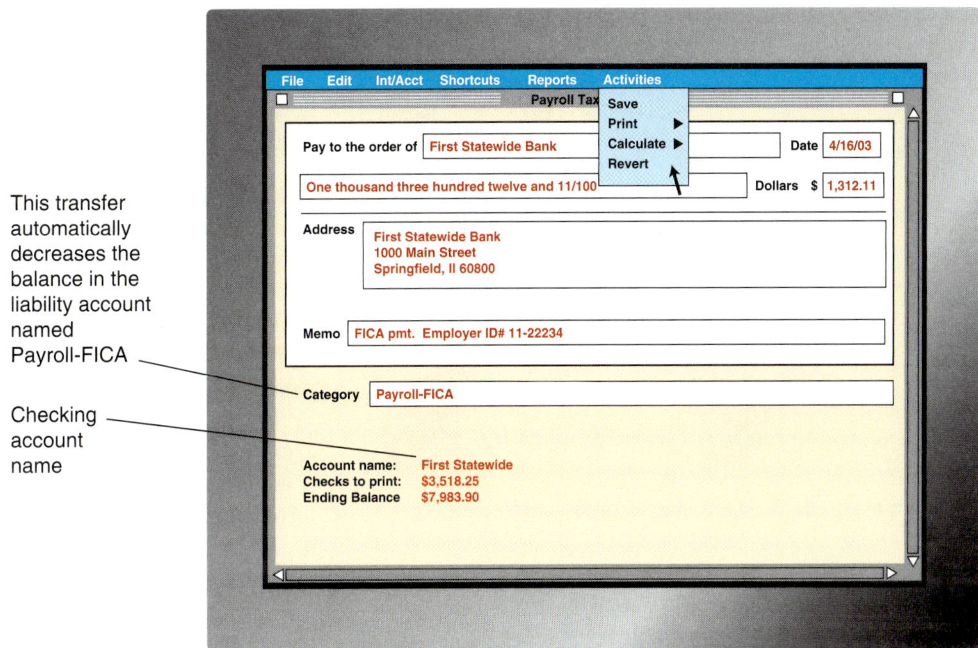

FIGURE 8-2. Computer screen showing a check for payroll taxes.

Paying bills by computer requires using the software to open the check-writing file. Checks are presented on the computer screen in the same way that a paper check would normally appear (Fig. 8-2), and the information that is required to appear on the check is entered on the computer keyboard. The information is stored and the check is printed out; the computer program automatically subtracts the amount of the check from the account's balance. The bookkeeper can print one check at a time or a batch of checks together.

The computer can "memorize" checks so that the information on them can be recalled and reprinted without reentering it; this is especially helpful with payroll checks. A good accounting program also allows for bill reminders and disk or magnetic tape backup reminders. Of course, it is essential to back up financial data on magnetic tapes or floppy disks in case of computer problems.

Checkpoint Question

2. Whether using a manual, pegboard, or computer accounts payable system, two steps must always occur when ordering and receiving supplies. What are they?

PAYROLL

Types of Payroll Systems

The medical office will have payroll obligations to its staff, and federal, state, and, possibly, local payroll taxes will be due. The administrative medical assistant may issue payroll checks for the practice's entire staff, including the physician, or just for the office staff. Or an outside payroll service may be retained to issue the checks and keep the records. These payroll services specialize in computing, withholding, and paying taxes and payroll for businesses. Such a firm can provide all of these services for considerably less than it would cost for office time and personnel or for an accountant. The larger the practice's staff, the more economical a payroll service becomes. Firms that provide payroll services are especially cost effective, in that they are highly accurate, aware of changes in tax laws, and legally liable.

Generally, payroll checks for the medical office will be issued at one of the following intervals:

- Weekly (52 pay periods per year)
- Biweekly (26 pay periods per year)
- Monthly (12 pay periods per year)

The pay period is set up by your employer and is the same for all employees.

There are various ways to record payroll expenditures, depending on what type of bookkeeping system is used by the office.

Manual Payroll Systems

When payroll checks are issued manually without a pegboard system, separate payroll records must be kept. The check stub will indicate to whom the check was issued, in what amount, and on what date. A separate record or log book must be maintained to keep track of gross income and tax withholdings for each employee. These withholdings should be totaled monthly, quarterly, and annually; for this reason, it is advisable to maintain payroll records in a timely manner throughout the year.

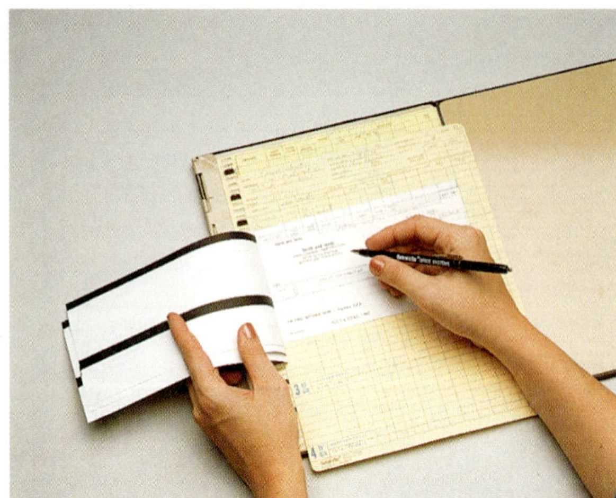

FIGURE 8-3. Sample pegboard payroll journal. (Courtesy of Control-o-fax, Waterloo, IA.)

Pegboard Payroll Systems

The pegboard system allows for payroll entries as well as the accumulation of payroll data by using an employee payroll record form and the correlating back page of each check register, called the **payroll journal** (Fig. 8-3). Procedure 8-1 outlines the steps in issuing a payroll check using the pegboard system.

Computer Payroll Systems

Payroll records can be maintained with various software packages; many such packages integrate payroll with other accounting functions, such as accounts receivable and accounts payable. Computer programs can calculate tax withholdings automatically, record payroll data, and print payroll checks. In most cases, a computer program provides substantial time savings over manual and pegboard payroll systems.

Employee Records

Regardless of the payroll system used, it is necessary to maintain an individual file for each employee that contains pertinent employment information. The personnel file should include the following information:

- Employee's original résumé or completed job application
- Job references
- Hourly rate or salary at the time of hire
- Dates and amounts of pay raises
- Job evaluations
- All employee withholding authorization forms, such as W-4 forms (discussed later)
- Pension plan, health, and life insurance paperwork
- Vital facts about the employee (e.g., date of birth, name of spouse, Social Security number, address and telephone number, name and daytime phone number of emergency contact person)

Tax Withholdings

Federal, state, and, possibly, local taxes must be withheld from employees' paychecks; for this reason, each employee must complete a W-4 form on the first day of hire. This form must be completed by the employee before the first pay period; otherwise, you are required to withhold taxes at the highest rate, which classifies the person as single with no dependents. The W-4 form lists the employee's name, Social Security number, address, marital status, and the number of exemptions to be used in the calculation of tax withholding. If any of the information contained on an employee's W-4 form changes, the employee must fill out a new form, which is placed in the personnel file.

The federally mandated taxes are Social Security (**FICA**), Medicare, and federal income tax. Each of these taxes is based on a percentage of total gross income; the federal income tax also factors in marital status and the number of withholding exemptions claimed on the W-4 form.

Box 8-2 features the information needed to calculate employee withholding manually by using the combination method found on the IRS website. Procedure 8-2 outlines the steps for calculating the amount of an employee's paycheck.

The employer must match the amount withheld from each employee's paycheck for Social Security and Medicare taxes. For example, if $150 is withheld from an employee's paycheck for Medicare and Social Security taxes, the employer must pay $300 to the IRS ($150 withheld from the employee plus $150 matching amount). The employer does not match federal, state, or local taxes. The practice's accountant should inform the office bookkeeper of tax rates and withholdings. Usually, each pay period or at least monthly you will deposit the federal taxes withheld from all employees plus doubled FICA in an account at a federal depository (normally the facility's bank). Your accountant normally will send you the estimated federal depository slips for this purpose.

The employer must also pay a **federal unemployment tax** (FUTA) for each employee based on that employee's gross income. The amount of this tax is calculated by the practice's accountant and paid either quarterly or annually. Individual states may levy their own unemployment tax. The practice's accountant calculates this tax.

Other withholdings from an employee's paycheck might include health, life, or disability premiums; pension plan contributions; or court-ordered garnishment of wages owed to a third party.

Checkpoint Question

3. What taxes must be withheld from an employee's paycheck?

Box 8-2

CALCULATING PAYROLL WITHHOLDING USING THE COMBINATION METHOD

Combined Income Tax, Employee Social Security Tax, and Employee Medicare Tax Withholding Tables

If you want to combine amounts to be withheld as income tax, employee Social Security tax, and employee Medicare tax, you may use the combined tables found in the IRS publications for businesses. Combined withholding tables for single and married taxpayers are provided for weekly, biweekly, semimonthly, monthly, and daily or miscellaneous payroll periods. The payroll period and marital status of the employee determine the table to be used.

If the wages are greater than the highest wage bracket in the applicable table, you must use one of the other methods for figuring income tax withholding described in the publication or in circular E. For wages that do not exceed $84,900, the combined Social Security tax rate and Medicare tax rate is 7.65% each for the employee and the employer for wages paid in 2002. You can figure the employee Social Security tax by multiplying the wages by 6.2%, and you can figure the employee Medicare tax by multiplying the wages by 1.45%.

The combined tables give the correct total withholding only if wages for Social Security and Medicare taxes and income tax withholding are the same. When you have paid more than the maximum amount of wages subject to Social Security tax ($84,900 in 2003) in a calendar year, you may not use the combined tables.

If you use the combined withholding tables, use the following steps to find the amounts to report on your form 941, employer's quarterly federal tax return:

1. Employee Social Security tax withheld: Multiply the wages by 6.2%.
2. Employee Medicare tax withheld: Multiply the wages by 1.45%.
3. Income tax withheld: Subtract the amounts from steps 1 and 2 from the total tax withheld.
4. You can figure the amounts to be shown on form W-2, wage and tax statement, in the same way.

Courtesy of the IRS website.

Payment of Taxes

Payroll taxes are paid according to different schedules as determined by the IRS and the state and local tax authorities. Federal taxes, such as Social Security, Medicare, and federal income tax, must be paid monthly, bimonthly, or more frequently, depending on the size of the gross payroll. Always remember to match the Medicare and Social Security payments withheld from the employee's check (the amount withheld × 2). These payments are made on IRS form 941 for deposit requirements; the IRS furnishes these forms free of charge.

If the total federal taxes due are more than $3000, these payroll taxes must be paid within 3 calendar days of the time the payroll check was issued. State taxes that are withheld from the employee's pay check are usually paid by mail and must be paid and mailed before the tax due date to avoid penalties.

The IRS also requires the employer to file quarterly returns for all federal taxes withheld; these returns are due by April 30, July 31, October 31, and January 31 each year. This quarterly return is a summary of the Social Security, Medicare, and federal wage taxes paid. State quarterly returns have the same due dates and are usually paid by mail. Your accountant will keep you informed of taxes due.

W-2 Forms

At the end of the calendar year, all pertinent payroll information should be summarized for each employee and made available to the practice's accountant. The W-2 statement provided to the employee by January 31 of each year should list the following information:

- Total gross income for the previous year
- Total federal, state, and local taxes withheld
- Any taxable fringe benefits
- The employee's total net income

Checkpoint Question

4. What information does the employee list on the W-4 form? What happens if this information changes?

PREPARATION OF REPORTS

The bookkeeper must also prepare reports for the practice's accountant or the IRS, based on financial data stored in the office's bookkeeping system. For this reason, care should always be taken when recording financial data.

WHAT IF

The medical practice where you work did not pay its payroll taxes. What can happen?

The IRS charges penalties and interest on all unpaid taxes. The IRS can attach the business and its assets and close the business.

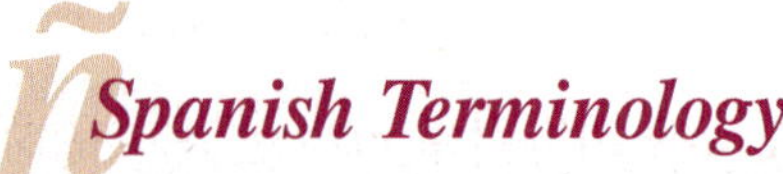

Spanish Terminology

Los impuestos deben ser sacados de su cheque.	Taxes must be taken out of your paycheck.
Usted necesita completar estas formas.	You need to complete these forms.
Gracias para su pago.	Thank you for your payment.
Gracias para su cheque.	Thank you for your check.
Esto es su recibo.	This is your receipt.

The manual system, when assisted by the use of a log or record book, should be able to provide monthly, quarterly, and annual summaries for income, expenditures, and payroll. It is advisable to have subtotals and totals for these periods for tax payment purposes.

The pegboard system is also practical for providing summaries of income, expenses, and payroll and can be totaled monthly, quarterly, and yearly. Each day sheet, check register, and payroll journal is individually totaled, with all balances forwarded to the next page. These records are stored in binders and kept for future reference.

A computer system of accounting offers all of the previously mentioned reports along with other more complicated reports that generally require more advanced accounting skills. The great advantage with report generating by computer is that the computer will perform all of the mathematical calculations for the time frame requested.

ASSISTING WITH AUDITS

An **audit** may be informal (in-house) and used to assist the practice's accountant with tax preparation, or it may be formal audits by the IRS. If meticulous attention to record keeping has been paid throughout the year, the preparation time needed for such an audit should be minimal. It is important to save all bank statements, copies of annual and quarterly tax returns, and receipts for expenditures. Canceled checks and payroll records should be readily available.

Manual and pegboard systems can provide spending category and payroll summaries in addition to examination of the actual entries for the period being audited. A computer accounting system can provide all of this plus reports such as profit-and-loss statements, which normally would be compiled by an accountant.

Procedure 8-1

Issuing a Payroll Check Using the Pegboard System

Equipment/Supplies

- Pegboard with checks
- Carbon paper
- Payroll register
- Tax tables
- Calculator
- Time card

Steps	Reason
1. Align the carbon or transfer strip at the top of the check on the employee's payroll record, then align both on the payroll journal.	The write-it-once system will eliminate the need to post information more than one time.
2. Enter the employee's name first, followed by the check number, the payroll period, and the **gross income** (the amount of money an employee earned before taxes are withheld) plus any additional earnings.	The employee's name must be entered to issue a payroll check. The pay period indicates to the employee the time frame of the checks.
3. From the gross income, subtract federal, state, and local taxes and Social Security; this is called tax **withholding**. See Procedure 8-2.	Witholdings must be subtracted from gross income to issue a payroll check.
4. Enter the **net pay** (amount of money an employee is paid after taxes are withheld) on the detachable payroll slip. Fold this slip behind the check.	When the check is placed in the envelope, this information will not be visible, which will protect the employee's privacy.
5. Total the payroll journal as each page is completed.	Total amounts of income and tax withholdings should be accrued for each quarter for tax-reporting purposes.

Procedure 8-2

Calculate the Amount of an Employee's Payroll Check

Equipment/Supplies

- Calculator
- W-4 form

Steps	Reason
1. Calculate the number of hours worked from the employee's time card or record.	The employee's payroll check is based on the number of hours worked.
2. Calculate the employee's annual gross wage using this formula: Hourly wage × number of hours worked per week × 52 (number of weeks in a year) = gross annual wage Assume an employee earns \$7 per hour and works 40 hours per week: \$7 × 40 × 52 = \$14,560 annual gross wage	The annual gross wage must be calculated to determine the employee's payroll check amount.
3. If your pay period is • Biweekly, then ÷ this sum by 26 • Monthly, then ÷ this sum by 12 • Weekly, then ÷ this sum by 52	This converts the gross wage into paycheck amounts.
4. Divide by 52 weeks in a year and then divide by 5 (work days in a week) to get the amount of a day's pay.	Always go to the yearly gross wage when figuring deductions or increases to gross wages; you will get the exact amount.
5. Deduct this amount from the gross wage to get the adjusted gross wage from which you will withhold taxes. Using the example above, the calculation would be as follows: (\$14,560 ÷ 52) = \$280 = week's pay \$280 ÷ 5 = \$56 = day's pay \$280 − \$56 = \$224 (adjusted gross wage)	The adjusted gross wage is needed to calculate withholding taxes.
6. Calculate any overtime worked.	Overtime is defined as hours worked over the normal for the pay period. Overtime is calculated by paying 1.5 times the normal hourly wage. If the employee earns \$7 per hour, overtime pay would be calculated by dividing \$7 in half (\$3.50) and adding that amount to the hourly wage: the hourly pay rate for overtime would be \$10.50.
7. Refer to the appropriate tax tables (e.g., federal, FICA, Medicare, state taxes) for the deductions for taxes.	The tax tables will specify the amount of withholdings.
8. Subtract the taxes from the gross or adjusted gross wages to obtain net pay.	The net pay amount is the result of the gross wages minus the withholdings
9. Write the payroll check for this amount.	The net pay is the amount of the payroll check.

SUMMARY

Accounting is a complex process involving many legal issues. As a medical assistant, you must keep neat and well-organized accounting records. You also will be expected to understand how to order goods and services efficiently and economically and how to pay invoices. In addition, you must understand the payroll process. With the computer being used for many administrative medical office functions, it is imperative that you keep abreast of changes and new opportunities to make this process more efficient and up-to-date.

Critical Thinking Challenges

1. Explain the advantages of manual, pegboard, and computer accounting systems. In what instances would each be the preferred method?
2. A vendor continually mixes up your orders, and the physician asks you to look for a new vendor. How do you decide which one to recommend? What factors influence your choice of one office supply vendor over another?
3. An employee gets divorced. She is irate when she gets her W-2 form and discovers that her deductions were still being based on her married filing status. What is your response? What should you do now?
4. The physician asks you, the office manager, how much money is owed to him. How do you gather the information needed to answer his question?

Answers to Checkpoint Questions

1. Besides cost, consider delivery charges and product quality when purchasing office supplies.
2. The bookkeeper must write out a purchase order and compare the packing slip and final invoice to the purchase order.
3. Social Security, Medicare, and federal, state, and local wage taxes must be withheld from an employee's paycheck.
4. The employee provides his or her name, Social Security number, marital status, current address, and number of withholding exemptions. If any of this information changes, the employee must complete a new W-4 form.

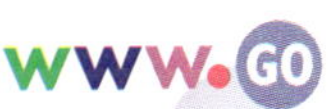

Websites

The Accounting Library (TAL)
www.accountinglibrary.com

Quickbooks Online
www.quickbooks.com

Microsoft Business Solutions
www.microsoft.com/businesssolutions

Internal Revenue Services
www.irs.gov

Payroll Taxes
www.payroll.com

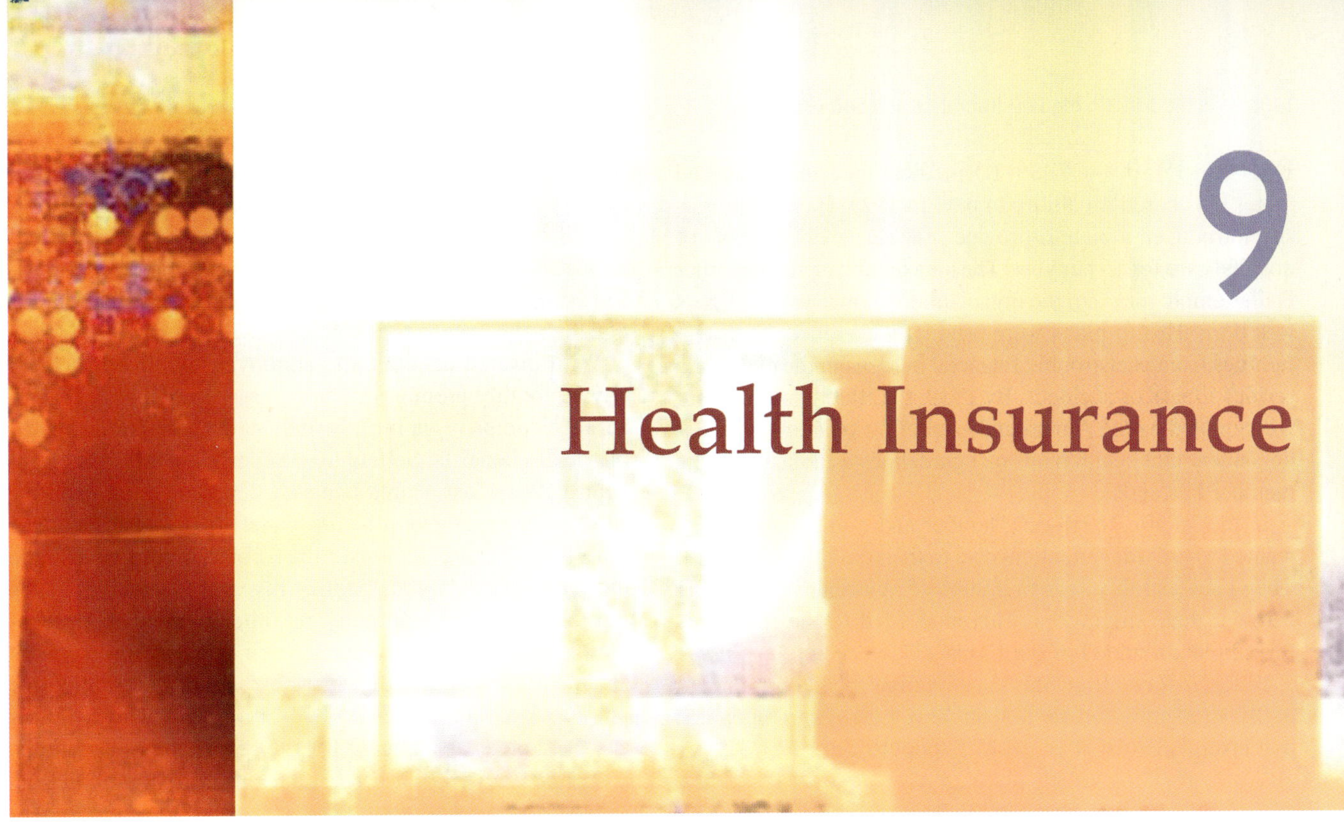

9 Health Insurance

CHAPTER OBJECTIVES

In this chapter, you'll learn:

1. To spell and define the key terms.
2. To describe group, individual, and government-sponsored (public) health benefits and explain the differences between them.
3. To explain the differences between Medicare and Medicaid.
4. To list the information required on a medical claim form and explain why each piece of information is needed.
5. To name two legal issues affecting claims submissions.
6. To explain how managed care programs work.
7. To explain the differences between health maintenance organizations, preferred provider organizations, and physician hospital organizations.

PERFORMANCE OBJECTIVES

In this chapter, you'll learn:

1. To fill out a CMS-1500 claim form.

KEY TERMS

assignment of benefits
balance billing
birthday rule
capitation
carrier
claims
claims administrator
coinsurance
coordination of benefits
co-payments
crossover claim
deductible
dependent
eligibility
employee
explanation of benefits (EOB)
fee-for-service
fee schedule
group member
health maintenance organization (HMO)
independent practice association (IPA)
insurance
insured
managed care
Medicare
peer review organization
physician hospital organization
plan maximum
preexisting condition
preferred provider organization (PPO)
third-party administrator
unbundling
usual, customary, and reasonable (UCR)
utilization review

BEFORE 1930, ACCESS TO medical care in the United States was based on ability to pay. In 1929, Baylor University introduced a plan to provide schoolteachers 21 days of hospital care for $6 per year. The idea quickly spread to other Dallas employers, and the organization known as Blue Cross was born. Health plans were originally designed to protect families from catastrophic financial burdens in the event of a serious illness or accident. By 1939, the Blue Cross symbol was adopted by the American Hospital Association as an endorsement that health plans met guidelines established by its member hospitals.

In the Pacific Northwest, lumber and mining companies wanted to provide outpatient care to their employees as well. They paid monthly fees to groups of physicians to provide care for their employees. This model led to the first Blue Shield plan, founded in California.

Blue Cross and Blue Shield as we know them today are actually a federation of more than 42 independent companies that insure about 30% of the U. S. population.

While the **insurance** industry was developing in the United States, other countries took a different approach to providing health care to their residents. Canada, for example, established publicly funded universal health insurance. This type of coverage provides hospital and physician services with no deductibles, **co-payments**, or dollar limits on coverage for insured services and is funded by tax revenues.

In the United States, health insurance is funded by a combination of employer and employee contributions and tax-funded coverage.

Today, virtually every state has a Blue Cross and a Blue Shield plan. Health benefits also are provided by insurance companies, self-funded group plans, and government plans such as Medicare and Medicaid. The benefits vary with each plan and from state to state. Approximately 80% of Americans are enrolled in health benefits plans of one sort or another. Consequently, most of the patients you will encounter in the physician's office have some type of health insurance. As a medical assistant, you will need to understand the differences in health benefits plans and the requirements of each so that you can complete and file claim forms appropriately. You will also need to learn the special terminology associated with health insurance claims. In addition, you may need to instruct patients about insurance matters.

HEALTH BENEFITS PLANS

Group Health Benefits

Group health benefits are sponsored by an organization, such as an employer, a union, or an association. A person covered by group health benefits is either an **employee** or a **group member**, who by virtue of employment or membership in an organization may participate in and receive benefits from a health plan. Coverage in health plans differs greatly, so you need to know the **eligibility** of the patient for services being provided by your office. For example, birth control is frequently not covered unless there is medical necessity.

Benefits may be either **insured** or self-funded. Commonly, health benefits are referred to as insurance. It is, however, important to distinguish between the actual benefits and the vehicle used to fund and provide them.

With insured benefits, the employer, employee, or both pay a monthly premium to an insurance company. The insurance company, in turn, is obligated to pay for any eligible health benefits. Self-funded benefits on the surface appear the same as insured benefits. They are paid for in the same manner as group health benefits, but instead of the employer paying the insurance company to invest the money to cover payments, they invest it themselves. They pay an insurance company or other agency to process **claims** and make payments on their behalf. Any payment for medical services that are not paid by the patient or physician is said to be paid by a *third-party payer*. In this case, the payer is an agent for the self-funded plan and is, therefore, known as a **third-party administrator** (TPA). Many employers now choose to self-fund their group benefit plans rather than insure them.

You will need to be aware of these funding differences as they relate to state and federal regulations. For instance, insured benefit plans are subject to state regulations. Many states mandate that certain types of benefits be included in any insurance plan. These mandated benefits vary from state to state but often include such medical services as childhood immunizations, routine diagnostic care, and treatment for substance abuse.

Although it would seem that these are routine medical services, many insurance companies consider them outside the scope of treating physical illness. Screening for illness, psychiatric illness, and prevention of illness by immunization are not routinely covered.

For a group benefit plan to cover (pay for) eligible expenses, the patient must meet several criteria, called eligibility requirements. These are defined in the policy or plan document and may include a minimum number of hours worked per week and a waiting period from the date of employment before benefits become effective.

The eligibility of a **dependent** (spouse, children) is based on the employee's eligibility. Certain eligibility limitations apply to dependent children. For example, children are usually eligible until they reach the limiting age defined by the plan. The age limitation is usually extended if the child is a full-time student. Eligibility usually requires that children be the unmarried natural or adopted children of the employee, unmarried stepchildren, or children for whom the employee has legal guardianship.

To confirm a patient's eligibility, call the **claims administrator** for the health benefits plan. A provider inquiry telephone number is commonly included on the patient's identification (ID) card (Fig. 9-1).

Group and individual health benefits describe contractual agreements and how the policies are paid. Both group and

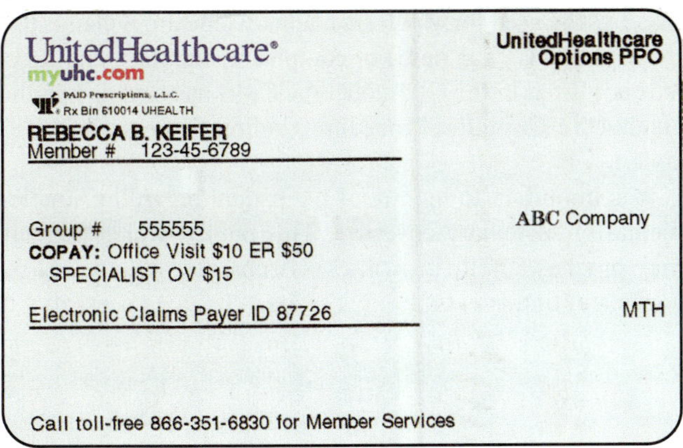

This card does not prove membership nor guarantee coverage.
For verification of benefits, please call Member Services.

IMPORTANT MEMBER INFORMATION
For authorization of health care services specific to your plan, you must call the number on the front of this card prior to the service to receive the highest level of benefits (see your benefit description for details). In emergencies, call Member Services within 48 hours.

Claim Address: PO BOX 740800, Atlanta, GA 30374-0800

United HealthCare Insurance Company Issued:01/04/03

FIGURE 9-1. Sample identification card for a managed care plan.

individual policies can be many different types of plans, such as traditional, HMO, and PPO. These types are further discussed later in this chapter.

Checkpoint Question

1. What is the difference between an insured benefits plan and one that is self-funded?

Individual Health Benefits

Individual health benefits policies are purchased by an individual from an insurance company. The individual pays premiums directly to the insurance company, and the insurance company pays either the doctor or the hospital directly if they are a participating provider or reimburses the individual for eligible medical expenses.

For patients with individual health benefits, the criteria for completing and filing claims are the same as for patients with group health benefits. Individual health policies commonly have less generous coverage, however, than group health plans have. An individual policy may also have a rider that limits or eliminates benefits for certain illnesses or injuries, based on the determination of the underwriter at the time the policy was issued. Box 9-1 outlines the requirements of the Health Insurance Portability and Accountability Act of 1996 (HIPAA), which include a provision to protect employees changing jobs from being denied benefits for preexisting conditions.

With the cost of health care skyrocketing and more insurance companies limiting what they will cover, many people have more than one health care insurance policy. It is extremely important that you know which insurance you bill first (primary) and which to bill the remainder of the charges (secondary).

Government-Sponsored (Public) Health Benefits

Government-sponsored benefit programs are funded and regulated by the federal government or individual states. Government programs have been developed over the years to assist persons who do not otherwise have health benefits, such as the elderly, the indigent, and others unable to obtain benefits. Government programs include Medicare, Medicaid, TRICARE/CHAMPVA, and workers' compensation.

Box 9-1

REQUIREMENTS OF HIPAA

As discussed in earlier chapters, the Health Insurance Portability and Accountability Act of 1996 brought about changes in the health care industry that protect patients and health care providers. According to the HIPAA website, www.cms.gov/hipaa, the following provisions are now in effect:

- HIPAA contains provisions for insured persons enrolled in employer-sponsored insurance programs without regard to their health status if they change employment.
- HIPAA prohibits the use of genetic testing information to deny health insurance coverage.
- HIPAA provides tax incentives for the purchase of long-term care insurance.
- HIPAA requires the adoption of new standards for financial and administrative electronic transmission of claims, new standards for claims attachments, and standardization of diagnostic and procedure coding.
- HIPAA strengthens existing regulations for fraud and abuse in the system.
- HIPAA Administrative Simplification: These HIPAA requirements, which are separate from the insurance portability requirements, are intended to reduce the costs and administrative burdens of health care by making possible the standardized electronic transmission of many administrative and financial transactions.
- HIPAA adds guidelines for confidentiality issues in electronic medical records.

Medicare

In 1965, the Social Security Act established **Medicare** to provide health insurance for the elderly. Elderly persons were defined as Social Security recipients age 65 or older. In 1972, amendments to the Social Security Act expanded Medicare coverage to two additional high-risk groups: disabled persons who have been receiving Social Security benefits for 24 months and persons suffering from end-stage renal disease.

Medicare Part A covers hospital expenses and is provided at no additional charge to persons eligible for Social Security benefits. Medicare Part B pays for physician fees, both inpatient and outpatient, diagnostic testing, certain immunizations (influenza and pneumonia), and specific screening tests (PSA, mammograms, Pap smears, bone density testing, colorectal screening). Part B Medicare is optional, and the participant is charged a monthly fee. The fee is deducted from the monthly Social Security payment.

Persons signing up for or receiving Social Security benefits are automatically enrolled in both Part A and Part B Medicare when they reach 65. If they do not wish to participate in Part B, they must decline it. Both Part A and Part B of Medicare have deductibles and co-payments, and as with most health insurance policies, these generally increase yearly.

A patient with Medicare coverage who is actively employed and covered by the employer's plan will have secondary Medicare benefits. A retired person age 65 or over who has health insurance in addition to Medicare will have primary Medicare benefits. Physicians are required to submit claims to Medicare on behalf of Medicare patients. These claims must be filed within 1 year of the time the service is incurred. (See section on filing claims for more information.)

After the **deductible** has been met, Medicare Part B reimburses the physician 80% of the Medicare-approved charges. The patient is responsible for the remaining 20% of the Medicare-approved fee. Under certain circumstances, if paying the 20% causes undue financial hardship, the physician may not charge the remaining 20%. The Centers for Medicare & Medicaid Services (CMS) can provide forms with the requirements, and the forms should always be used. In addition to Medicare, the Social Security Act of 1965 established Medicaid, a program of health care coverage for the poor. If patients are financially unable to pay the 20%, they may be eligible for Medicaid. This is referred to as a **crossover claim** because the patient is eligible under both Medicare and Medicaid and the claim crosses over automatically from one coverage to the other. In this situation, Medicare is primary and Medicaid is secondary. Medicare will accept original claims (no copies) filed on CMS-1500 universal claim forms only.

The CMS, which was known as the Health Care Financing Administration (HCFA) prior to July 1, 2001, is a government agency that oversees the financial aspects of health care in the United States (Box 9-2). The CMS has adopted a revised Current Procedural Terminology (CPT) coding system that must be used for Medicare claims. Medicare B claims use the standard CPT codes. For equipment, supplies, and services not listed in the CPT code, the CMS has established the Healthcare Common Procedure Coding System (HCPCS) codes.

It is important to inquire of the patient regarding supplemental or secondary coverage. This policy, which patients may purchase on their own, covers charges not covered by Medicare. In this case, filing a second claim is necessary.

Checkpoint Question

2. What is the difference between parts A and B of Medicare coverage?

Medicaid

Medicaid provides health benefits to low-income or indigent persons of all ages. Often, eligibility for Medicaid is based on a patient's eligibility for other state programs, such as welfare assistance. The federal government provides funds to each state for Medicaid costs; each state is required to provide a Medicaid program. Although the federal government

Box 9-2

WHAT IS THE CMS?

In 1977, the administration of the Medicare and Medicaid programs were combined under a single administrative agency. The administrator is appointed by the president of the United States and reports directly to the Secretary of Health and Human Services. Formerly known as HCFA, the CMS has become a big influence in the health care industry.

According to its website, **www.cms.gov**, the CMS is the federal agency that administers Medicare, Medicaid, and the State Children's Health Insurance Program (SCHIP). It provides health insurance for more than 74 million Americans. It also performs quality-focused activities, including regulation of laboratory testing, development of coverage policies, and quality-of-care improvement. The CMS maintains oversight of the survey and certification of nursing homes and continuing care providers, including home health agencies and intermediate-care facilities for the mentally retarded. It makes available to beneficiaries, providers, researchers, and state surveyors information about these activities and nursing home quality.

To ensure public and expert involvement in running their programs, the HCFA maintains a number of chartered advisory committees. These committees, whose meetings are open to the pubic, provide advice or make recommendations on a variety of issues relating to HCFA's responsibilities and activities.

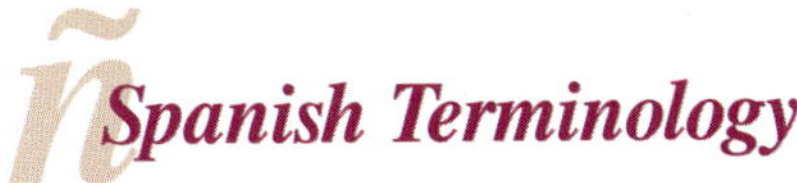

Spanish Terminology

¿Tiene usted seguro médico?	*Do you have medical insurance?*
¿Qué es el nombre del seguro?	*What is the name of the insurance?*
¿Qué es el número de su póliza?	*What is the number of your policy?*
¿Va a pagar el hospital?	*Will it pay for the hospital?*
¿Tiene Medicare?	*Do you have Medicare?*
¿Tiene su tarjeta de Medicare?	*Do you have your Medicare card?*

stipulates the minimum health care coverage, states can provide coverage beyond the minimum. Therefore, Medicaid eligibility and benefits vary from state to state. At a minimum, Medicaid provides 100% coverage for the following:

- Inpatient hospital care
- Outpatient treatment and services
- Diagnostic services
- Family planning
- Skilled nursing facilities
- Diagnostic screenings for children

Many states have gone to a managed care type of Medicaid coverage in which recipients make a co-payment based on their income and are assigned a primary care physician as a gatekeeper.

Since circumstances that make recipients eligible for coverage change from month to month (i.e., employment), Medicaid patients receive a new ID card each month. Make a photocopy of the card for the patient's file on the first visit of each month. Most states require prior authorization by the Medicaid **carrier** before any services are rendered. Because reimbursement is considerably less than other insurances, not all physicians accept Medicaid patients, nor are they required to do so. If Medicaid patients are accepted, you need to be familiar with Medicaid as administered in your state.

Checkpoint Question

3. How often do Medicaid recipients receive a new card?

TRICARE/CHAMPVA

TRICARE, the new name for CHAMPUS, is administered by the U. S. Department of Defense and provides medical coverage for dependents of active service personnel, dependents of service personnel who died during active duty, and retired service personnel. When Congress realized that CHAMPUS costs could be controlled with managed care, they mandated that HMOs and PPOs (discussed later in this chapter) be added to the coverage. This three-part system is now called TRICARE. This system requires that participants be assigned a primary care manager (PCM). The PCM is named on the beneficiary's card.

If a patient lives within 40 miles of a uniformed services hospital and that facility is unable to handle the needs of patients covered by TRICARE, a statement of unavailability is required for treatment by a physician's office or civilian hospital. Patients who live more than 40 miles from a uniformed services hospital do not need this statement to be treated in a physician's office or civilian hospital and for the physician or hospital to be reimbursed.

The Civilian Health and Medical Program of the Veterans Administration (CHAMPVA) covers dependents of veterans who have total and permanent service-connected disabilities. CHAMPVA is administered by the area Veterans Administration hospital. Once admitted to the CHAMPVA program, patients select their own physician; this allows them the same benefits as private insurance.

MANAGED CARE

Over the past 3 decades, health care costs in the United States have grown at about twice the general rate of inflation. As a result, the United States now spends more for health care services than any other industrialized nation, both as a percentage of gross national product and per person. At the same time, a smaller percentage of our population has health insurance coverage than in other advanced nations.

In the United States, most people obtain health coverage through their employer. The exceptions are Medicare for the

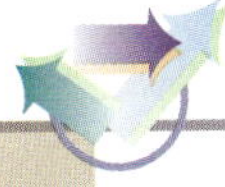

ETHICAL TIP

All patients must be treated equally and fairly. Financial issues regarding the patient's type of insurance or lack of insurance should have no bearing on the care provided. As a medical assistant, you must avoid stereotyping and care for the patient in an objective, professional manner.

elderly, TRICARE for the retired military and their dependents, Medicaid for low-income Americans, and those who do not have access to group coverage and buy coverage directly from insurers. In total, these programs cover fewer people than employment-based health plans.

The rapid rate of health care inflation has encouraged employers to begin offering **managed care** programs, which are typically less costly than traditional insurance coverage systems. Managed care programs vary greatly, but all involve a different relationship between the insurer, health care provider, and covered individual from that of traditional insurance programs. To understand this difference, we first discuss the traditional insurance system.

In traditional insurance systems, the covered patient may seek care from any provider. Normally, the patient and physician decide what care is needed. Then, services are rendered and the insurer pays a portion of the provider's bills (after deductibles and coinsurance). The insurer has no relationship with the provider.

In managed care systems, however, the insurer has a contractual relationship with the provider. The contract usually establishes what prices will be charged for each service and the conditions under which a service would be covered. Most managed care programs contain the following elements:

- *Precertification of hospital admissions* (often also called utilization management [UM] or utilization review [UR]). A patient can be admitted to a hospital for certain conditions only if that admission has been certified (approved) by the insurer. The goal of this requirement is to ensure that a patient's care is provided in the most cost-effective setting. For example, many surgical procedures that used to require an inpatient hospital stay can now be performed in an outpatient setting if proper education and support are available to the patient. Conflict between a UR guideline and the physician's requirements for the patient should be appealed to an impartial **peer review organization** composed of physicians and specialists who will review the case and make the final recommendation.
- *Approved referrals.* In many managed care plans a specialty physician can provide services to a managed care patient only on referral from the patient's primary care physician. The purpose is to ensure that the services provided by the specialist are medically necessary and, again, provided in the most cost-effective setting.
- *Network.* A network consists of providers (physicians, hospitals, pharmacies, and other providers and suppliers) who have signed contracts with the insurer or **health maintenance organization (HMO)** to provide services to covered persons in individual, group, or public health plans. A patient is normally required to use network providers to receive full coverage. The financial penalties (lost coverage) are often very high if a patient does not use these providers.
- ***Assignment of benefits.*** By contract, the network provider cannot bill the patient for any amounts not paid by the insurer (no **balance billing**) except for copayments, coinsurance, and deductibles. If payment for a service provided by a network physician or hospital is denied by the insurer because it was not properly authorized, the provider cannot bill the patient for these services unless the contract does not contain a hold-harmless clause for the patient. This puts teeth in the control features of the managed care program.

Most physicians have contracts with more than one managed care program, and each of these programs has its own requirements and reimbursement schedules. So that the physician can provide the patient with needed health care services, while ensuring that the physician is paid for his or her services, it is necessary to consider the requirements of each patient's program. UM or precertification requirements are extremely important. Check the patient's ID card for details. UM requirements may apply to inpatient services or to a variety of outpatient and doctor office services.

Until you are very familiar with the requirements of each of your patient's managed care programs, you should call the number on the ID card before a patient is admitted to a hospital (on a nonemergency basis), referred to another physician, or scheduled for specific laboratory, radiological, or other test or evaluation. For inpatient admissions, the UM firm may ask for the diagnosis, the procedure or procedures to be performed, and other related information before approving the admission. Once the procedure is approved, the UM firm may only approve a specified length of stay in the hospital. Failure to comply with the precertification requirements results in a financial penalty for the patient and possibly also for the physician and the hospital.

It is important to be familiar with physicians within the network. The physician, hospital, laboratory, or other provider you normally refer a patient to may not be in the patient's managed care network. By calling the UM number to check, you can avoid penalties and improve the satisfaction of the patient with your services.

Checkpoint Question

4. What are the four key elements of a managed care program?

Health Maintenance Organizations

It is easiest to understand how a HMO functions if we contrast it with a traditional health insurance program. In the traditional insurance system, the relationship between the covered individual and the insurer or self-insurer is purely financial. In return for receiving a paid monthly premium, the insurer promises to reimburse (indemnify) the individual if he or she incurs certain types of covered medical expense. There are often limits to coverage (exclusions and limitations), and normally the coverage has a **deductible** (amount below which services are not reimbursable) and **coinsurance** (the patient pays a percentage of the medical expense after the deductible is satisfied). For example, the patient pays the first $200 (deductible) in physician charges each year starting January 1; then insurance pays 80% of covered charges, and the patient must pay the other 20%.

The covered individual seeks medical services and thereby incurs an expense. The individual, not the insurer, must pay for this expense. If the medical treatment is covered as defined in the insurance policy, the insurer will reimburse the patient a portion of the amount incurred after deductibles and coinsurance.

In contrast to traditional insurance companies, a HMO promises to provide covered services rather than pay for them. In this respect, the HMO acts as both an insurer and a provider of service. HMO policies are written differently from insurance policies. The HMO policy lists the medical services that the member is entitled to receive and the physicians and hospitals that will provide these services. The HMO has a contract with both the patient and provider. It must provide covered services to the member either directly from its own physician staff and hospitals or indirectly from physicians and hospitals contracted to provide the services promised to the member. The HMO, rather than the patient, is responsible for the costs of medical services, and providers bill the HMO rather than the patient when a reimbursable service is rendered to a HMO member.

This is one reason HMOs do not normally use deductibles and coinsurance, which are standard features of health insurance programs. A patient does not receive a provider's bill, so deductibles and coinsurance cannot apply. Instead, HMOs use predetermined co-payments (e.g., $10 per physician office visit) to reduce premium prices.

Health maintenance organizations come in many forms. Kaiser Permanente Health Plan is generally recognized as the nation's first HMO (there were earlier organizational forms but none that lasted into the modern era). In the early 1930s, Kaiser Industries needed to provide physician services for its employees in remote areas where no physicians were available. Kaiser sought the services of a physician to build a medical group that would provide the necessary services. Rather than paying for these services on a **fee-for-service** basis, the company paid the physicians per employee (as the company did for workers' compensation coverage).

Over time, the physician group grew and became the Permanente Medical Group. Coverage was expanded first to include non–work-related illness and injury for employees and then services for the dependents and spouses of employees. Finally, the program was expanded to allow other employers to purchase care for their employees from the Permanente Medical Group. The organization was restructured into three mutually dependent entities: Kaiser Permanente Health Plan, Permanente Medical Group (a very large multispecialty group practice), and Kaiser Foundation Hospitals. This company, the best example of the group model HMO, serves more than 6 million members. The HMO contracts with employers to cover their employees. The medical group and hospitals contract with the health plan to provide the services required in the health plan's contract with employers.

Consistent with its history, the health plan does not pay the medical group a fee for each service provided. Instead, it pays each party based on the number of members enrolled in the health plan. This is often called **capitation** because there is one payment per capita. Capitation payments are also used by other types of HMOs.

As group model HMOs developed (they were called prepaid group practices until 1973 federal legislation changed their names), nongroup physicians organized into an entity called an **independent practice association (IPA)**. The early IPA HMOs were often sponsored by a local medical society and were developed to allow independent physicians to compete with prepaid group practices.

IPA HMOs contract with employers in the same manner as group model HMOs, and their members receive covered services from IPA physicians. The HMO's contracts with physicians are different, however, because these physicians are not organized into a single multispecialty group practice. IPA physicians are paid in a number of ways. Some are paid on a capitation basis, and some may be paid on a fee-for-service basis using a **fee schedule** established by the HMO. Often, a portion of any reimbursement is withheld by the HMO and paid only if the HMO's total medical expense is within budget; this encourages the physician to be cost conscious in caring for patients.

In some of these HMOs, the IPA is a separate corporation, often owned by physicians. With this structure (still called an IPA HMO), the IPA contracts with physicians, and the HMO contracts with the IPA instead of directly with each physician.

Over the years, HMOs have continued to evolve, and many are now a mixture of these discussed models. As a medical assistant, you must know what type of relationship the practice has with a HMO before you can determine how the practice is reimbursed. Most HMOs require claims to be submitted even if payment is capitation rather than fee-for-service. Many HMOs also require the collection and transmission of other patient information, which is not required in the traditional insurance industry.

Checkpoint Question

5. How does a HMO differ from a traditional health insurance program?

Preferred Provider Organizations

Whereas HMOs promise to provide services and have a financial risk in their relationships with subscribers, a **preferred provider organization (PPO)** is a type of health benefit program whose purpose is simply to contract with providers, then lease this network of contracted providers to health care plans. The PPO network is not risk bearing; it does not have any financial involvement in the health plan.

PPOs are typically developed by hospitals and physicians as a vehicle to attract patients, although some are developed and managed by insurance carriers.

PPOs contract with participating providers, including hospitals and physicians. These contracts allow the PPO to contract with insurers and other purchasers of health care services on behalf of the participating providers, who typically accept less than their normal charges and agree to follow the UM and other administrative protocols as specified by the PPO.

Typically, a health plan with a PPO offers benefits at two levels, commonly referred to as in network and out of network. Unlike in a HMO, patients may visit any provider they wish for services. If the provider is in network (a participating provider), the levels of benefits for the patient are greater than if the patient receives services from an out-of-network (nonparticipating) provider.

A typical health plan with a PPO may look like the breakdown shown in Figure 9-2.

As you can see from the example, each time the patient sees an in-network provider, he or she receives significantly better benefits. A primary difference between a HMO and PPO, therefore, is that patients can see any physician of their choice and receive benefits; they simply have an incentive in the form of higher benefits when they see an in-network provider.

As part of your responsibilities, you should identify the PPOs with which the physician has contracted and determine the administrative requirements set forth by each PPO in the contract. To understand the necessary administrative procedures agreed to by the physician, review all managed care contracts carefully. Also be aware that most PPOs have a provider relations representative who works with the contracted providers (physicians) to answer questions and clarify procedures. The PPO is typically operated by a group of hospitals or physicians or by an insurance company or independent organization. Physicians agree to participate in PPOs to serve their existing patients who now have PPO plans and sometimes to gain additional patients who seek the services of a PPO physician.

Participating physicians have agreed to perform certain administrative services for PPO patients. Commonly, the physician's office must accept assignment of benefits and provide claims filing services for the patient. The physician agrees to accept the reimbursement by the claims administrator as payment in full and agrees not to bill the patient for any difference between the physician's usual charge and the PPO-negotiated charge for the service. The participating physician is responsible for collecting any co-pay amount at the time of service. The physician also agrees to comply with any precertification requirements stipulated by the plan.

Example of a Health Plan With a PPO

Benefit	In-network	Out-of-network
Deductible	$100	$300
Coinsurance	90%	70%
Routine care	$200 per calendar year	-0-
Mental health	80%	50%
Office visit	$10 co-pay; no deductible	70%

FIGURE 9-2. A health plan with a PPO.

Checkpoint Question

6. What is the primary difference between a HMO and a PPO?

Physician Hospital Organizations

Physicians and hospitals have become more active in developing managed care alternatives. A **physician hospital organization (PHO)** is a coalition of physicians and a hospital contracting with large employers, insurance carriers, and other benefits groups to provide discounted health services. There are numerous variations of PHOs. A PHO may look much like a PPO with no risk-bearing elements, in which case the network of providers constituting the PHO are under no financial obligation to subscribers. A PHO may be more like a HMO, wherein the participating providers in the PHO do have a risk-bearing contract and assume responsibility for the overall medical budget of subscribing units. Physician organizations (POs) are such groups consisting of physicians only. As with any managed care program, it is important to know and understand the particulars of each managed care contract and requirements of the provider and obligations to patients and the managed care entity.

Other Managed Care Programs

Although HMOs, PPOs, and increasingly PHOs are the most common managed care programs, many others cover patients today and still more are being developed.

Although requirements vary, a gatekeeper provision is common. A gatekeeper is a primary care physician. Participants are required to see a primary care physician for all nonemergency services. That physician will either treat the patient or, if necessary, refer the patient to a specialist. The physician must complete and submit a referral form or call the claims administrator for approval of the referral.

The gatekeeper provision seeks to reduce the plan cost of specialists. For example, without such a provision, a patient might see a specialist first at a more costly fee, even though the condition may have been adequately treated by a less costly primary care physician. The gatekeeper approach also encourages patients to establish a relationship with a primary care physician, who is then in a position to manage the patient's care.

The Future of Managed Care

Managed care has changed the organizational structure of medicine. To form risk-bearing organizations, physicians and hospitals are combining into new relationships. Hospitals are buying physician practices, and small-group or solo-practice physicians are combining into larger group practices. Some of these are forming public companies and raising investment capital to foster even more rapid growth in size and geographic scope. The size of medical practices is increasing and is expected to continue to increase in the foreseeable future.

The role of primary care physicians is changing relative to subspecialty physicians. In many managed care programs, primary care physicians act as patient care managers. Services authorized by these gatekeepers are covered, whereas those not authorized by the patient's primary physician may be denied or paid at a lower rate. Patients often join managed care organizations only if their primary care physician is a participant in a particular plan.

As coverage changes from an insured fee-for-service system to a managed care system with incentives to decrease the cost of patient care, employers and other purchasers have become much more interested in measuring the quality of care provided by managed care organizations. The very largest employers worked with leading HMOs to develop a report called HEDIS (Healthplan Employer Data Information Set). This uniform data set (reporting many indicators of health care quality, such as immunization rates and cesarean section rates) is now required of any HMO that wishes to serve the largest employers in the nation. HEDIS is upgraded continually and is being adopted by governmental agencies and many smaller employers as a prerequisite for a HMO to cover employees and governmental populations. This is only a start. Demands for increasingly sophisticated medical information will intensify.

The new demands to reduce the cost of care while measuring quality and improving it over time have led many organizations to develop increasingly sophisticated patient care protocols. These require documentation of efficacy and quality using information contained in patients' medical records. These demands are leading to increased automation of medical records. With automated medical records, a patient's medical history can be immediately available to any provider in virtually any location. Not only will it be easier to document quality and measure improvement over time, but a complete medical record that is available to any provider (with the patient's permission) will improve coordination among physicians and reduce illness. This alone can lead to substantial improvement in the quality of care.

Physicians are no longer isolated practitioners but are continuously involved with and accountable to community standards of practice. Protocols for patient care are becoming common and will change further as knowledge increases. Quality measurement and reporting will become more public, and the best medical care systems may be rewarded with higher patient volume for attaining the highest standards of patient care quality and satisfaction.

How does the progression of managed care affect you as a medical assistant? Managed care will continue to evolve and be refined. These trends in managed care will continue to affect individual physician practices as the face of health care continues to change. There will be increasing cooperative efforts by groups of physicians contracting together, with or without hospitals, carriers, or other parties. Family practice physicians will accept expanded responsibilities in managing the total care of a patient, managing specialist care and hospitalizations. These coalitions of providers will result in more uniform protocols of care and the application of outcome measurements in physician practices. The collection of data will become increasingly important to the practice. That collection and the management of the data will be a vital responsibility for you.

WORKERS' COMPENSATION

Employees in every state are covered by a workers' compensation program administered by the state. Workers' compensation benefits were developed to cover the expenses resulting from a work-related illness or injury. In the event of

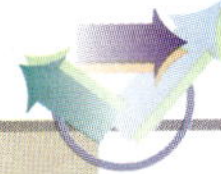

ETHICAL TIP

The following scenario may occur in a medical office:

> While you are filing an insurance claim, the physician tells you to "readjust" the laceration length from 4 cm to 9 cm. (The physician can bill more for a 9-cm laceration.) When you question him about this, he says, "Don't worry. The patient isn't paying the difference, the insurance company is, and they have plenty of money." How should you handle this situation?

Ethically and legally, you cannot change the length of a laceration on the medical record or the bill. This is fraud. You must explain to the physician that you are uncomfortable with this request and that you are ethically and legally bound to truthful billing. Any requests to alter or misrepresent the medical records or claims of a patient must be firmly denied.

A physician who operates in an unethical manner should be reported. If he or she is a partner in a practice, alert the other physicians about the suspect actions. You can also contact your state medical association, the American Medical Association, or the institutional review board at the hospital where your physician is affiliated.

PLEASE DO NOT STAPLE IN THIS AREA

CARRIER

PICA

HEALTH INSURANCE CLAIM FORM

PICA

1. MEDICARE (Medicare #) MEDICAID (Medicaid #) CHAMPUS (Sponsor's SSN) CHAMPVA (VA File #) GROUP HEALTH PLAN (SSN or ID) FECA BLK LUNG (SSN) OTHER (ID)

1a. INSURED'S I.D. NUMBER (FOR PROGRAM IN ITEM 1)

2. PATIENT'S NAME (Last Name, First Name, Middle Initial)

3. PATIENT'S BIRTH DATE MM | DD | YY SEX M F

4. INSURED'S NAME (Last Name, First Name, Middle Initial)

5. PATIENT'S ADDRESS (No., Street)

6. PATIENT RELATIONSHIP TO INSURED Self Spouse Child Other

7. INSURED'S ADDRESS (No., Street)

CITY STATE

8. PATIENT STATUS Single Married Other

CITY STATE

ZIP CODE TELEPHONE (Include Area Code) ( )

Employed Full-Time Student Part-Time Student

ZIP CODE TELEPHONE (INCLUDE AREA CODE) ( )

9. OTHER INSURED'S NAME (Last Name, First Name, Middle Initial)

10. IS PATIENT'S CONDITION RELATED TO:

11. INSURED'S POLICY GROUP OR FECA NUMBER

a. OTHER INSURED'S POLICY OR GROUP NUMBER

a. EMPLOYMENT? (CURRENT OR PREVIOUS) YES NO

a. INSURED'S DATE OF BIRTH MM | DD | YY SEX M F

b. OTHER INSURED'S DATE OF BIRTH MM | DD | YY SEX M F

b. AUTO ACCIDENT? PLACE (State) YES NO

b. EMPLOYER'S NAME OR SCHOOL NAME

c. EMPLOYER'S NAME OR SCHOOL NAME

c. OTHER ACCIDENT? YES NO

c. INSURANCE PLAN NAME OR PROGRAM NAME

d. INSURANCE PLAN NAME OR PROGRAM NAME

10d. RESERVED FOR LOCAL USE

d. IS THERE ANOTHER HEALTH BENEFIT PLAN? YES NO *If yes,* return to and complete item 9 a-d.

READ BACK OF FORM BEFORE COMPLETING & SIGNING THIS FORM.

12. PATIENT'S OR AUTHORIZED PERSON'S SIGNATURE I authorize the release of any medical or other information necessary to process this claim. I also request payment of government benefits either to myself or to the party who accepts assignment below.

SIGNED ______ DATE ______

13. INSURED'S OR AUTHORIZED PERSON'S SIGNATURE I authorize payment of medical benefits to the undersigned physician or supplier for services described below.

SIGNED ______

PATIENT AND INSURED INFORMATION

14. DATE OF CURRENT: MM | DD | YY ◄ ILLNESS (First symptom) OR INJURY (Accident) OR PREGNANCY(LMP)

15. IF PATIENT HAS HAD SAME OR SIMILAR ILLNESS. GIVE FIRST DATE MM | DD | YY

16. DATES PATIENT UNABLE TO WORK IN CURRENT OCCUPATION FROM MM | DD | YY TO MM | DD | YY

17. NAME OF REFERRING PHYSICIAN OR OTHER SOURCE

17a. I.D. NUMBER OF REFERRING PHYSICIAN

18. HOSPITALIZATION DATES RELATED TO CURRENT SERVICES FROM MM | DD | YY TO MM | DD | YY

19. RESERVED FOR LOCAL USE

20. OUTSIDE LAB? YES NO $ CHARGES

21. DIAGNOSIS OR NATURE OF ILLNESS OR INJURY. (RELATE ITEMS 1,2,3 OR 4 TO ITEM 24E BY LINE)

1. ___ . __
2. ___ . __
3. ___ . __
4. ___ . __

22. MEDICAID RESUBMISSION CODE ORIGINAL REF. NO.

23. PRIOR AUTHORIZATION NUMBER

24. A DATE(S) OF SERVICE From MM DD YY To MM DD YY	B Place of Service	C Type of Service	D PROCEDURES, SERVICES, OR SUPPLIES (Explain Unusual Circumstances) CPT/HCPCS | MODIFIER	E DIAGNOSIS CODE	F $ CHARGES	G DAYS OR UNITS	H EPSDT Family Plan	I EMG	J COB	K RESERVED FOR LOCAL USE
1										
2										
3										
4										
5										
6										

25. FEDERAL TAX I.D. NUMBER SSN EIN

26. PATIENT'S ACCOUNT NO.

27. ACCEPT ASSIGNMENT? (For govt. claims, see back) YES NO

28. TOTAL CHARGE $

29. AMOUNT PAID $

30. BALANCE DUE $

31. SIGNATURE OF PHYSICIAN OR SUPPLIER INCLUDING DEGREES OR CREDENTIALS (I certify that the statements on the reverse apply to this bill and are made a part thereof.)

SIGNED DATE

32. NAME AND ADDRESS OF FACILITY WHERE SERVICES WERE RENDERED (If other than home or office)

33. PHYSICIAN'S, SUPPLIER'S BILLING NAME, ADDRESS, ZIP CODE & PHONE #

PIN# GRP#

PHYSICIAN OR SUPPLIER INFORMATION

(APPROVED BY AMA COUNCIL ON MEDICAL SERVICE 8/88) ***PLEASE PRINT OR TYPE*** APPROVED OMB-0938-0008 FORM CMS-1500 (12-90), FORM RRB-1500, APPROVED OMB-1215-0055 FORM OWCP-1500, APPROVED OMB-0720-0001 (CHAMPUS)

FIGURE 9-3. CMS-1500 claim form. This is the most commonly used insurance claim form. On the facing page you will find a detailed list explaining how to complete each line of the form. The form should be clearly and neatly typed.

Box Number	Information to Be Entered	Comments
1	Where the claim is being submitted	Confirm the patient's coverage and accuracy of your file information. A change in the patient's coverage will change how the claim is filed.
1a	The insured's ID number	Important: Enter the ID number of the insured (or employee), not the patient. This frequent filing error will cause rejection of the claim. The ID number is often the SSN, but check the ID card; the ID number may differ from the SSN.
2	Name of patient	The correct order (last, first, middle initial) is important.
3	Patient's date of birth	
4	Name of insured	Again, be sure to enter the name of the insured (or employee), not the patient.
5	Address of patient	
6	Patient's relationship to the insured	
7	Address of the insured	Check and update regularly.
8	Patient's status	Check and update frequently.
	Name of other insured	If the patient is covered under more than one plan, enter second plan here. For example, if a patient's claim is being submitted for her employer but she is also covered under her husband's plan, list the husband's name here.
9	Other insured's name	
9a	Other insured's policy or group number	Husband's policy number
9b	Other insured's date of birth	Husband's date of birth and sex
9c	Employer's name or school	Husband's employer
9d	Insurance plan name or program name	Husband's insurance company
10	Patient's condition	
10a	Patient's condition related to employment?	If yes, claim should be submitted to the workers' compensation carrier.
10b	Related to an auto accident?	If yes, the claim will not be processed unless a police report is attached.
10c	Other accident?	If yes, details of that accident must be attached.
11	Insured's policy group or FECA number	Very important. Some payers automatically return claim if group number is not indicated here. Group number is on patient's ID card.
11a	Insured's date of birth	Again, this is insured person, not patient.
11b	Employer's name	The insured's employer or school.
11c	Insurance plan name or program name	
11d	Is there another health plan?	If the patient is covered under more than one plan, check yes. If yes, the coverage will be coordinated between the plans covering the patient.
12	Patient's or authorized person's signature	This signature authorizes the release of information necessary to process the claim. If the patient's signature is in his or her file in your office, "signature on file" may be entered here.
13	Insured's signature	
14	Date of current	This is not date of service but the date the illness began or accident occurred.
15	If patient has had same or similar illness	If the patient has had this illness before, enter the date of the first occurrence.
16	Is patient unable to work	This information is required for the patient to receive disability payments.
17	Name of referring physician	If this patient was referred by another physician, enter name here.
17a	ID number of referring physician	EIN of the physician who referred the patient
18	Hospitalization dates	If the patient has been hospitalized for this illness or reason for visit, enter dates here.
20	Outside lab	If charges were incurred by an outside lab, check yes and enter amount. If not, check no.
21–24	Codes	Accuracy of this information determines accuracy of reimbursement. Thorough understanding of coding is essential for completing this section.
25	Tax ID number	Enter the EIN of the physician
26	Patient's account number	If you have assigned an account number to the patient, enter it here.
27	Accept assignment?	If you will accept assignment of the benefits, check yes. If not, check no.
28	Total charge	Enter the total amount of charges for this visit or service
29	Amount paid	Enter here any amount paid by the patient.
30	Balance due	Subtract any amount paid from the total charge and enter that amount here.
31	Signature of physician	
32	Name and address of facility where service was rendered	If the service was rendered outside of the physician's office, enter that address here.
33	Physician's billing name, address, zip code, and phone	This information will be used to mail reimbursement. Be sure it is current. The physician's billing name is required; may be a practice or corporate name.

SSN, Social Security number; FECA, Federal Employee Compensation Act; EIN, employer ID number.

a work-related illness or injury, claims submitted to the group or individual health benefits plan will be returned with instructions to file with the workers' compensation administrator, who determines the validity of the claim and reimburses accordingly. Because your practice will likely be taking care of the patient for both routine medical care and work-related illness or injury, it is important to determine at the time services are rendered whether the illness or injury is work-related and, if so, to account and file for those services separately.

You are responsible for knowing your state's workers' compensation regulations and procedures. Consult your state's office for workers' compensation or your state's designated claims administrator of the workers' compensation program for specific information.

FILING CLAIMS

If the provider requires patients to make full payment at the time of the visit, the physician may still submit a claim on the patient's behalf; however, the patient may need to submit claims to the claims administrator for reimbursement. Most providers accept assignment of benefits, however. To do this, the patient must give written authorization for the claims administrator to reimburse the physician for billed charges. As a medical assistant, you may be responsible for obtaining all necessary claims information from the provider and the patient and then submitting a claim for payment to the claims administrator.

The patient's ID card is a source of information necessary for complete and accurate claims submission. Keep a copy of this card in the patient's file and be sure to update it at least yearly and preferably at each visit, since the patient's employment and eligibility may change.

In addition, a patient may be covered by more than one group plan. For example, a patient may be covered both on an employer's group plan and as a dependent on his or her spouse's group plan. The primary plan—the one that pays first—is the plan provided by the patient's employer. Any unpaid amount is then considered for payment by the spouse's group plan, which is considered secondary. This is called **coordination of benefits**.

Dependent children may be covered under one or two parents' plans. Unless the plans state otherwise, the plan of the parent whose birthday occurs first each calendar year (not necessarily the oldest parent) is the primary plan. This is known as the **birthday rule**. This rule is commonly used by benefit plans and claims administrators to coordinate the benefits of dependent children covered by two plans. If the parents are legally separated or divorced, however, the primary plan is the plan of the parent who has custody or, in some instances, is subject to a court order or divorce decree.

After establishing the primary plan and the claims submission destination, you prepare the claim for filing. The CMS-1500 was developed by the American Medical Association to standardize an acceptable claim form for different plans and different claims administrators. It is the most widely used method of filing a health claim (Fig. 9-3). The CMS-1500 is accepted by most claims administrators, including Blue Shield, Medicare, Medicaid, and TRICARE/CHAMPVA.

Most plans include a clause that excludes coverage for a stated period (usually 12 months) for a condition, called a **preexisting condition**, that existed before the plan's effective date. For example, a patient with a diagnosis of depression before the effective date of his or her plan would be covered for all other conditions from the effective date forward but would not be covered for services related to the diagnosis or treatment of depression for the preexisting exclusion period (in this example, 12 months).

Many pieces of information are necessary for timely and efficient claims processing. The insurance company or managed care plan cannot process claims with incomplete or inaccurate information and will return them to the provider for completion, correction, and resubmission. This lengthens the time the provider must wait for reimbursement, making accurate claims submission a critical aspect of your responsibilities. The most frequent causes for denial of a claim and the corrective actions that you can take are as follows:

1. The patient cannot be identified as a covered person. Confirm that coverage information on file is current, including insurance company and group number, and that the Social Security number is accurate.
2. Coding is deemed inappropriate for services provided. Review provided services and recode as necessary.
3. The patient is no longer covered by the plan. Bill the patient for the charges. The patient may provide confirmation of new coverage.
4. The data are incomplete. Complete the required data and resubmit the claim.
5. Services are not covered by the plan. Bill the patient for the charges unless there is a basis for an appeal.

Electronic Claims Submission

Although some practices continue to submit claims on paper through the mail and most claims administrators continue to accept this practice, most practices submit at least their

WHAT IF

The reason for a rejection or denial of a claim is not clear. What should you do?

If the reasons for denial of the claim are not clear, telephone the claims administrator and ask for clarification. Be sure to have the claim and papers with you when you make the telephone call.

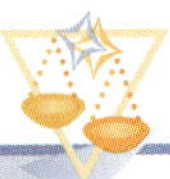

Legal Tip

Keeping patient information confidential is a primary concern in all medical practices. You should not release any information about the patient to any party, including the claims administrator, without the written authorization of the patient or the patient's guardian. Obtain a written authorization to release information from each patient on his or her first visit to the practice. Keep this information in the patient's file. Any claims submitted by the physician's office must have "signature on file" on the claim form. With written authorization for the release of information, only such information as is pertinent to the claim and necessary for the processing of that claim should be released. Releasing any patient information without written consent is a breach of confidentiality.

Medicare and Medicaid claims electronically. As of October 2003, HIPAA requires nearly all, with very few exceptions, to be submitted electronically. The physician's office computer software includes the CMS-1500 format for convenient and automated claims filing. With a computer and a modem, health claims can be filed immediately, reducing the time for the reimbursement cycle. You will need to work closely with your practice's software vendor to ensure compatibility with the insurance companies' computer systems.

Several regional and national clearinghouses receive health benefits claims and electronically direct them to the appropriate claims administrators. This system allows you to file all electronic claims through one clearinghouse rather than filing separately with each claims administrator. The system requires that all fields on the electronic claim form be completed and in the required format. If the claim is incomplete or inaccurate, the system will not transmit the form. You can complete or correct the form online, allowing the form to be transmitted. Claims submitted electronically that do not meet the plan's criteria will be rejected by the clearinghouse and must be submitted by mail. In addition, claims that are particularly complicated or cumbersome, have attachments, or are otherwise unsuitable for electronic submission should be filed on paper with the claims administrator.

Explanation of Benefits

When the claims administrator settles a claim, that is, makes a payment, an **explanation of benefits (EOB)** is issued to both the provider and the patient (Fig. 9-4). The EOB tells how the payment was made, including deductible and coinsurance information. Some EOBs include information for several claims on several patients that may have been processed during a particular period. You may be responsible for checking the EOB to be sure that all payments made to the physician are for the appropriate procedures and in the correct amounts.

POLICIES IN THE PRACTICE

Managed care contracts and negotiated services affect many practice policies. You must be knowledgeable and precise in administering practice policies, especially with regard to assignment of benefits and balance billing.

Assignment of benefits is a service the practice may provide. If assignment of benefits is accepted, the patient's signature must be on file, authorizing the claims administrator to reimburse the physician. Managed care plans require physicians to accept assignment, although many physicians do not accept assignment for non–managed care patients. If assignment is not accepted, the patient is responsible for paying all charges and filing a claim with the claims administrator for reimbursement directly to the patient.

Balance billing is prohibited by most managed care contracts. The physician cannot charge the patient the difference between the physician's usual charge and the allowable charge specified by the contract. For other types of plans, however, balance billing is not restricted, and the practice may bill the patient for any difference between the physician's charged fee and the amount allowable by the plan according to **usual, customary, and reasonable (UCR)** tables.

A few national firms provide UCR data to claims administrators who use that information to determine the maximum amount payable for any given service (the **plan maximum**). UCR data are calculated from surveys of the amount physicians charge for each service or procedure. That amount is calculated on a geographic basis to reflect regional variations in health care costs. Non–managed care plan physician reimbursements are based on a maximum allowable charge as specified in the UCR data. The physician may choose to bill the patient for the difference between the amount charged and the UCR amount.

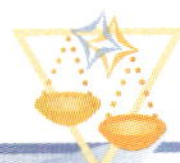

Legal Tip

It is fraudulent to misrepresent or expand the services rendered on the coding of a claim so as to receive additional reimbursement. Unbundling procedures so as to receive a greater reimbursement is also fraudulent. **Unbundling** is the practice of submitting a claim with several separate procedure codes rather than the single code that represents the services performed. Most payers now have software that detects such practices and rejects the claim.

Explanation of Benefits

Employee Name: Joe Doe
SSN: 555-55-5555 (1)
Group No. 55555
Patient Name: Joe Doe

Date of Service: 6-15-2004
Provider: Dr. Jones
Provider TIN: 35-5555555

Date of Service (2)	Comment Code (3)	Amount of Charge (4)	Amount Allowed (5)	At (6)	Amount Paid (7)
6-15-2004	57	87.00	82.00	80%	65.60
			Total (8)		65.60
			Less Deductible (9)		25.00
			Amount Paid (10)		40.60

Payable to: Dr. Jones
Address

Comment Code:
57 - The amount charged exceeds Usual and Customary

Reading the EOB (Explanation of Benefits)
After the claim has been processed, an EOB will be issued. Although each payer has his or her own EOB format, this sample EOB illustrates the key points included in an EOB. The terms used may differ, and the formats differ widely.

1. The top section typically includes the name of the employee and the Social Security number (SSN) or other identifying number, as well as the name of the patient, the group number, the date of service and provider name, and employer identification number (EIN) (Federal identification number assigned to the physician).
2. The date of service is included and is shown as the date the service is actually rendered, not the date that was posted or billed.
3. The Comment Code is a tool used on many EOBs to indicate a coded comment that is either on the bottom as exceeding "Usual and Customary." In this situation, the claim will be processed on the Usual and Customary amount. The difference between the amount charged ($87.00) and the amount allowed ($82.00) is $5.00. Unless the physician is contractually bound by an agreement with a managed care plan that forbids the practice of balance billing, that difference of $5.00 may be billed to the patient.
4. Amount of Charge shows the amount that the physician's office billed for the service.
5. Amount Allowed shows the amount of charge upon which the claim processing will be based (in this example, it is the amount of Usual and Customary).
6. This indicates the percentage of co-insurance payable by the plan.
7. Amount Paid shows the amount payable by the plan after co-insurance has been applied, but is not necessarily the amount that is actually paid (see #10).
8. The Total shows the total submitted and payable after the claim has been processed.
9. After all processing on the claim has been completed, any deductible is applied. In this example, Joe still had $25.00 to be applied to his annual deductible. Therefore, $25.00 is deducted from the amount paid and the actual reimbursement to the physician is $40.60. The amount applied to the deductible should be billed to the patient.
10. The amount actually reimbursed.

FIGURE 9-4.

Procedure 9-1

Processing Insurance Claim Forms

Equipment/Supplies: CMS-1500 claim form, patient's file, dates and names of services performed, medical dictionary, CPT-4, ICD-9-CM Volumes 1 and 2, computer software for insurance processing.

Steps

1. Using the ICD-9-CM index, locate a code or code range for each service or procedure performed for the patient.
2. Find that code or code range in the CPT-4 book.
3. Read the descriptor up to the semi-colon for codes that are not stand alone codes.
4. Review the documentation (operative report, x-ray report, lab report, etc.) to match the appropriate code.
5. If necessary, confirm your choice with the provider who performed the service.
6. Place the selected code in block 21of the CMS-1500 claim form.

SUMMARY

Most patients in the physician's office have some type of health care plan. Types of plans include group, individual, and government-sponsored health benefits, such as Medicare or Medicaid. Many physicians have contracts with managed care plans, such as HMOs and PPOs. Each type of plan has certain requirements regarding eligibility and claims submission, and you must be knowledgeable about those requirements. In particular, one of your primary duties is to file claims in a timely and accurate manner to ensure appropriate reimbursement for the physician. When filing claims, you must be careful to maintain patient confidentiality and to avoid fraud.

Critical Thinking Challenges

1. Jane and Joe are married, and both are employed and cover themselves and their two children on their health plans. Jane's birthday is July 23 and Joe's birthday is August 9. Joe is 2 years older than Jane. When claims are submitted for their two children, which spouse's plan is primary? Show which plan is primary and secondary for each family member.

	Primary	Secondary
Jane		
Joe		
Child 1		
Child 2		

2. The requirements for Medicaid vary from state to state. How do you determine the Medicaid requirements for your particular state? Locate the name, address, and telephone number of your state's resource.

Answers to Checkpoint Questions

1. With insured benefits, a monthly premium is paid by the employer or organization to an insurance company. The insurance company in turn is obligated to pay for any eligible health benefits. In contrast, self-funded benefits are provided to eligible employees or members by their employer or organization. Claims are processed by a professional claims administrator, such as a third-party administrator.
2. Persons enrolled in Social Security are automatically enrolled in Medicare Part A, which covers hospital services and expenses only, and Medicare Part B, which covers the physician's charges for inpatient or outpatient care as well as diagnostic services. Part B does not cover routine examinations, well care, routine immunizations, or cosmetic surgery. Part A is provided at no charge to Social Security recipients, and Part B caries a monthly fee. If Part B is not wanted, it must be declined.
3. Medicaid patients receive a new ID card each month.
4. The four elements of managed care programs are precertification of hospital admissions (often also called utilization management or **utilization review**—UM or UR), approved referrals, network, and assignment of benefits.
5. In a traditional insurance system, the individual, not the insurer, seeks medical services and thereby incurs the expense. An HMO promises to provide covered services rather than pay for them.
6. A primary difference between a HMO and a PPO is that patients with PPO coverage can see any physician of their choice and receive benefits; they simply have an incentive in the form of higher benefits when they see an in-network provider.

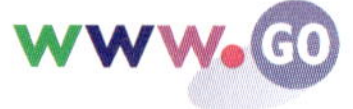

Websites

Medicare for providers and recipients
www.CMS.gov

Medicare for recipients
www.Medicare.gov

Blue Cross Blue Shield
www.bluecares.com

Local medical review policies
www.LMRP.net

American Medical Association
www.AMA-assn.org

All government agencies, federal and state
www.firstgov.gov

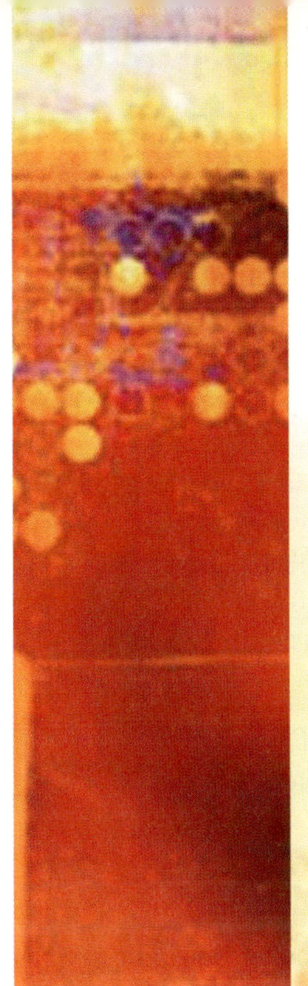

10

Diagnostic Coding

CHAPTER OBJECTIVES

In this chapter, you'll learn:

1. To spell and define the key terms.
2. To name and describe the coding system used to describe diseases, injuries, and other reasons for encounters with a medical provider.
3. To give four examples of ways diagnostic coding is used.
4. To describe the relationship between coding and reimbursement.
5. To explain the format of the ICD-9-CM.
6. To list the steps in identifying a proper code.
7. To name common errors in outpatient diagnostic coding.

KEY TERMS

advance beneficiary notice
audits
conventions
cross-reference
E-codes
eponym
etiology
inpatient
International Classification of Diseases, Ninth Revision, Clinical Modification
late effects
main terms
medical necessity
outpatient
primary diagnosis
service
specificity
V-codes

CODING, AT ITS SIMPLEST, is the assignment of a number to a verbal statement or description. Medical coding is anything but simple. The ***International Classification of Diseases, Ninth Revision, Clinical Modification*** is a system for transforming verbal descriptions of disease, injuries, conditions, and procedures into numeric codes. It is essential that the physician and medical assistant work together to achieve accurate documentation, code assignment, and reporting of diagnoses and procedures. Use of standardized codes makes it easier for third-party payers to understand the reason for the patient's encounter with the health care provider and increases the likelihood of timely processing of claims and prompt payment when appropriate.

Coding is a way to standardize medical information for purposes such as collecting health care statistics, performing a medical care review, and indexing medical records. It is also used for health insurance claims processing. Because coding is the basis for reimbursement, it is imperative that you code patient visits accurately and precisely. Incorrect, insufficient, or incomplete coding on claims forms can lead to nonpayment for the physician as well as incorrect information in the insurance companies databases, which may effect the patient's insurability. For example, if a patient complaining of chest pain is coded as having "acute myocardial infarction" instead of "chest pain rule out myocardial infarction," that patient may be incorrectly labeled as having heart disease. The Current Procedural Terminology (CPT) codes, used to report services and procedures performed by health care providers, determine the amount paid, but the code assigned to the diagnosis or reason for the service or procedure proves the medical necessity for the services or procedures so that claims are paid. The third-party payer needs to know why the service was performed to assess **medical necessity**. Medical necessity means the procedure or service would have been performed by any reasonable physician under the same or similar circumstances. The ICD-9 diagnostic codes convey this information. Is a chest radiograph medically necessary for a patient who has gout? No, but it may be necessary for a patient with acute bronchitis. The diagnosis justifies the procedure.

Since Medicare considers certain procedures medically necessary only at certain intervals, having the patient sign an **advance beneficiary notice** (ABN) will ensure payment of treatments and procedures that will likely be denied by Medicare. An example is a Pap smear for a low-risk woman, which will be paid for once every 2 years. If the physician considers it *not* to be medically necessary, but the patient wants a Pap test, the patient will be responsible for payment and must sign an ABN.

Checkpoint Question

1. What is meant by medical necessity?

DIAGNOSTIC CODING

International Classification of Diseases, Ninth Revision, Clinical Modification (ICD-9-CM) is a statistical classification system based on the International Classification of Diseases, Ninth Revision (ICD-9), developed by the World Health Organization (WHO). The CM, which stands for clinical modification, addresses the intent of these codes to describe the clinical picture of the patient. These codes are much more precise than those needed for statistical grouping and trend analysis found in the ICD-9 and used in hospital coding.

The ICD-9-CM, which is now mandated by Health Insurance Portability and Accountability Act of 1996 (HIPAA), is the most current and comprehensive statistical classification of its kind. Containing more than 10,000 diagnostic codes and 1,000 procedure codes, it consists of three volumes:

- Volume 1: Tabular List of Diseases
- Volume 2: Alphabetic Index of Diseases
- Volume 3: Tabular List and Alphabetic Index of Procedures

The ICD-9-CM code books are available from several publishers, and although the presentation of the material may be different, the content must be the same. Depending on the publisher, these three volumes may be included within one book. In the physician's office, only Volumes 1 and 2 are used. Volume 3 is used by hospitals.

The diagnostic classification systems in Volumes 1 and 2 are maintained by a federal government agency, the National Center for Health Statistics (NCHS); the procedure classification (Volume 3) is maintained by the Centers for Medicare & Medicaid Services (CMS), the federal agency that regulates health care financing. All three volumes are updated regularly, with codes being added, revised, and sometimes deleted. Changes in the ICD-9-CM are published by NCHS and CMS with the approval of WHO. Both the American Health Information Management Association (AHIMA) and the American Hospital Association (AHA) advise and assist in keeping the classification system current.

Checkpoint Questions

2. What are the three volumes of the ICD-9-CM system?
3. What organization must approve any changes in the disease classification system?

Inpatient Versus Outpatient Coding

There is a big difference between coding medical claims in a hospital or other inpatient facility and coding for the physician in an outpatient medical practice. The systems and references used to assign codes to third-party claims is only one difference in the coding requirements and practices of the physician and the inpatient medical facility. Volumes 1 and 2 of the ICD-9 CM are used to report the diagnostic code that justifies physician services whether those services are provided in the office or in the hospital. Hospital coders use Volume 3 to report inpatient procedures, services, and supplies, as well as the reasons for the services.

The UB-92 (uniform bill) is used by institutions to report inpatient admissions and outpatient and emergency department services and procedures. These charges are for nursing services, building maintenance, and all costs associated with running the institution. These charges do not include physician services. The CMS-1500 (universal claim form) is used to report physician services, whether the physician sees the patient in the office, emergency department, hospital, or nursing home, because even though the physician may have been in the hospital, it is his **service** for which we are billing in the medical office.

The term **outpatient** is used to describe patients treated in the following places:

- Health care provider's office
- Hospital clinic
- Emergency department
- Hospital same-day surgery unit or ambulatory surgical center that releases the patient within 23 hours
- Observation status in a hospital (the patient is admitted for a short time for observation only, and the physician bills for his or her service during the stay)

The term **inpatient** refers to a patient who is admitted to the hospital for treatment with the expectation that the patient will remain in the hospital for 24 hours or more.

Hospital coders code only services provided by the hospital and hospital employees. Coders who are employed by the physician practice are concerned with the services provided by the physician no matter where the services are provided. For example, the hospital room, meals, and laboratory testing that a patient receives are billed and coded by the hospital billing department. The daily visits the physician makes to the patient are billed and coded by the physician's office.

Since the focus of this textbook is medical assisting, we concentrate on outpatient coding.

Checkpoint Question

4. Define the terms *inpatient* and *outpatient.*

ICD-9-CM: THE CODE BOOK

Coding books are available from several publishers, such as Ingenix and Medicode. The AMA (American Medical Association) Press also publishes coding books and training materials. The classification system is also available as part of a medical software package; one of these packages is CodeManager from the AMA. Although each publisher offers special features and helpful aids, the format remains the same. Some coders become comfortable with certain special features (i.e., AMA publications are spiral bound) and, since the content is the same, can choose among the various publications based on organization, illustrations, tabs, bullets, and color coding.

To become an expert medical coder, you need general knowledge of human anatomy and medical terminology. In addition to using a code book, you will need reference materials such as a medical dictionary and/or medical dictionary software.

To ensure accurate coding, update your ICD-9-CM coding books and software as needed. (Updates and addenda can be purchased from the publisher of your coding book.) You must update codes on superbills (preprinted bills listing a variety of procedures) or any other forms you use. Experts have estimated that millions of dollars in reimbursement have been lost because an incorrect code was taken from a standardized form that had not been updated. New codes are published each October, and most third-party payers require their use after January 1.

Checkpoint Question

5. How often is the ICD-9-CM updated?

Volume 1: Tabular List of Diseases

Volume 1 contains the classification of diseases (conditions) and injuries by code numbers. Figure 10-1 shows the table of contents from this volume. These 11 chapters cover groupings of diseases and injuries by **etiology** or cause (e.g., infectious diseases) and by anatomic system (e.g., digestive, respiratory). Each chapter has a heading or title (e.g., 16, Symptoms, Signs, and Ill-defined Conditions (780–799). Following the title in parentheses is the range of three-digit categories included in that chapter. In each chapter you will find subtitles in large type followed by a range of three-digit categories in parentheses (e.g., 16, Symptoms (780–789). These sections describe general disease. Three-digit codes followed by a title, the category codes, describe specific diseases (e.g., 780, general symptoms). The fourth digit further breaks down the category (e.g., 780.0, alteration of consciousness), and the fifth digit is the highest level of definition (e.g., 780.01, coma). Figure 10-2 is a sample page from the tabular list showing each level of classification.

Volume 1 is always used to code a diagnosis to its highest definition. This volume tells you how many digits are required to code a diagnosis correctly and to a level that most third-party payers will accept. Volume 1 also includes five appendices, outlined in Box 10-1.

Supplementary Classifications

Supplementary classifications in Volume 1 include V- and E-codes.

V-codes. **V-codes**, which range from V01 to V82, provide a means of indexing the reason for hospital or physician office care for other than current or genuine illness, such as a history of illness, immunizations, or live-born infants according to type of birth. An example of a V-code is V10.04, used for a person with a personal history of a malignant neoplasm of the stomach. Because of this history, it would be

TABLE OF CONTENTS

FIGURE 10-1. Table of contents from ICD-9-CM, Volume 1.

important for this patient to have regular checkups. You would not want to code the visit 230.2, neoplasm of the stomach, because that would imply the patient has the malignant neoplasm at this visit. The ICD-9-CM offers a variety of codes for HIV testing. The patient who is simply afraid carries one V-code, while the patient who has known exposure carries another. V-codes may be used alone if no disease diagnosis is appropriate or as the second or third code to help better explain the reason for the visit.

E-codes. **E-codes**, which range from E800 to E999, are used to classify external causes of injuries and poisoning. Specificity is limited to the fourth digit level. E-codes are used in conjunction with codes in Chapters 1 to 11. They help to provide information of interest to industrial medicine, insurance underwriters, national safety programs, public health agencies, and others concerned with causes of injuries (e.g., auto accidents, accidents caused by heavy industrial machinery). These codes do not affect reimbursement.

✓5th 780.5 **Sleep disturbances**
EXCLUDES *that of nonorganic origin (307.40-307.49)*
780.50 **Sleep disturbance, unspecified**
780.51 **Insomnia with sleep apnea**
DEF: Transient cessation of breathing disturbing sleep.

780.52 **Other insomnia**
Insomnia NOS
DEF: Inability to maintain adequate sleep cycle.

780.53 **Hypersomnia with sleep apnea**
DEF: Autonomic response inhibited during sleep; causes insufficient oxygen intake, acidosis and pulmonary hypertension.

780.54 **Other hypersomnia**
Hypersomnia NOS
DEF: Prolonged sleep cycle.

780.55 **Disruptions of 24-hour sleep-wake cycle**
Inversion of sleep rhythm
Irregular sleep-wake rhythm NOS
Non-24-hour sleep-wake rhythm
780.56 **Dysfunctions associated with sleep stages or arousal from sleep**
780.57 **Other and unspecified sleep apnea**
780.59 **Other**

✓4th 780 **General symptoms**
✓5th 780.0 **Alteration of consciousness**
EXCLUDES *coma:*
diabetic (250.2-250.3)
hepatic (572.2)
originating in the perinatal period (779.2)
780.01 **Coma**
DEF: State of unconsciousness from which the patient cannot be awakened.

780.02 **Transient alteration of awareness**
DEF: Temporary, recurring spells of reduced consciousness.

780.03 **Persistent vegetative state**
DEF: Persistent wakefulness without consciousness due to nonfunctioning cerebral cortex.

780.09 **Other**
Drowsiness
Semicoma
Somnolence
Stupor
Unconsciousness

780.1 **Hallucinations**
Hallucinations:
NOS
auditory
gustatory
Hallucinations:
olfactory
tactile
EXCLUDES *those associated with mental disorders, as functional psychoses (295.0-298.9)*
organic brain syndromes (290.0-294.9, 310.0-310.9)
visual hallucinations (368.16)
DEF: Perception of external stimulus in absence of stimulus; inability to distinguish between real and imagined.

✓5th 779.8 **Other specified conditions originating in the perinatal period**
779.81 **Neonatal bradycardia**
EXCLUDES *abnormality in fetal heart rate or rhythm complicating labor and delivery (763.81-763.83)*
bradycardia due to birth asphyxia (768.5-768.9)
779.82 **Neonatal tachycardia**
EXCLUDES *abnormality in fetal heart rate or rhythm complicating labor and delivery (763.81-763.83)*
779.89 **Other specified conditions originating in the perinatal period**

FIGURE 10-2. Sample page from ICD-9-CM, Volume 1, showing categories, subheadings, and so on.

Box 10-1

ICD-9-CM APPENDICES

The following five appendices are found in Volume I

- Appendix A: Morphology of Neoplasms
  This appendix is used in conjunction with Chapter 2 in ICD-9-CM when coding neoplasms. It lists the five-digit alphanumeric codes used to identify the morphology of a neoplasm. For example, in the morphology code M8070/3, the 8070 indicates the morphology is squamous cell carcinoma. The /3 indicates that it is the primary site.
- Appendix B: Glossary of Mental Disorders
  Alphabetic list of mental disorders, including detailed descriptions of each disease.
- Appendix C: Classification of Drugs by American Hospital Formulary Service (AHFS) List Number and the ICD-9-CM Equivalents
  This appendix lists the AHFS list number (e.g., 24:04 for cardiac drugs) and the ICD9-CM code number for each one (e.g., 24.04 cardiac drugs would be equivalent to category 972.9, the ICD9-CM category "other and unspecified agents primarily affecting the cardiovascular system").
- Appendix D: Classification of Industrial Accidents by Agency
  This includes codes that can be used as a supplement to describe types of equipment or materials that may be responsible for an industrial accident or illness.
- Appendix E: List of Three-Digit Categories
  This is a list of all three-digit categories in ICD-9-CM.

Appendices A through D are not recognized by most government programs, such as Medicare and Medicaid. As previously mentioned, ICD-9-CM has other uses, however, and you may find that you need the appendices to track such things as disorders treated.

Volume 2, Section 3, has a separate index to access E-codes, the Alphabetic Index to External Causes of Injury and Poisoning.

Checkpoint Question

6. List four reasons for using E-codes.

Volume 2: Alphabetic Index to Diseases

Volume 2, the alphabetic index to diseases, contains many diagnostic terms that do not appear in Volume 1. For example, itch, barbers, beard, and scalp are all listed under Itch in Volume 2. In Volume 1 they are all listed under code 110.0. The index is arranged by condition. Always check all indentations in the index under the condition to ensure that you have the one most appropriate to the diagnosis you intend to code.

The alphabetic index is organized into three sections:

- Section 1, Alphabetic Index to Diseases and Injuries, is organized by **main terms** printed in boldface type. Section 1 is used for reporting the reason for patient encounters for most insurance claims. Following the main term is a code number, which refers you to the tabular listing (Volume 1). You must not accept this number as the correct code without a **cross-reference** or check of the tabular list. Never code directly from the alphabetic index. This could result in an incomplete or incorrect coding assignment. For example, if you have a patient with fluid overload and you look under fluid, it may seem logical to code the first code under fluid, which is abdomen, 789.5, but your patient is generally retaining fluid. If you use the alphabetic index only, you do not know that the correct code is 276.6, fluid overload, which excludes ascites, 789.5, and localized edema, 782.3. Box 10-2 lists several exceptions to the main term rule.
- Section 2, Table of Drugs and Chemicals, includes an extensive listing of drugs, chemical substances, and toxic agents. It also shows E-codes and American Hospital Formulary Service (AHFS) list numbers, which are in the table under the main term *drug*.
- Section 3, Alphabetic Index to External Cases of Injuries and Poisonings, leads you to codes that describe circumstances of injuries, accidents, and violence. These codes are not used for medical diagnoses. Main entries in this section usually are a type of accident or violence (e.g., assault, fall, collision). These codes can supplement the diagnostic code, but they should never be used alone or as principal diagnosis codes. E-codes

Box 10-2

EXCEPTIONS TO THE MAIN TERM RULE

Keep in mind the following exceptions to this rule:

1. Obstetric conditions may be found under the main terms *delivery*, *pregnancy*, and *puerperal*.
2. Complications of medical or surgical procedures can be found under *complication*.
3. Late effects are found under *late effect*.
4. V-codes are found under main entries such as *admissions*, *examination*, *history of observation*, *problem* (with), *status*, *vaccination*, *encounter for*, and *follow-up*.

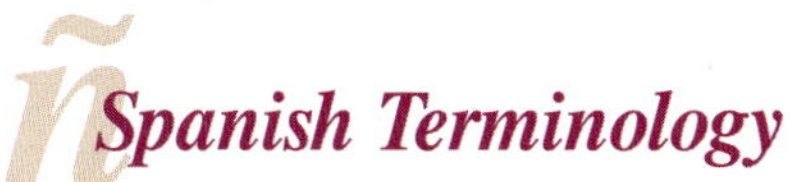

Spanish Terminology

¿Qué son todo estos números?	*What are all these numbers? Is that my bill?*
No, estos números se utilizan para su seguro.	*No, these numbers are used for your insurance.*
Estos se llaman los números de codificación.	*These are called coding numbers.*

are frequently used with these codes. For example, a person who fractured a tibia in a fall off a sidewalk curb would be given a code from chapter 10, Volume 1, in the ICD-9-CM for the injury (e.g., fracture of tibia, closed, is 823.80), and an additional code, E880.0, indicates that the accident was a fall off a sidewalk curb.

Checkpoint Question

7. What are V-codes used for?

Volume 3: Inpatient Coding

Volume 3, the Tabular List and Alphabetic Index of Procedures, is used in inpatient facilities and is based on anatomy, not surgical specialty. There are no alphabetic characters in these procedure codes. The codes are two-digit categories with a maximum of two decimal digits where necessary. Most refer to surgical procedures, and the rest cover miscellaneous diagnostic and therapeutic procedures. An example of a procedure code is 31.61, larynx laceration suture. Volume 3 is used for inpatient coding only.

LOCATING THE APPROPRIATE CODE

Box 10-3 outlines CMS guidelines for diagnostic coding. These are explained next.

Using the ICD-9-CM Conventions

Figure 10-3 lists the conventions used in the ICD-9-CM indexes. **Conventions** are rules that apply to the assignment of the ICD-9 codes. They are found throughout both the Index to Diseases and the Tabular List and include general notes using specific terms, cross-references, abbreviations, punctuation marks, symbols, typeface, and format. They direct and guide the coder to the appropriate code and should be strictly adhered to. Each publisher uses these same conventions, and many add more to assist coders in providing the most complete and accurate reason for the encounter. For example, when you locate the word itch, you will find "see pruritus," the medical term for severe itching. This is a helpful tool for coders who are unfamiliar with medical terminology.

Box 10-3

CMS DIAGNOSTIC CODING GUIDELINES

CMS defines specific guidelines that provide the basic knowledge necessary to apply the correct ICD-9 codes. Although these guidelines were developed for use in submitting government claims, most insurance companies have also adopted them. Many variations exist among the private insurance companies; therefore, care must be taken in recognizing the different requirements for each third-party payer. Most coders operate on the assumption that the government regulations are the strictest, and following those guidelines will satisfy most third-party payers.

1. Identify each service and procedure, or supply with an ICD-9 code from 001.0 through V82.9 to describe the diagnosis, symptom, complaint, condition, or problem.
2. Identify services or visits for circumstances other than disease or injury, such as follow-up care after chemotherapy, with V-codes provided for this purpose.
3. Code the reason for the visit first and code any coexisting conditions that affect the treatment of the patient for that visit or procedure as supplementary information. Do not code a diagnosis that is no longer applicable.
4. Code to the highest degree of specificity. Carry the numeric code to the fourth or fifth digit when necessary.
5. Code a chronic diagnosis as often as it is applicable to the patient's treatment.
6. When only ancillary services are provided, list the appropriate V-code first and the problem second. For example, if a patient is receiving only physical therapy, list the V-code first, followed by the code for the condition on line 24E on the CMS-1500 form.
7. For ambulatory or outpatient surgical procedures, code the diagnosis applicable to the procedure. If the postoperative diagnosis is different from the preoperative diagnosis, use the postoperative diagnosis.

Conventions

Braces { } These are used in the Tabular List to connect a series of terms to a common stem. Each term on the left of the brace is incomplete without one of the terms to the right of the bracket.

Brackets [ ] Brackets enclose synonyms, alternate wording, or explanatory phrases

Colon : A colon is used after an incomplete term that needs one or more of the modifiers that follow to make it assignable to a given category

Parentheses ( ) Parentheses enclose supplementary words that may be present or absent in the statement of a disease or procedure, without affecting the code number to which it is assigned.

NEC (not elsewhere classifiable) Alerts the coder that the specified form of the condition is classified differently. Codes following NEC should be used only when the coder lacks the information necessary to code the term in a more specific category.

NOS (not otherwise specified) The coder should continue to look for a more specific code

Note Used to define terms and give coding instructions. Found most often with list of fifth digits.

"Includes" Indicates separate terms as adjectives that further modify sites and conditions or to further define or give examples of the content of a certain category.

"Excludes" A box with "excludes" in italics draws the reader's attention to instructions that direct the coder to the proper code. This convention is found in the Tabular List.

"See," "See Also," and "See Category" Direct the coder to other terms or sections that should be considered. ALWAYS follow these instructions.

"Use additional code" This directs the coder to add another code to further explain and give the third-party payer a better understanding of a diagnosis.

"Code First Underlying Disease" This direction is used in the tabular list when a reason for an encounter results from another disorder. The coder is instructed to indicate the underlying disease that caused the current problem or symptom that brought the patient to the office.

Index to Disease Example

478.1 Other diseases of nasal cavity and sinuses

Abscess }
Necrosis } Of nose (septum)
Ulcer }

422.92 Septic myocarditis
Myocarditis, acute or subacute:
Pneumococcal
Staphylococcal
Use additional code to identify infectious organism [e.g., Staphylococcus 041.1]

See above example 478.1 (septum) may or may not be present in the diagnosis given.

Infection
Streptococcal NEC 041.00
Group
A 041.01
B 041.02

As soon as the bacterium is identified, code for specific infection.

At the time of the service, it has not been established whether a neoplasm is benign or secondary, for example. Remember, you are coding for a date of service with the information documented for that date of service.

	Allergic rhinitis (nonseasonal)
INCLUDES	477 Allergic rhinitis (seasonal)
	Hay fever
EXCLUDES	Allergic rhinitis with asthma (bronchial) (493.0)

Itch (see also Pruritus) 698.9

See 422.92 examples above.

362.72 Retinal dystrophy in other systemic disorders and syndromes
Code first underlying disease, as:
Bassen-Kornzweig syndrome (272.5)
Refsum's disease (356.3)

FIGURE 10-3. Conventions used in ICD-9.

Main Term

When trying to locate a diagnosis with more than one word, look first under the main term or condition. Often, a diagnosis may be an **eponym** (e.g., Ménière's disease or syndrome). These terms can be found under the main term *disease* or *syndrome*. In the diagnosis breast cyst, the main term is *cyst*. Find the condition, not the location. Remember the exceptions to the rules of using the main term.

Fourth and Fifth Digits

In many instances, a fourth digit has been added to a category to provide more detail, or **specificity**. These are subcategory

Box 10-4

STEPS IN LOCATING A DIAGNOSTIC CODE

1. Choose the main term within the diagnostic statement.
2. Locate the main term in Volume 2.
3. Refer to all notes and conventions under the main term.
4. Find the appropriate indented subordinate term.
5. Follow any relevant instructions, such as "see also."
6. Confirm the selected code by cross-referencing to Volume 1. Make sure you have added any fourth or fifth digits necessary.
7. Assign the code.

codes. Some codes also have a fifth digit because of the need to code to a higher specificity. For example, diabetes mellitus is category 250. It is necessary to use one of the fourth-digit subcategories to indicate the specific complications that may accompany the diabetes and then add a fifth digit to indicate whether the diabetes is insulin dependent or non–insulin dependent. Those codes requiring a fifth digit are identified in both Volumes 1 and 2. Incomplete coding here affects reimbursement and causes data errors. Figure 10-4 shows samples of fifth-digit classifications from the ICD-9-CM, Volumes 1 and 2. The code 807.1 tells the third-party payer that the patient was seen for an open fracture of a rib. The fifth digit is added to describe how many ribs. A patient who fractured two ribs would be assigned the code 807.12. This gives a more thorough picture of the patient's problem and enables the payer to determine whether the treatment is medically necessary.

Primary Codes

In outpatient coding, the **primary diagnosis** is simply the patient's chief complaint or the reason the patient sought medical attention today. It may be a routine follow-up visit, or there may be a new problem. The primary code is listed first on the CMS-1500 (Box 10-4).

When More Than One Code Is Used

In many cases, more than one code is used for a single patient visit. When patients have more than one diagnosis, it is necessary to convey an accurate picture of the patient's total condition. For example, an elderly patient may have the following diagnoses listed each time she visits the doctor: degenerative arthritis, type II diabetes mellitus, macular degeneration, hypertension, and pernicious anemia. If any of these conditions is related to or affects her treatment, they should be listed as supplementary information. If she visits the doctor because she has influenza and her other diagnoses are not addressed at the visit, it is not necessary to list all the diagnoses given. The primary diagnosis is her reason for coming to the office (symptoms of influenza). But the fact that she is diabetic will affect her treatment and makes her visit medically necessary. Multiple codes should be sequenced with the proper service or procedure code on the proper line of the CMS-1500. Figure 10-5 shows the proper sequencing for another patient's CMS-1500. On line 1 of Section 24 on the CMS-1500 you place the code and charge for the visit. In Block 24E, the diagnosis code for the ankle injury appears first because that is what brought the patient to the office today. One Line 2 of 24A, the laboratory work is listed but is also referenced to the diagnosis on Line 21, Item 2, which is the proper code for the patient's diabetes; this is referenced to Item 2 on Line 24. If the patient did not have diabetes, the laboratory work would not be considered reasonable for a patient with an ankle injury. If this procedure were not followed, the laboratory work would be seen as medically unnecessary, and the physician would not be reimbursed.

Late Effects

Late effects are symptoms or conditions arising from an acute illness. The effects are present after treatment for the acute illness or injury has ended. Proper coding sequence requires that you list the code number identifying the residual or current condition first, with the code number identifying the cause or original illness or injury listed second. Key words used in the patient's medical records defining late effects include late, due to an old injury, due to a previous illness/injury, due to an illness or injury occurring a year or more ago, sequela of . . . , as a result of . . . , resulting from . . . , and so on. Patients who are status post cerebrovascular accident (CVA) may have residual effects from their original stroke, for example, and may have a diagnosis of left hemiparesis as a result of CVA 3 years ago. Figure 10-6 is a sample listing of a late effect from the ICD-9-CM.

LEGAL TIP

Remember that the ICD-9 codes placed on the CMA-1500 are confidential and should be protected as much as any other medical information. Forms left lying in common areas in the office may be seen by other patients. Keep printers and copies of these forms in a private place and share the diagnosis codes only with those who need the information to carry out their duties. Patients have the right to keep their diagnoses private.

INJURY AND POISONING **807–808.49**

✓4th **807 Fracture of rib(s), sternum, larynx, and trachea**

The following fifth-digit subclassification is for use with codes 807.0-807.1:

0 rib(s), unspecified
1 one rib
2 two ribs
3 three ribs
4 four ribs
5 five ribs
6 six ribs
7 seven ribs
8 eight or more ribs
9 multiple ribs, unspecified

✓5th **807.0 Rib(s), closed** MSP

✓5th **807.1 Rib(s), open** MSP

807.2 Sternum, closed MSP

DEF: Break in flat bone (breast bone) in anterior thorax.

807.3 Sternum, open MSP

DEF: Break, with open wound, in flat bone in mid anterior thorax.

807.4 Flail chest MSP

807.5 Larynx and trachea, closed MSP

Hyoid bone Trachea
Thyroid cartilage

A **807.6 Larynx and trachea, open** MSP

Fracture — *continued*
multiple — *continued*
skull, specified or unspecified bones, or
face bone(s) with any other bone(s) —
continued

Note — Use the following fifth-digit subclassification with categories 800, 801, 803, and 804:

0 unspecified state of consciousness
1 with no loss of consciousness
2 with brief [less than one hour] loss of consciousness
3 with moderate [1-24 hours] loss of consciousness
4 with prolonged [more than 24 hours] loss of consciousness and return to pre-existing conscious level
5 with prolonged [more than 24 hours] loss of consciousness, without return to pre-existing conscious level
Use fifth-digit 5 to designate when a patient is unconscious and dies before regaining consciousness, regardless of the duration of the loss of consciousness
6 with loss of consciousness of unspecified duration
9 with concussion, unspecified

with
contusion, cerebral 804.1 ✓5th
epidural hemorrhage 804.2 ✓5th
extradural hemorrhage 804.2 ✓5th
hemorrhage (intracranial) NEC 804.8 ✓5th
intracranial injury NEC 804.4 ✓5th
laceration, cerebral 804.1 ✓5th
subarachnoid hemorrhage 804.2 ✓5th
subdural hemorrhage 804.2 ✓5th

B

FIGURE 10-4. Samples of fifth-digit classifications from ICD-9-CM. **(A)** Volume 1. **(B)** Volume 2.

PLEASE DO NOT STAPLE IN THIS AREA

PICA

HEALTH INSURANCE CLAIM FORM

PICA

CARRIER

1. MEDICARE [X] (Medicare #) MEDICAID (Medicaid #) CHAMPUS (Sponsor's SSN) CHAMPVA (VA File #) GROUP HEALTH PLAN (SSN or ID) FECA BLK LUNG (SSN) OTHER (ID)

1a. INSURED'S I.D. NUMBER (FOR PROGRAM IN ITEM 1): 000-00-0000A

2. PATIENT'S NAME (Last Name, First Name, Middle Initial): Naomi A Dishman

3. PATIENT'S BIRTH DATE MM DD YY: 04 14 24 SEX M [ ] F [X]

4. INSURED'S NAME (Last Name, First Name, Middle Initial): Same

5. PATIENT'S ADDRESS (No., Street): 405 Carolina Ave

6. PATIENT RELATIONSHIP TO INSURED: Self [ ] Spouse [ ] Child [ ] Other [ ]

7. INSURED'S ADDRESS (No., Street)

CITY: Danville STATE: VA

8. PATIENT STATUS: Single [ ] Married [X] Other [ ]

CITY STATE

ZIP CODE: 24540 TELEPHONE (Include Area Code): (434) 555-5555

Employed [ ] Full-Time Student [ ] Part-Time Student [ ]

ZIP CODE TELEPHONE (INCLUDE AREA CODE) ( )

9. OTHER INSURED'S NAME (Last Name, First Name, Middle Initial): NONE

10. IS PATIENT'S CONDITION RELATED TO:

11. INSURED'S POLICY GROUP OR FECA NUMBER

a. OTHER INSURED'S POLICY OR GROUP NUMBER

a. EMPLOYMENT? (CURRENT OR PREVIOUS) YES [ ] NO [X]

a. INSURED'S DATE OF BIRTH MM DD YY SEX M [ ] F [ ]

b. OTHER INSURED'S DATE OF BIRTH MM DD YY SEX M [ ] F [ ]

b. AUTO ACCIDENT? PLACE (State) YES [ ] NO [X]

b. EMPLOYER'S NAME OR SCHOOL NAME

c. EMPLOYER'S NAME OR SCHOOL NAME

c. OTHER ACCIDENT? YES [X] NO [ ]

c. INSURANCE PLAN NAME OR PROGRAM NAME

d. INSURANCE PLAN NAME OR PROGRAM NAME

10d. RESERVED FOR LOCAL USE

d. IS THERE ANOTHER HEALTH BENEFIT PLAN? YES [ ] NO [ ] *If yes*, return to and complete item 9 a-d.

READ BACK OF FORM BEFORE COMPLETING & SIGNING THIS FORM.

12. PATIENT'S OR AUTHORIZED PERSON'S SIGNATURE I authorize the release of any medical or other information necessary to process this claim. I also request payment of government benefits either to myself or to the party who accepts assignment below.

SIGNED Signature of File DATE 052803

13. INSURED'S OR AUTHORIZED PERSON'S SIGNATURE I authorize payment of medical benefits to the undersigned physician or supplier for services described below.

SIGNED

PATIENT AND INSURED INFORMATION

14. DATE OF CURRENT: MM DD YY 05 28 03 ◀ ILLNESS (First symptom) OR INJURY (Accident) OR PREGNANCY(LMP)

15. IF PATIENT HAS HAD SAME OR SIMILAR ILLNESS. GIVE FIRST DATE MM DD YY

16. DATES PATIENT UNABLE TO WORK IN CURRENT OCCUPATION FROM MM DD YY TO MM DD YY

17. NAME OF REFERRING PHYSICIAN OR OTHER SOURCE

17a. I.D. NUMBER OF REFERRING PHYSICIAN

18. HOSPITALIZATION DATES RELATED TO CURRENT SERVICES FROM MM DD YY TO MM DD YY

19. RESERVED FOR LOCAL USE

20. OUTSIDE LAB? YES [ ] NO [ ] $ CHARGES

21. DIAGNOSIS OR NATURE OF ILLNESS OR INJURY. (RELATE ITEMS 1,2,3 OR 4 TO ITEM 24E BY LINE)

1. 845.03

2. 250.00

3. ___ . ___

4. ___ . ___

22. MEDICAID RESUBMISSION CODE ORIGINAL REF. NO.

23. PRIOR AUTHORIZATION NUMBER

24.	A DATE(S) OF SERVICE From MM DD YY	To MM DD YY	B Place of Service	C Type of Service	D PROCEDURES, SERVICES, OR SUPPLIES (Explain Unusual Circumstances) CPT/HCPCS MODIFIER	E DIAGNOSIS CODE	F $ CHARGES	G DAYS OR UNITS	H EPSDT Family Plan	I EMG	J COB	K RESERVED FOR LOCAL USE
1	05 28 03	05 28 03	11		99213	1	100 00	1				
2	05 28 03	05 28 03	11		82947	2	25 00	1				
3												
4												
5												
6												

25. FEDERAL TAX I.D. NUMBER SSN EIN: 54-0000000

26. PATIENT'S ACCOUNT NO.: 1234

27. ACCEPT ASSIGNMENT? (For govt. claims, see back) YES [X] NO [ ]

28. TOTAL CHARGE: $ 125 00

29. AMOUNT PAID: $

30. BALANCE DUE: $ 125 00

31. SIGNATURE OF PHYSICIAN OR SUPPLIER INCLUDING DEGREES OR CREDENTIALS (I certify that the statements on the reverse apply to this bill and are made a part thereof.)

SIGNED DATE

32. NAME AND ADDRESS OF FACILITY WHERE SERVICES WERE RENDERED (If other than home or office)

33. PHYSICIAN'S, SUPPLIER'S BILLING NAME, ADDRESS, ZIP CODE & PHONE #

JOSEPH G NORTH, MD
1111 GRAYSON STREET
DANVILLE VA

PIN# GRP#

PHYSICIAN OR SUPPLIER INFORMATION

(APPROVED BY AMA COUNCIL ON MEDICAL SERVICE 8/88) ***PLEASE PRINT OR TYPE*** APPROVED OMB-0938-0008 FORM CMS-1500 (12-90), FORM RRB-1500, APPROVED OMB-1215-0055 FORM OWCP-1500, APPROVED OMB-0720-0001 (CHAMPUS)

FIGURE 10-5. Sample CMS-1500 claim form indicating proper sequencing.

LATE EFFECTS OF INJURIES, POISONINGS, TOXIC EFFECTS, AND OTHER EXTERNAL CAUSES (905-909)

Note: These categories are to be used to indicate conditions classifiable to 800-999 as the cause of late effects, which are themselves classified elsewhere. The "late effects" include those specified as such, or as sequelae, which may occur at any time after the acute injury.

✓4th **905 Late effects of musculoskeletal and connective tissue injuries**

905.0 Late effect of fracture of skull and face bones
Late effect of injury classifiable to 800-804

905.1 Late effect of fracture of spine and trunk without mention of spinal cord lesion
Late effect of injury classifiable to 805, 807-809

905.2 Late effect of fracture of upper extremities
Late effect of injury classifiable to 810-819

905.3 Late effect of fracture of neck of femur
Late effect of injury classifiable to 820

905.4 Late effect of fracture of lower extremities
Late effect of injury classifiable to 821-827

905.5 Late effect of fracture of multiple and unspecified bones
Late effect of injury classifiable to 828-829

905.6 Late effect of dislocation
Late effect of injury classifiable to 830-839

905.7 Late effect of sprain and strain without mention of tendon injury
Late effect of injury classifiable to 840-848, except tendon injury

905.8 Late effect of tendon injury
Late effect of tendon injury due to:
open wound [injury classifiable to 880-884 with .2, 890-894 with .2]
sprain and strain [injury classifiable to 840-848]

905.9 Late effect of traumatic amputation
Late effect of injury classifiable to 885-887, 895-897
EXCLUDES *late amputation stump complication (997.60-997.69)*

A

Late

Late — *continued*
effect(s) (of) — continued
tuberculosis — *continued*
genitourinary (conditions classifiable to 016) 137.2
pulmonary (conditions classifiable to 010-012) 137.0
specified organs NEC (conditions classifiable to 014, 017-018) 137.4
viral encephalitis (conditions classifiable to 049.8, 049.9, 062-064) 139.0
wound, open
extremity (injury classifiable to 880-884 and 890-894, except .2) 906.1
tendon (injury classifiable to 880-884 with .2 and 890-894 with.2) 905.8
head, neck, and trunk (injury classifiable to 870-879) 906.0

B

FIGURE 10-6. Sample section of late effects in ICD-9-CM. **(A)** Volume 1. **(B)** Volume 2.

Coding Suspected Conditions

In the inpatient setting, coders list conditions after the patient's testing is complete. In other words, they are coding with complete information. In outpatient settings, however, the coder reports the reason for the patient visit as it occurs. When filing claims, the coder is limited by the information and documentation on hand at the time of the patient visit. If at the end of the visit the diagnosis is not confirmed, the physician may indicate "rule out," "suspected," or "probable." For example, a patient who comes in complaining of headache may be sent for magnetic resonance imaging (MRI) of the head because the physician suspects a serious disorder. On the patient's encounter form, the physician may list the diagnosis as "rule out brain tumor." It is not accurate to code the visit as brain tumor before it is confirmed by MRI. On this first visit to the physician's office, the reason for being seen is headache. The patient's symptom (headache) is the only

WHAT IF

You need to code a condition described as acute, chronic, or both. What code should you use?

When a particular condition is described as both acute and chronic, code it according to the subentries in the alphabetic index (Volume 2) for the condition. If there are separate entries listed for acute, subacute, and chronic, use both codes. The first code listed should be for the acute condition, the reason the patient came to the office today. Respiratory and orthopedic conditions tend to be acute and chronic. That is, a patient with emphysema will always have underlying symptoms of progressive disease, but during the spring, pollen may aggravate the condition and cause acute breathing problems.

confirmed reason for the encounter at this point. On the second visit to the doctor, the MRI has confirmed a glioma in the frontal lobe. For the second and all subsequent visits, glioma is coded as the reason for the encounter. Figure 10-2 shows a page from the ICD-9-CM that includes many of the symptom codes.

Checkpoint Question

8. Before a definitive diagnosis is made, what is coded?

Documentation Requirements

As discussed throughout this chapter, you should choose the code assigned to any given claim for a service or procedure based on the documentation available in the patient's record at the time of the service. An **audit** is conducted by the government, a managed care company, and a health care organization to determine compliance and to detect fraud. Remember, if it's not in the chart, it did not happen. Auditors verify the codes used based on information recorded in the chart on the date of service.

THE FUTURE OF DIAGNOSTIC CODING: *INTERNATIONAL CLASSIFICATION OF DISEASES, TENTH REVISION*

A new edition of the ICD, the *International Classification of Diseases, Tenth Revision* (ICD-10), is scheduled to be introduced sometime between 2003 and 2005. The WHO is responsible for revising the ICD to improve the quality of data input into clinical databases. The ICD-10-CM will include more codes and will be used by every type of health care provider for all encounters, including hospice and home health care. The new codes are alphanumeric, but the format of the index is similar to the ICD-9-CM. Two new chapters relating to disorders of the eye and the ear are being added to the ICD-10. Computer software will be revised, and the ICD-9-CM code books will be obsolete.

Checkpoint Question

9. List two reasons for a chart audit.

SUMMARY

Medical outpatient diagnostic coding involves the use of numbers to describe diseases, injuries, and other reasons for seeking medical care. ICD-9-CM provides an index to report and track diseases. Diagnostic coding is linked to reimbursement because it assures that the physician's service or procedure was medically necessary. As a medical assistant, you must understand the format and guidelines for assigning a code or reason for each encounter, treatment, and/or service.

Critical Thinking Challenges

Tom Barksdale has been seen by the physician for controlled non–insulin-dependent type 2 diabetes mellitus for about 10 years. While being seen for a routine check of his blood sugar, he complains of numbness and tingling in his left lower leg and foot. An x-ray of both legs is performed, since poor circulation in the extremities can be a complication of diabetes. The x-ray confirms the diagnosis of peripheral neuropathy.

1. Which ICD-9 code should be listed with the office visit?
2. Which code indicates the reason for the x-ray?
3. Which code should be placed on the CMA-1500 first as the primary diagnosis or reason for the visit?

Answers:

1. 250.60
2. 337.1
3. 250.60

Answers to Checkpoint Questions

1. Medical necessity means a particular service or procedure is reasonable.
2. The three volumes of ICD-9-CM are Volume 1, the Tabular List of Diseases; Volume 2, the Alphabetic Index of Diseases; and Volume 3, the Tabular List and Alphabetic Index of Procedures.
3. The World Health Organization must approve any changes in the ICD-9-CM system.

4. Inpatient refers to a patient who is admitted to the hospital for a stay anticipated to be longer than a day. An outpatient is one who is seen in the physician's office or for 1-day surgery and will stay in the inpatient facility for less than 24 hours.
5. ICD-9-CM is updated annually in October.
6. E-codes are used to provide information to (1) industry, (2) insurance underwriters, (3) national safety programs, and (4) public health agencies and others concerned with injuries and poisonings.
7. V-codes are used to report reasons for receiving services other than illness.
8. Before a definitive diagnosis is assigned to a patient, services must be coded with the patient's symptoms at the time he or she was seen.
9. Chart audits are conducted to assess compliance and to detect fraud.

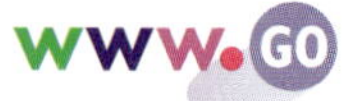

Websites

World Health Organization
www.who.int

Health and Human Services
www.hhs.gov

Centers for Medicare & Medicaid
www.cms.gov

American Health Information Management Association
www.ahima.org

American Hospital Association
www.aha.org

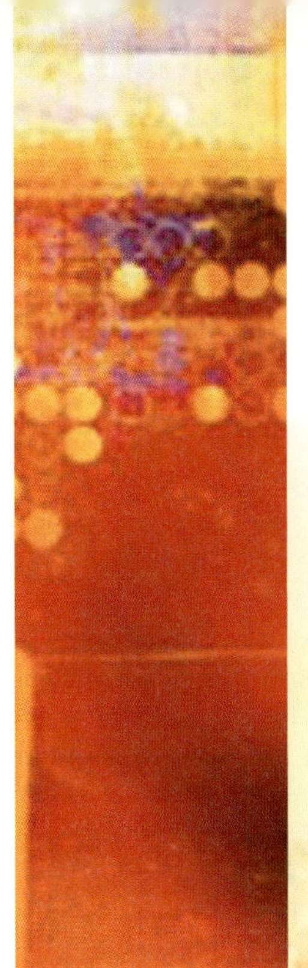

11

Outpatient Procedural Coding

CHAPTER OBJECTIVES

In this chapter, you'll learn:

1. To spell and define the key terms.
2. To explain the format of Current Procedural Terminology (CPT-4) and its use.
3. To explain the Healthcare Common Procedure Coding System (HCPCS) and level 2 and 3 codes.
4. To explain what diagnostic related groups (DRGs) are and how they are used to determine Medicare payments.
5. To discuss the goals of resource-based relative value system (RBRVS).
6. To describe the relationship between coding and reimbursement.

KEY TERMS

Current Procedural Terminology
descriptor
diagnostic related group
Healthcare Common Procedure Coding System
key component
modifiers
outlier
procedure
resource-based relative value scale
upcoding

Coding is a way to standardize medical information for purposes such as collecting health care statistics, performing a medical care review, and indexing medical records. It is also used for health insurance claims processing. Because coding is linked to reimbursement, you must code accurately and precisely. Incorrect, insufficient, or incomplete coding on claims forms can lead to improper reimbursement for the physician as well as recording and possibly passing along inaccurate patient information.

PHYSICIAN'S CURRENT PROCEDURAL TERMINOLOGY

Physician's **Current Procedural Terminology** (CPT) is a comprehensive listing of medical terms and codes for the uniform coding of procedures and services provided by physicians. First published in 1966 by the American Medical Association (AMA), CPT initially focused mainly on surgical procedures, with a limited number of other codes to describe medical, radiology, laboratory, and pathology procedures. New editions were published in 1970, 1973, and 1977. The fourth edition, CPT-4, contains more than 7000 new codes. Although there has not been a major revision of the CPT since 1977, CPT-4 is updated annually, with the newest version available each December.

CPT-4 contains a listing of all current U.S. Food and Drug Administration–approved physicians' procedures and services. The AMA developed it in collaboration with various other health organizations. In the early 1980s, Congress decided to use CPT-4 to code all physicians' procedures and services for Medicare patients. The aim of CPT-4 was to establish a way in which interested parties would know what procedures and services had been provided to the patient without reading a lengthy report. For example, the CPT-4 allows insurance companies to:

- Communicate easily with one another
- Compare reimbursable amounts for procedures
- Speed claims processing

CPT-4 is a system of five-digit numeric codes and corresponding meanings, as illustrated in Figure 11-1, a sample page from the CPT-4 book.

Every code means something unique and is used only to describe a specific **procedure**, service, or medical supply provided by physicians to their patients. This is true for inpatients and outpatients. Codes and descriptions are updated, revised, or changed yearly. If your physician's office uses a superbill or preprinted routing slip that lists the procedures performed, you must update this form yearly and work with your software vendor to update your computer software. The CPT-4 code selected will be placed on the CMS-1500 universal claim form in Section 24, Box D, along with any modifiers used. Figure 11-2 is a sample universal claim form showing the proper placement of codes for consultation and chest radiography.

The CPT-4 book is divided into six major sections:

1. Evaluation and management
2. Anesthesia
3. Surgery
4. Radiology
5. Pathology and laboratory
6. Medicine

Reading Descriptors

When reading a code's **descriptor**, or description, you will read up to the semicolon and then look down for any indentations using the same words before the semicolon. For example, the code 25065 carries the following descriptor: Biopsy, soft tissue of forearm and/or wrist; superficial. The CPT code for a soft tissue biopsy of the forearm and/or wrist is 25065. If the tissue sample was taken from the superficial skin, 25065 is used. Look at the indented line that bears the code 25066. Because it is indented, you must look at the lines above to find the category. Then read up to the semicolon. The description of this code is Biopsy, soft tissue of forearm and/or wrist; deep superficial or intramuscular. Use of the indentation and the semicolon saves space and keeps the CPT books from becoming too long.

Guidelines

Each section begins with its own specific guidelines and a listing of specific procedures and services applicable in that field. The guidelines contain definitions, explanatory notes, a listing of the previously unlisted procedures found in that particular section, directions on how to file a special report, modifiers for use in that particular section, and definitions to assist the coder.

Unlisted Procedures and Special Reports

Occasionally, a physician will perform a service that is not listed in the CPT-4 book. CPT provides unlisted codes at the beginning of each section for use when an unusual, variable, or new procedure is done. When an unlisted code is used, however, you must submit a copy of the procedure report with the claim. This special report should include the following information:

1. Definition or description of the nature, extent, and need for the procedure
2. Time, effort, and equipment necessary to provide the service
3. Complexity of symptoms
4. Final diagnosis
5. Pertinent physical findings
6. Diagnostic and therapeutic procedures
7. Concurrent problems
8. Follow-up care

27556—27615 Surgery / Musculoskeletal System

(27554 has been deleted. To report, see 27550, 27552, 27556, 27557, 27558)

27556 Open treatment of knee dislocation, with or without internal or external fixation; without primary ligamentous repair or augmentation/ reconstruction

27557 with primary ligamentous repair

27558 with primary ligamentous repair, with augmentation/reconstruction

27560 Closed treatment of patellar dislocation; without anesthesia

(For recurrent dislocation, see 27420-27424)

27562 requiring anesthesia

(27564 has been deleted. To report, see 27560, 27562, 27566)

27566 Open treatment of patellar dislocation, with or without partial or total patellectomy

Manipulation

27570* Manipulation of knee joint under general anesthesia (includes application of traction or other fixation devices)

Arthrodesis

▲27580 Arthrodesis, knee, any techniques

Amputation

27590 Amputation, thigh, through femur, any level;

27591 immediate fitting technique including first cast

27592 open, circular (guillotine)

27594 secondary closure or scar revision

27596 re-amputation

27598 Disarticulation at knee

Other Procedures

27599 Unlisted procedure, femur or knee

Leg (Tibia and Fibula) and Ankle Joint

Incision

27600 Decompression fasciotomy, leg; anterior and/or lateral compartments only

27601 posterior compartment(s) only

27602 anterior and/or lateral, and posterior compartment(s)

(For incision and drainage procedures, superficial, see 10040-10160)

(For decompression fasciotomy with debridement, see 27892-27894)

27603 Incision and drainage, leg or ankle; deep abscess or hematoma

27604 infected bursa

▲27605* Tenotomy, percutaneous, Achilles tendon (separate procedure); local anesthesia

27606 general anesthesia

27607 Incision (eg, osteomyelitis or bone abscess) leg or ankle

(27608 has been deleted)

▲27610 Arthrotomy, ankle, including exploration, drainage, or removal or foreign body

(27611 has been deleted)

▲27612 Arthrotomy, posterior capsular release, ankle, with or without Achilles tendon lengthening

(See also 27685)

Excision

27613 Biopsy, soft tissue of leg or ankle area; superficial

▲27613 deep (subfascial or intramuscular)

(For needle biopsy of soft tissue, use 20206)

27615 Radical resection of tumor (eg, malignant neoplasm), soft tissue of leg or ankle area

FIGURE 11-1. Sample page from CPT 2003.

Evaluation and Management Codes

Evaluation and management (E/M) codes are five-digit numbers that begin with the number 9. These are the most frequently used codes. E/M codes describe various patient histories, examinations, and decisions physicians must make in evaluating and treating patients in various settings (e.g., office, outpatient, hospital). In essence, the E/M codes address what the physician does when interacting with the patient. For this reason, the physician's documentation must meet standards so the physician and coder (medical assistant) can decide which code to use for a specific patient–physician encounter.

To code the services described in the E/M section, you must be sure that the patient's medical record indicates that **key components** are present. Two of three key components are required for established patients and three of three for new patients. These components are the elements that make up the visit. All E/M codes contain the following components:

- History
- Physical examination
- Medical decision making
- Counseling
- Coordination of care

PLEASE
DO NOT
STAPLE
IN THIS
AREA

CARRIER

PICA **HEALTH INSURANCE CLAIM FORM** PICA

1. MEDICARE MEDICAID CHAMPUS CHAMPVA GROUP HEALTH PLAN FECA BLK LUNG OTHER
X (Medicare #) (Medicaid #) (Sponsor's SSN) (VA File #) (SSN or ID) (SSN) (ID)

1a. INSURED'S I.D. NUMBER (FOR PROGRAM IN ITEM 1)
654321987A

2. PATIENT'S NAME (Last Name, First Name, Middle Initial)
Labosky, Theodore P

3. PATIENT'S BIRTH DATE MM DD YY SEX
05 10 1901 M X F

4. INSURED'S NAME (Last Name, First Name, Middle Initial)
Same

5. PATIENT'S ADDRESS (No., Street)
1313 Mockingbird Lane

6. PATIENT RELATIONSHIP TO INSURED
Self X Spouse Child Other

7. INSURED'S ADDRESS (No., Street)

CITY Philadelphia STATE PA

8. PATIENT STATUS
Single Married Other X
Employed Full-Time Student Part-Time Student

CITY STATE

ZIP CODE 19103 TELEPHONE (Include Area Code) (215)123-3456

ZIP CODE TELEPHONE (INCLUDE AREA CODE) ( )

9. OTHER INSURED'S NAME (Last Name, First Name, Middle Initial)
Labosky, Theodore P

10. IS PATIENT'S CONDITION RELATED TO:

11. INSURED'S POLICY GROUP OR FECA NUMBER

a. OTHER INSURED'S POLICY OR GROUP NUMBER
Medigap 67891237777

a. EMPLOYMENT? (CURRENT OR PREVIOUS) YES X NO

a. INSURED'S DATE OF BIRTH MM DD YY SEX M F

b. OTHER INSURED'S DATE OF BIRTH MM DD YY SEX M F

b. AUTO ACCIDENT? PLACE (State) YES X NO

b. EMPLOYER'S NAME OR SCHOOL NAME

c. EMPLOYER'S NAME OR SCHOOL NAME
Retired

c. OTHER ACCIDENT? YES X NO

c. INSURANCE PLAN NAME OR PROGRAM NAME
Medicare

d. INSURANCE PLAN NAME OR PROGRAM NAME

10d. RESERVED FOR LOCAL USE

d. IS THERE ANOTHER HEALTH BENEFIT PLAN?
YES NO *If yes,* return to and complete item 9 a-d.

READ BACK OF FORM BEFORE COMPLETING & SIGNING THIS FORM.
12. PATIENT'S OR AUTHORIZED PERSON'S SIGNATURE I authorize the release of any medical or other information necessary to process this claim. I also request payment of government benefits either to myself or to the party who accepts assignment below.

SIGNED Signature on File DATE 8/12/03

13. INSURED'S OR AUTHORIZED PERSON'S SIGNATURE I authorize payment of medical benefits to the undersigned physician or supplier for services described below.

SIGNED SOF

PATIENT AND INSURED INFORMATION

14. DATE OF CURRENT: MM DD YY ILLNESS (First symptom) OR INJURY (Accident) OR PREGNANCY(LMP)
08 12 2003

15. IF PATIENT HAS HAD SAME OR SIMILAR ILLNESS. GIVE FIRST DATE MM DD YY

16. DATES PATIENT UNABLE TO WORK IN CURRENT OCCUPATION FROM MM DD YY TO MM DD YY

17. NAME OF REFERRING PHYSICIAN OR OTHER SOURCE
John Mahan MD

17a. I.D. NUMBER OF REFERRING PHYSICIAN
54-0000000

18. HOSPITALIZATION DATES RELATED TO CURRENT SERVICES FROM MM DD YY TO MM DD YY

19. RESERVED FOR LOCAL USE

20. OUTSIDE LAB? YES NO $ CHARGES

21. DIAGNOSIS OR NATURE OF ILLNESS OR INJURY. (RELATE ITEMS 1,2,3 OR 4 TO ITEM 24E BY LINE)
1. 466.0
2. ___._
3. ___._
4. ___._

22. MEDICAID RESUBMISSION CODE ORIGINAL REF. NO.

23. PRIOR AUTHORIZATION NUMBER

24.	A DATE(S) OF SERVICE From MM DD YY	To MM DD YY	B Place of Service	C Type of Service	D PROCEDURES, SERVICES, OR SUPPLIES (Explain Unusual Circumstances) CPT/HCPCS | MODIFIER	E DIAGNOSIS CODE	F $ CHARGES	G DAYS OR UNITS	H EPSDT Family Plan	I EMG	J COB	K RESERVED FOR LOCAL USE
1	08 12 03	08 12 03			99243	1	150 00	1				
2	08 12 03	08 12 03			71020	1	110 00	1				
3												
4												
5												
6												

25. FEDERAL TAX I.D. NUMBER SSN EIN
54-0111111 X

26. PATIENT'S ACCOUNT NO.
1234

27. ACCEPT ASSIGNMENT? (For govt. claims, see back) X YES NO

28. TOTAL CHARGE $ 260 00

29. AMOUNT PAID $ 00 00

30. BALANCE DUE $ 260 00

31. SIGNATURE OF PHYSICIAN OR SUPPLIER INCLUDING DEGREES OR CREDENTIALS (I certify that the statements on the reverse apply to this bill and are made a part thereof.)

SIGNED DATE

32. NAME AND ADDRESS OF FACILITY WHERE SERVICES WERE RENDERED (If other than home or office)

33. PHYSICIAN'S, SUPPLIER'S BILLING NAME, ADDRESS, ZIP CODE & PHONE #
215 123-0000
Donald Myers MD PC
233 South Sixth Street
Philadelphia PA 19106
PIN# GRP#

PHYSICIAN OR SUPPLIER INFORMATION

(APPROVED BY AMA COUNCIL ON MEDICAL SERVICE 8/88) *PLEASE PRINT OR TYPE* APPROVED OMB-0938-0008 FORM CMS-1500 (12-90), FORM RRB-1500, APPROVED OMB-1215-0055 FORM OWCP-1500, APPROVED OMB-0720-0001 (CHAMPUS)

FIGURE 11-2. Sample insurance claim form for consultation and chest radiography.

- Nature of presenting problem
- Time

History, physical examination, and medical decision making are key components for a visit. The others are contributing elements.

Four classifications of histories and physical examinations are described in CPT-4. These include the following:

- Problem-focused
- Expanded problem-focused
- Detailed
- Comprehensive

Table 11-1 describes these classifications in greater detail. The provider must pick one of these based on information provided by the physician and documented in the patient's record.

The third key component, medical decision making, is defined in CPT-4 as one of the following:

- Straightforward
- Low complexity

Table 11-1 History and Physical Examinations

The physician or provider must select which history and physical examination code to use. You, however, should have a basic understanding of each category. It is important to note that there are separate codes for each category and separate codes for both new and established patients.

Type of History and Physical Examination	Patient Problems and Physician Time Required	Examples
Problem focused	Patient problems are self-limited and minor. Physician time: usually 10 minutes	• 9-month-old patient with diaper rash • 40-year-old patient with sunburn • 18-year-old patient with poison ivy • 60-year-old patient with a routine blood pressure check
Expanded problem focused	Patient problems are mild to moderate. Physician time: between 15–20 minutes	• 55-year-old patient with recurrent urinary tract infections • 16-year-old patient with chronic asthma presents with a cold • 76-year-old patient with osteoarthritis • 56-year-old patient with a stomach ulcer
Detailed	Patient problems are moderate to severe. Physician time: usually 30 minutes	• 18-year-old patient with first Pap smear and contraceptive education • 67-year-old patient with new onset of dysuria • 18-month-old patient with delayed motor skill development. • 34-year-old patient with diabetes requiring insulin dose changes
Comprehensive	Patient problems are moderate to severe. Physician time: usually 45 minutes	• 36-year-old patient with infertility • 8-year-old patient with new onset of diabetes • 65-year-old patient with history of left-sided weakness and confusion

- Moderate complexity
- High complexity

Medical decision making refers to the kinds of things the physician must do to establish a diagnosis for the patient (e.g., determine the management options available, the amount and complexity of the data to be reviewed, the risk of complications, or other problems, such as worsening of the illness or death). To qualify for a particular decision-making level, the physician must meet or exceed two of the three elements for an established patient and all three for a new patient.

Time spent with a patient (e.g., counseling or coordinating care) is sometimes the key component in determining E/M codes. When time spent with the patient is more than 50% of the typical time for the visit, time becomes the deciding factor in choosing an E/M code. For example, if a physician spends an additional 15 minutes counseling a patient in what would normally be only a 10-minute expanded problem-focused history and physical examination, the counseling was more than 50% of the typical 25-minute face-to-face time. The appropriate E/M code is one with a 25-minute time frame (10 minutes and an extra 15 minutes for counseling).

There are other special considerations regarding E/M codes. Initial hospital care codes can be used only by the admitting physician. All other physicians must use consultation codes for a first visit and then subsequent hospital care codes. Box 11-1 outlines the difference between a consultation and a referral. Emergency department service codes are to be used only when the service is rendered in a 24-hour hospital-based facility that specializes in providing treatment of unscheduled events.

Checkpoint Question

1. To code for a service in the E/M section, two of the three key components must be present for an established patient, and all three must be present for a new patient. What are the three key elements?

Anesthesia Codes

Anesthesia codes are five-digit codes that begin with 0. Anesthesia codes are divided by anatomic site and by specific type of procedure. For example, head, neck, and thorax

Box 11-1

IS IT A REFERRAL OR A CONSULTATION?

There are four subcategories of consultations: office, initial inpatient, follow-up inpatient, and confirmatory (in any setting). Each subcategory has specific reporting instructions. When a physician asks another provider to offer an opinion or advice regarding evaluation and management of a specific problem, the second provider becomes a consultant for the patient. The initial encounter is coded as a consultation, and the documentation must support the encounter. A letter should accompany the patient seeing a consulting physician, and the advising physician should send a letter back to the patient's primary physician outlining the findings. If the consulting physician takes over part or all of the patient's care, follow-up or subsequent visits are coded as regular subsequent visits. A confirmatory consultation is considered a second opinion, and the physician should offer only an opinion or advice. A confirmatory consultant does not take over the treatment of the patient. A referral is defined as passing on a patient to another physician. Referrals are coded as new patients, not consultations. Consider this scenario: A 17-year-old girl sees her family physician for recurrent sore throats. When the family physician realizes that the girl probably needs a tonsillectomy, the patient is *referred* to an otorhinolaryngologist for evaluation and possible surgery. The patient has been referred to the surgeon, who will take over that part of her care. When she has recovered from the procedure, she is discharged from the care of the surgeon and returns to her family physician for continued care.

In another example, a patient may be seen by an orthopedic surgeon for arthritis. When it is determined that the patient's problem may be rheumatoid arthritis, he may be sent to a rheumatologist for consultation. The rheumatologist advises the orthopedic surgeon on a treatment plan, but the orthopedic surgeon continues to see the patient and carries out that plan. Written communications between the two physicians are kept in the chart. The significant difference between a consultation and a referral is whether the patient's treatment is transferred to another physician for that problem.

are anatomic sites, and the codes in each section represent the specific procedure, such as plastic repair of cleft lip. Medical assistants in an anesthesiology practice code anesthesia procedures provided in the hospital setting, even though the office is an outpatient facility.

Two types of **modifiers** (letters or numbers added to a code to add detail to the code) are used in the anesthesia section. One type is the standard modifier that is found in all sections of CPT. The other type is the physical status modifier, a two-digit code beginning with the letter P and ending in a number from 1 to 6. These physical status modifiers indicate the patient's condition at the time of anesthesia and the corresponding complexity of services (e.g., P1 indicates a normal, healthy patient and P5 indicates a patient who is not expected to survive without the procedure).

Surgery Codes

Surgery codes begin with numbers 1 through 6. You need to be aware of the following elements, which are discussed in the guidelines of the surgery section.

Unstarred Codes

The CPT-4 codes in this section that do not have a star (*) refer to codes that include a surgical package. The code that follows identifies the surgical package including normal, uncomplicated follow-up care. The surgical package means that local infiltration, metacarpal, metatarsal, or digital block or topical anesthesia, the operation itself, and normal uncomplicated follow-up care are all included in the code that covers the operation itself.

If there is no star next to the code, it means that you cannot bill separately for preoperative and postoperative components.

The Centers for Medicare & Medicaid Services (CMS) has defined the surgical package for Medicare recipients somewhat differently. According to CPT-4, no complications or problems related to the surgery are included in the surgical package. If additional procedures are performed to correct or alleviate these problems, they should be coded separately. According to CMS, however, complications that do not require a revisit to the operating room are included in the price of surgery.

Some insurance carriers have a set number of follow-up days that is consistent for all unstarred surgical services. Check with your carrier to learn what these are so you can bill for the additional office, outpatient, or hospital visits.

Starred Codes

Codes with a star (*) are for the surgical service itself. The surgical package does not apply. You should code any preoperative anesthesia and postoperative components separately. Figure 11-1 includes several starred codes, for example, of repair—simple superficial wounds of scalp, neck, axilla, external genitalia, and so forth:

12001*—2.5 cm or less
12002*—2.6 cm to 7.5 cm
12004*—7.6 cm to 12.5 cm
12005—12.6 cm to 20.10 cm (notice no star)

If a patient came in for routine follow-up care of a scalp wound coded 12001, 12002, or 12004, the coder could also code for both office visits (99212). There is a corresponding fee for this service. If, however, the patient was returning for routine follow-up care for a wound repair that was originally coded 12005, the code 99024 (postoperative follow-up visit) could be used, but there is no charge for this because the service was already included in the surgical package. Remember, 12005 is not a starred procedure. Third-party payers have different rules about what constitutes a surgery package, so the coder must check with the relevant third-party payers.

Integumentary System

This section has codes for which a measurement is necessary. It is important that both the size of the defect and the size of the specimen be measured before they are sent to the laboratory. All excisions listed in the integumentary section include simple closure.

Repairs

CPT-4 defines three types of repairs: simple, intermediate, and complex. Repairs should be measured and recorded in centimeters to be coded appropriately.

Cast Reapplication

You cannot assign the same code for cast replacement as you did for the original cast application because the code for replacement does not include treatment of the fracture, as the original cast application code did; it, therefore, carries a lower reimbursement rate.

Multiple Procedures Furnished on the Same Day

Unless these are part of the overall service, they should be coded separately and placed on the claims form in order from major to minor.

Checkpoint Question

2. What items are included in a surgical package?

Radiology Codes

The radiology section of CPT-4 is divided into the following four subsections:

- Diagnostic radiology/diagnostic imaging
- Diagnostic ultrasound
- Radiation oncology
- Nuclear medicine

WHAT IF

You need help coding a chart. What should you do?

If you have a question about coding, never guess; find the correct answer. For example, you can ask colleagues, the office manager, or the physician. Insurance companies may have a help line. If you are a member of a professional health care organization, network with fellow members. The American Medical Association (AMA) publishes various books to assist in ICD and CPT coding. The AMA also has a magazine, *CPT Assistant*, that is written by CPT experts. It contains many articles designed to make coding easier. In addition, this magazine will keep you current with updates and changes. For further information on the *CPT Assistant* or other works the AMA publishes on coding, call 800-621-8335 or visit the website at www.amapress.org.

All radiology codes are five-digit numbers that begin with 7. They are generally arranged by anatomic site, from the top of the body to the bottom. Many radiology codes indicate the number of views for a particular study. Obviously, the facility must be reimbursed for film, developer, and the radiology technologist's time and service.

Some radiological tests require the administration of a contrast medium that enhances the image. The descriptors for such tests specify "with contrast" or "without contrast." "With contrast" refers to contrast medium that is given intravascularly. If the contrast medium is given orally or rectally, you use the code "without contrast."

If a physician performs the procedure and supervises and interprets a procedure (e.g., injects contrast medium and then supervises and interprets), two codes should be used. A written report in the patient's medical record is necessary for billing these codes. The code for the procedure can be found in the surgery, medicine, or radiology section, and the code for supervision and interpretation is found in the radiology section. If two physicians are participating (e.g., a surgeon and radiologist), the radiology portion is billed by the radiologist.

Pathology and Laboratory Codes

All codes in pathology and laboratory work are five-digit numbers that begin with 8. These codes are divided into sections for panels of tests, drug testing, consultations with pathologists, urinalysis, chemistry testing, antibody testing, cytopathology, and so on. The last part of the pathology and laboratory section includes services and procedures provided by a pathologist, including gross (can be seen by the naked eye) and microscopic examination of tissue removed in surgery. Each tissue specimen is submitted under a different identifying code for diagnosis by the pathologist. The codes represent the level of the physician's work. Postmortem examination or autopsy is performed by a pathologist, and CPT-4 provides codes to report such examinations.

A subsection, automated multichannel tests, deserves a special note. When coding, check that the tests performed are included in the lists under this subsection. For example, the physician may perform the following three tests for a patient: bilirubin, direct; cholesterol; and blood urea nitrogen (BUN). To code this, you assign the code 80003, three clinical chemistry tests, because all of these tests are listed under the automated multichannel test subsection. If the tests performed were bilirubin, direct; cholesterol; and blood acetaldehyde, however, you would code 80002, two clinical chemistry tests, and 82000, blood acetaldehyde. That is because blood acetaldehyde was not on the list of clinical chemistry tests in the automated multichannel test subsections.

Medicine Codes

Like the E/M codes, medicine codes are five-digit numbers that begin with 9. Like the other five sections of the CPT-4, this section includes guidelines for appropriate coding.

Pay particular attention to the information related to the immunization injections subsection, which includes codes from 90701 to 90749.Typically, immunization injections are given when the patient comes to the physician's office for either a routine physical examination or for a minor problem, such as a sore throat. When the injection is given at the time of such a visit, use two codes: one for the service (usually an E/M code) and one for the immunization injection. For example, an established patient may come into the physician's office for a brief examination for a minor problem (e.g., controlled hypertension blood pressure check). The patient may be examined briefly by a nurse or medical assistant while the physician is in the office and may also be given an immunization for poliomyelitis. The coding for this is:

1. 99211, office and other outpatient visit for the evaluation and management of an established patient, which may not require the presence of a physician. Usually, the presenting problems are minimal. Typically, 5 minutes are spent performing or supervising services. (This code is generally used for examination by employees of the practice while a physician is in the office but not performing the examination.)
2. 90713, poliomyelitis vaccine.

For therapeutic or diagnostic injections (codes 90782–90799), you need to specify what was injected (90281–90399). For example, consider the code 90782, therapeutic injection of medication (specify); subcutaneous or intramuscular. This code is the same for a number of injectable therapeutic substances, making the additional, more specific code necessary. A code for administration should also be added (90471–90472). If a significant separately identifiable E/M service is performed, the appropriate E/M service code should be reported in addition to the injection code.

In Medicare claims, the cost of administering injections is included in the price of office and outpatient visits and other procedures furnished on the same day. Supplying the drug is a separate billable service, however, and should be assigned the appropriate code. (This may not be true of other carriers, so you need to check with them.)

Using the most specific codes for different injectable substances and supplies while keeping invoices to document actual cost helps verify charges submitted for these services.

The medicine section also includes cardiac diagnostic testing, such as electrocardiography and echocardiography. This section also lists the codes for performing cardiopulmonary resuscitation and dialysis treatment.

Checkpoint Question

3. A patient comes in for a tetanus booster, and the physician gives the booster and completes a routine physical examination. How many codes do you use for this visit?

CPT-4 Modifiers

CPT-4 provides a way to give additional information about a procedure through the use of additional numbers called modifiers.

There are several ways to write modifiers:

- Write the five-digit code with a hyphen followed by the two-digit modifier (e.g., 28702-22).
- Write the code without a hyphen separating it from the modifier (e.g., 2870222).
- Write the five-digit code that needs multiple modifiers with the first modifier as −99 (multiple modifiers), followed by the additional modifiers (e.g 28702-9922 . . .)

Of course, the modifier can never appear on the claim form by itself because it refers to the procedure and must be directly below it on the claim form (Fig. 11-2).

Box 11-2 provides a few examples of modifiers. A separate listing of available modifiers can be found in Appendix A of CPT-4. Check Appendix A first; then go to the appropriate section to verify that the modifier may be used with the specific CPT code. Failure to use an appropriate modifier causes database and billing errors.

Checkpoint Question

4. Where can a coder find a list of all CPT modifiers?

Box 11-2

EXAMPLES OF CPT-4 MODIFIERS

Here are just a few examples of CPT-4 modifiers. A complete list can be found in Appendix A of CPT-4.

- *20 microsurgery or 09920:* This modifier signifies that the surgeon used an operating microscope to perform a procedure.
- *23 unusual anesthesia or 09923:* This modifier signifies that anesthesia was used in a procedure that normally would not require it.
- *26 professional component or 09926:* This modifier signifies that there are two components to the procedure, a professional and a technical one. For example, when a physician requests a radiograph, the radiology technologist takes the radiograph and the physician reads it. This modifier lets the insurance carrier know that the physician did not provide both service components.

HEALTHCARE COMMON PROCEDURE CODING SYSTEM

Because the AMA's CPT-4 codes do not include such items as ambulance service, wheelchairs, or injections, CMS designed another coding system based on the CPT-4. This system is referred to as the **Healthcare Common Procedure Coding System** or HCPCS.

The HCPCS uses codes contained in CPT-4 (now known as HCPCS Level 1) plus expanded codes developed by CMS and fiscal intermediaries to classify physician and nonphysician patient care services on the national level (now known as HCPCS Level 2). Level 2 HCPCS codes are most commonly referred to as the HCPCS codes, and Level 1 HCPCS codes are referred to as CPT. Since 1985, physicians have had to use the HCPCS to bill for services provided to Medicare patients either in the medical office or in the hospital. Since October 1986, physicians also have used the HCPCS to bill for services provided to Medicaid patients.

As of July 1, 1987, federal law requires hospitals to use the HCPCS to report outpatient surgery services to patients receiving health benefits sponsored by the federal government. By October 1, 1987, federal law had extended ambulatory surgical center (ASC) prospective payment methodology to hospital outpatient surgery payments. The purpose of this was twofold:

- To permit identification of ASC procedures so a blended payment rate could be applied to ambulatory surgery performed in the hospital outpatient department
- To provide a database for future payment amounts for all hospital outpatient services

The HCPCS includes three levels of codes, discussed in the following sections.

HCPCS Level 1 Codes

The HCPCS Level 1 codes are in CPT-4. This is a listing of terms and codes that provide a means to report physician procedures and services under both private and government-sponsored health insurance programs.

HCPCS Level 2 Codes: National Codes

The HCPCS Level 2 code listing comes out once a year in the *National Coding Manual*, which can be ordered from the American Hospital Association, American Medical Association, or other publishers of the CPT coding book. It includes codes for the following:

- Chemotherapeutic drugs
- Dental services
- Durable medical equipment
- Injections
- Ophthalmology services
- Orthotics
- Some pathology and laboratory and rehabilitation supplies
- Vision care

National codes are five-digit alphanumeric codes that begin with the letters A to V (e.g., L8100 is elastic support, elastic stocking, below knee, medium weight, each).

HCPCS Level 3 Codes: Local Codes

The HCPCS Level 3 codes were developed to address regional coding—the ability to code something performed or offered in one state that may or may not be performed or offered in another state. These codes, which are produced and made available through your state Medicare carrier, may vary from state to state. Local codes begin with letters W to Z. CMS takes full responsibility for the codes in the *National Coding Manual*, leaving local codes up to Medicare carriers in each state.

Checkpoint Question

5. Where do you find codes for dental services?

REIMBURSEMENT

Diagnostic Related Groups

Diagnostic related groups (DRGs) are categories into which inpatients are placed according to the similarity of their diagnoses, treatment, and length of hospital stay. Initially, these categories were developed by Yale University researchers in the mid 1970s to aid the process of utilization review. Some 13,000 codes were run through a computer and grouped according to their clinical similarities (including similarities in resources used). Today, DRGs are used to determine reimbursement for Medicare patients' inpatient services. The fee attached to each DRG is based on the national average of all Medicare discharges and is adjusted for regional differences in hospital wages and updates. Hospitals are paid a set amount for each DRG regardless of actual costs for treating the patient. For example, if a hospital uses fewer resources to care for a patient and discharges that patient in less time, it may keep the difference between its actual cost and the DRG payment. Conversely, if the patient stays longer than usual and requires more services, the hospital absorbs the loss. A patient who has an unusually long stay or a complicated case is considered an outlier, and the hospital may be paid more than the standard DRG rate if the added expenses can be justified.The hospital coder uses ICD-9-CM codes to pick the appropriate DRG. The more information the hospital has prior to admission, the more accurate the coding; for example, for a patient admitted with chest pain, the hospital coder needs to know that the patient also has hypertension and diabetes.

You may be asked to schedule a patient for admission to the hospital. Assigning the correct ICD-9-CM code from the outpatient practice will influence the DRG to which the patient will be assigned. The hospital coder selects the proper DRG based on these factors:

- Principal diagnosis
- Surgeries
- Complications and comorbid conditions

Physicians can help with coding in thc following ways:

- Record the appropriate documentation to identify each patient's problems, complaints, or other reasons for the encounter or visit.
- Work with the medical records or the office coding and billing staffs to determine the proper diagnosis to code, using terminology that includes specific diagnoses, symptoms, problems, or reasons for the encounter (ICD-9-CM codes describe all of these).

Resource-Based Relative Value Scale

As part of the 1989 Omnibus Budget Reconciliation Act (OBRA), the U. S. Congress stipulated that reimbursement to physicians for Medicare services is based on a fee schedule. This fee schedule sets a maximal fee for each service based on the **resource-based relative value scale** (RBRVS). The goal of RBRVS is to reduce Medicare Part B costs and to establish national standards for payment based on CPT-4 codes. (Remember, Part B Medicare covers physicians' services; Part A covers hospital expenses.)

Fee calculations are based on the following factors:

- Intensity of the service
- Time required
- Skills needed
- Overhead expenses
- Malpractice premiums

The particular fee is adjusted by a geographical practice cost index (GPCI), which reflects the difference in health care costs in different parts of the country. These determine the relative value unit (RVU). Finally, a national conversion factor is assigned yearly. The formula looks like this:, CPT code 99205 has an RVU of 4.58, and the national conversion factor is 36.7856. The Medicare allowed charge would be $168.48.

Checkpoint Question

6. Why are DRGs used?

FRAUD AND CODING

Billing for services not performed, using another patient's coverage to receive reimbursement, and falsifying records are examples of blatant fraud. The attorney general of the United States has jurisdiction over such cases, and in most states the Office of the Inspector General investigates reports of possible fraud. Less severe and undeliberate fraudulent practices also cause misuse of health care dollars, and CMS remains vigilant by conducting audits. Even though the physician you work for may already have been paid for a claim, the medical office may still be audited. As a federal program, Medicare has the same authority as the Internal Revenue Service to audit claims and may do so retroactively. This means that an audit can occur even a couple of years after payment has been received for claims. If the medical

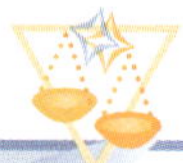

LEGAL TIP

When submitting Medicare or other insurance claims, do not bill for services the physician has not performed, and do not bill more for a service than it is worth. Billing high is called **upcoding**.

Millions of dollars have been budgeted to investigate fraud and abuse. Fiscal intermediaries (organizations under contract with the U. S. government to handle Medicare claims) randomly review and compare the documentation in the record and report their findings on the particular providers. Peer review organizations have been authorized by CMS to obtain medical records of Medicare beneficiaries for review.

practice is found to be in error, the physician may be required to repay an amount owed plus interest. Even worse, such errors can jeopardize the physician's ability to participate in Medicare-funded programs. To avoid costly errors, be certain that you can justify your coding:

- Keep adequate, accurate, and complete documentation in medical and billing records.
- Use the proper tools to code. Code books are updated yearly. Always use the most recent book.
- Follow the coding rules, becoming familiar with new rules and keeping up-to-date on any changes to existing ones. Medicare has regional updates, usually at no charge, and provides one of the best sources of changes.
- Work closely with the provider, and never code anything about which you are not sure.

SUMMARY

Medical coding involves the use of numbers to describe diseases, injuries, and procedures. It has several purposes, including indexing medical records, performing medical care reviews, deriving health statistics, and reimbursing physicians and hospitals for services. As a medical assistant, you are responsible for knowing the format and usage of CPT-4, the system used to report services and procedures by the physician. Accurate and thorough coding is essential to ensure appropriate reimbursement. You must assist the physician in making sure the proper documentation is available to substantiate the codes used on a claim. Because learning to code is an ongoing process, continuing education is vital. This can be accomplished by attending workshops in your geographic area or by joining a local association of coders, which may also sponsor coding clinics. Two such organizations are the American Academy of Professional Coders (AAPC) and the American Health Information Management Association (AHIMA). Other sources are local medical societies and your school. As in all other aspects of patient contact and care, coding of patients' records is covered by the Health Insurance Portability and Accountability Act of 1996 (HIPAA). Only those with a need to know should have access to patient records.

Critical Thinking Challenges

1. How would you handle a physician who you think overbills for procedures? To whom would you report this? How might you collect documentation of fraud?
2. Create a reminder card to be used when you are to assist with coding.
3. Assume you are working for a family practice physician. Identify three patient problems that you might encounter. Then use the CPT and ICD-9-CM coding books at your school library or the hospital library to find the correct codes.

Answers to Checkpoint Questions

1. The three key elements are history, physical examination, and medical decision making.
2. The surgical package consists of local infiltration, metacarpal, metatarsal, or digital blocks, topical anesthesia, the operation, and normal uncomplicated follow-up care.
3. There are two codes: one for the service and one for the immunization.
4. A list of all modifiers and their meanings is found in Appendix A of CPT-4.
5. Dental codes are found in the HCPCS Level 2 national codes.
6. DRGs are used to determine the reimbursement for Medicare patients' inpatient services.

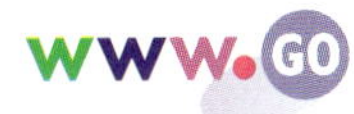

Websites

Coding Institute
 www.codinstitute.com

Compliant Billing Service
 www.compliantbilling.com

Medical Billing Association
 www.e-medbill.com

GLOSSARY OF KEY TERMS

A

accounting cycle a consecutive 12-month period for financial record keeping following either a fiscal year (starting on a specified date) or the calendar year (January to December).

accounts payable a record of all monies owed.

accounts receivable a record of all monies due.

acute abrupt in onset

adjustments changes in a posted account.

advance beneficiary notice document that informs covered patients that Medicare may not cover a certain service and the patient will be responsible for the bill.

agenda a brief outline of the topics to be discussed at a meeting.

aging schedule a form used to track outstanding balances.

Americans with Disabilities Act (ADA) a law designed to meet the needs of people with physical and mental challenges.

analogue pertains to use of dictation machine with a hand-held microphone to tape a report of a patient encounter or other correspondence.

annotation the process of reading, highlighting and summarizing a document for another person.

assignment of benefits transfer of the patient's legal right to collect third-party benefits for medical expenses to the provider of the services.

attitude a state of mind; how a person feels about a given subject or at a given time.

audit inspection of records to determine compliance and to detect fraud.

B

balance equality between the debit and credit sides of an accounting equation; that which is left over after additions and subtractions have been made to an account; remainder; amount due.

balance billing billing the patient for the balance or difference between the physician's charges and the Medicare-approved charges; prohibited by most managed care contracts.

BiCaps words or phrases with unusual capitalization.

birthday rule determination of which policyholder's insurance is the first to pay when a patient is covered by two policies. The policyholder whose birth month and day comes first in the calendar is primary.

block a type of letter format in which the date, subject line, closing and signatures are to the right margin; all other lines are justified left.

bookkeeping organized and accurate record keeping for financial transactions.

budget financial planning tool that helps an organization estimate its anticipated expenditures and revenues.

buffer extra time to accommodate emergencies, walk-ins, and other demands on the provider's daily time schedule that are not considered direct patient care

C

capitation managed care plan that pays a certain amount to a provider over a specific time for caring for the patients in the plan regardless of what or how many services are performed.

carrier person infected with a microorganism but without signs of disease; a company that assumes the risk of an insurance company.

charge slip a preprinted three-part form that can be placed on a day sheet to record the patient's charges and payments along with other information in an encounter form.

check register place to record checks that have been written.

check stub indicates to whom a check was issued, in what amount, and on what date.

chronic long-standing.

claims requests to an insurance company for reimbursement of costs.

claims administrator an individual who manages the third-party reimbursement policies for a medical practice.

closed captioning printed words displayed on a television screen to help people with hearing disabilities or impairments.

clustering grouping patients with similar problems or needs.

coinsurance the agreed-upon amount paid to the provider by a policyholder. Also called co-payment.

collection a process of acquiring funds that are due.

compliance officer person charged with ensuring that a facility follows laws, policies, and protocols.

constellation of symptoms a group of clinical signs indicating a particular disease process.

consultation request for assistance from one physician to another.

conventions general notes, symbols, typeface, format, and punctuation that direct and guide the coder to the most complete and accurate ICD-9 code.

coordination of benefits the method of designating the order in which multiple carriers pay benefits to avoid duplication of payment.

co-payments that part of an insured service the patient must pay.

credit balance in one's favor on an account; promise to pay a bill at a later date; record of a payment received.

crossover claim a claim that crosses over automatically from one coverage to another for payment.

cross-reference a note that tells the reader to look for additional information in another place

Current Procedural Terminology (CPT) a comprehensive list of codes used by physicians to bill for

D

day sheet/daily journal a daily business record of charges and payments.

debit a charge or money owed on an account.

deductible a specified amount paid by the policyholder before the carrier begins paying.

dependent spouse, children, and sometimes other individuals designated by the insured who are covered under a health care plan.

descriptor description of a service listed with its code number.

diagnostic related group (DRG) categories used to determine hospital and physician reimbursement for Medicare patients' inpatient services.

diction the style of speaking and enunciating words.

digital pertaining to, resembling, or performed with a finger; expressed in digits (0–9).

diplomacy the art of handling people with tact and genuine concern.

double booking the practice of booking two patients for the same period with the same physician

E

E-codes codes indicating the external cause or reason for an injury or illness.

eligibility the determination of an insured's right to receive benefits from a third-party payer based on such criteria as payment of premiums and date of start of coverage.

emergency medical service (EMS) a group of health care providers working as a team to care for sick or injured patients before they arrive at the hospital.

employee a person hired to perform given duties in return for financial compensation.

enclosure indication for the reader that an item is accompanying the letter.

encounter form a preprinted statement that lists codes for basic office charges and has sections to record charges incurred in an office visit, the patient's current balance, and next appointment.

eponym word derived from a personal name, e.g., Alzheimer disease.

ergonomic describes a workstation designed to prevent work-related injuries and to promote work efficiency.

etiology cause of disease.

explanation of benefits (EOB) a statement that accompanies a payment from an insurance carrier and outlines which dates and services are being paid.

F

Family and Medical Leave Act a law designed to allow an employee up to 12 weeks of unpaid leave from his or her job to meet family needs.

federal unemployment tax tax is used to finance all administrative expenses of the federal/state unemployment insurance system and the federal costs involved in extended benefits.

fee-for-service an established set of fees charged for specific services and paid by the patient or insurance carrier.

fee schedule a list of preestablished fee allowances set for specific services and procedures performed by a provider.

FICA Federal Insurance Contributions Act; the law that established Social Security and that mandates Social Security tax payments and benefits.

font a typeface; affects the way written messages look.

full block a type of letter format in which all letter components are justified left.

G

gross income the amount of money earned by an employee before taxes are withheld.

group member a policyholder who is a member of a group and covered by the group's insurance carrier.

H

health maintenance organization (HMO) an organization that provides a wide range of services through a contract with a specified group at a predetermined payment.

Healthcare Common Procedure Coding System AMA's coding system based on CPT-4; assigns alphabetic and numeric codes to items such as ambulance service, wheelchairs, and injections.

I

independent practice association (IPA) several independently practicing physicians contracted with a health maintenance organization to provide services to HMO members.

inpatient a medical setting in which patients are admitted for diagnostic, radiographic, or treatment purposes.

installment partial payment of a bill.

insurance a policy that promises to pay some or all of a customer's medical bills.

insured an individual who owns a policy that promises to pay some or all of his or her medical bills.

intercaps words or phrases with unusual capitalization.

Internal Revenue Service (IRS) a federal agency that regulates and enforces various taxes.

International Classification of Diseases (ICD) a classification system used to assign a numerical code to a disease.

International Classification of Diseases, Ninth Revision, Clinical Modification a system for transforming verbal descriptions of disease, injuries, conditions, and procedures to numeric codes.

invoice a statement of debt owed; a bill.

J

job description a statement that informs an employee about the duties and expectations for a given job.

K

key component the criteria or factors on which the selection of a CPT-4 evaluation and management is based.

L

late effects conditions that result from another condition. For example, left-sided paralysis may be a late effect of a stroke.

ledger card a record of the patient's financial activities.

liabilities amounts the practice owes.

M

main terms words in a multiple-word diagnosis that a coder should locate in the alphabetic listing. They represent the condition (not the location) to be coded.

managed care the practice of third-party payers to control costs by requiring physicians to adhere to specific rules as a condition of payment.

margin the blank space around the edges of a piece of paper, such as a letter or page of a book.

matrix a system for blocking off unavailable patient appointment times.

medical necessity a determination made by a third party that a certain service or procedure was necessary based on sound medical practice.

Medicare Social Security–established health insurance for the elderly.

memorandum a type of written documentation used for interoffice communication.

mission statement a statement describing the goals of the medical office and those it serves.

modifiers letters or numbers added to a code to clarify the service or procedure.

N

net pay the amount of money an employee is paid after all taxes are withheld.

O

organizational chart a flow sheet depicting the members of a team in a structured or hierarchical manner.

outlier a patient whose hospital stay is longer than allowed by the DRG.

outpatient a medical setting in which patients receive care but are not admitted.

P

packing slip a document that accompanies a supply order and lists the enclosed items.

participating providers those who agree to participate with managed care contracts and other third-party payers in exchange for building a solid patient base.

patient co-payment the part of an insured service that the patient must pay.

payroll the process of calculating employee salary.

payroll journal a method for keeping track of payroll data using the pegboard system.

peer review organization a group of physicians and specialists that conducts a review of a disputed case and makes a final recommendation.

physician hospital organization a coalition of physicians and a hospital contracting with large employers, insurance carriers, and other benefits groups to provide discounted health services.

plan maximum the highest amount paid by a third-party payer for any given service.

policy a statement that reflects the organization's rules on a given topic.

posting listing financial transactions in a ledger.

precertification approved documentation prior to referrals to specialists and other facilities

preexisting condition medical problem treated by a physician before an insurance plan's effective date. A third-party payer may exclude coverage for preexisting conditions.

preferred provider organization (PPO) an organization whose purpose is to contract with providers, then lease this network of contracted providers to health care plans.

primary diagnosis the condition or chief complaint that brings a person to a medical facility for treatment.

procedure a series of steps required to perform a given task; a medical service or test that is coded for reimbursement.

professional courtesy a discount fee given to healthcare professionals.

profit-and-loss statement statement of income and expenditures; shows whether in a given period a business made or lost money and how much.

proofread read the written draft for accuracy and clarity and correct errors.

providers a health care worker who delivers medical care.

purchase order a document that lists the required items to be purchased.

R

receptionist a person who greets patients as they arrive at a medical office and performs various administrative tasks.

referral instruction to transfer a patient's care to a specialist

resource-based relative value scale (RBRVS) a value scale designed to decrease Medicare Part B costs and establish national standards for coding and payment.

returned check fee amount of money a bank or business charges for a check written with insufficient funds.

S

salutation an introductory phrase that greets the reader of a letter.

semiblock a type of letter format that is styled the same as block, except the first sentence of each paragraph is indented five spaces.

service medical interventions completed by a provider.

service charge a charge by a bank for various services.

specificity relating to a definite result.

STAT immediately.

streaming a method of allotting time for appointments based on the needs of the individual patient to minimize gaps in time and backups

summation report any report that provides a summary of activities, such as a payroll report or a profit-and-loss statement.

T

teletypewriter (TTY) a special machine that allows communication on a telephone with a hearing-impaired person.

template a skeleton of a letter or document with preset and prespaced elements.

third-party administrator administrator who processes claims for the sponsor of self-funded benefit planning.

tickler file a file that provides a reminder to do a given task at a particular date and time.

transcription the process of typing a dictated message.

triage sorting of patients into categories based on their level of sickness or injury; to ensure that life-threatening medical conditions are treated immediately.

U

unbundling the practice of submitting a claim with several separate procedure codes rather than a single code that represents the services performed.

upcoding billing more for a patient care service than it is worth by selecting a code that is higher on the coding scale; this is an illegal practice.

usual, customary, and reasonable (UCR) the basis of a physician's fee schedule, the usual and customary cost of the same service or procedure in a similar geographic area and under the same or similar circumstances.

utilization review an analysis of individual cases by a committee to make sure services and procedures being billed to a third-party payer are medically necessary and to ensure compliance with its rules and regulations regarding reimbursement.

V

V-codes codes assigned to patients who receive service but have no illness, injury, or disorder, e.g., a vaccination or a screening mammogram.

W

wave scheduling system a flexible scheduling method that allows time for procedures of varying lengths and the addition of unscheduled patients, as needed.

withholding not initiating certain medical treatments.

write-off cancellation of an unpaid debt.

INDEX

Page numbers followed by a "f" indicate figures, those followed by a "t" indicate tables, those followed by a "b" indicate boxes, those followed by a "p" indicate procedures.

1

The First Contact: Telephone and Reception

CHAPTER COMPETENCIES

Review the information in your text that supports the following course objectives.

Learning Objectives

In this chapter, you'll learn:

1. To spell and define the key terms.
2. To explain the importance of displaying a professional image to all patients.
3. To list six duties of the medical office receptionist.
4. To list four sources from which messages can be retrieved.
5. To discuss various steps that can be taken to promote good ergonomics.
6. To describe the basic guidelines for waiting room environments.
7. To describe the proper method for maintaining infection control standards in the waiting room.
8. To discuss the five basic guidelines for telephone use.
9. To describe the types of incoming telephone calls received by the medical office.
10. To describe how to triage incoming calls.
11. To discuss how to identify and handle callers with medical emergencies.
12. To list the information that should be given to an emergency medical service dispatcher.
13. To describe the types of telephone services and special features.

CHAPTER OUTLINE	NOTES
Professional Image	
Importance of a Good Attitude	
The Medical Assistant as a Role Model	
Courtesy and Diplomacy in the Medical Office	
First Impressions	
Reception	
Definition of a Receptionist	
Duties and Responsibilities of the Receptionist	
Prepare the Office	
Retrieve Messages	
Prepare the Charts	
Welcome Patients and Visitors	
Register and Orient Patients	
Manage Waiting Time	

CHAPTER OUTLINE *continued*	NOTES
Ergonomics Concerns for the Receptionist	
The Waiting Room Environment	
General Guidelines for Waiting Rooms	
Guidelines for Pediatric Waiting Rooms	
Americans with Disabilities Act Requirements	
Infection Control Issues	
The End of the Patient Visit	
Telephone	
Importance of the Telephone in the Medical Office	
Basic Guidelines for Telephone Use	
Diction	
Pronunciation	
Expression	
Listening	
Courtesy	
Routine Incoming Calls	
Appointments	
Billing Inquires	
Diagnostic Test Results	
Routine and Satisfactory Progress Reports	
Test Results	
Unsatisfactory Progress Reports and Test Results	
Prescription Refills	
Other Calls	
Challenging Incoming Calls	
Unidentified Callers	
Irate Patients	
Medical Emergencies	
Triaging Incoming Calls	
Taking Messages	
Outgoing Calls	
General Guidelines for Outgoing Calls	
Calling Emergency Medical Services	
Services and Special Features	
Telecommunication Relay Systems	

LEARNING SELF-ASSESSMENT EXERCISES

Key Terms

Define the following key terms:

attitude ______________________________

closed captioning ______________________________

diction ______________________________

diplomacy ______________________________

emergency medical service (EMS) ______________________________

ergonomic ______________________________

receptionist ______________________________

teletypewriter (TTY) ______________________________

triage ______________________________

Matching

Match the phrase in part 1 with its association in part 2.

PART 1	PART 2
_____ 1. Acting as a role model	a. Personal appearance
_____ 2. Speak clearly	b. Confidentiality
_____ 3. Positive expression	c. Nonjudgmental
_____ 4. Listen attentively	d. Courtesy and diplomacy
_____ 5. Well-managed waiting time	e. Conversation focused
_____ 6. Fundamental to successful human relations	f. Pronunciation
_____ 7. Patient information not divulged	g. Keep patient informed
_____ 8. Acceptance of the patient as a unique individual	h. Friendly attitude

Multiple Choice

1. How you feel influences how you act; therefore
   a. Attitude shapes behavior
   b. Behavior shapes attitude
   c. Feelings do not affect attitude
   d. None of the above
2. Which of the following items of jewelry should not be worn by the medical professional?
   a. Small stud earrings
   b. Wedding rings
   c. Dangling earrings
   d. All of the above
3. Each morning the medical receptionist should
   a. Make coffee
   b. Review the appointment schedule
   c. Prepare charts
   d. *b* and *c* only
4. The patient registration may be completed
   a. During the interview with the patient
   b. After the patient leaves
   c. Over the telephone
   d. None of the above

5. Office policies and procedures may include
   a. How the bill will be paid
   b. When the bill will be paid
   c. Who will pay the bill
   d. *a* and *b* only

6. Preferred medical office color schemes are
   a. Primary colors
   b. Muted colors
   c. Bright colors
   d. Dark colors

7. The use of sofas in a medical office is
   a. Comfortable
   b. Preferred over chairs
   c. Not recommended
   d. Esthetically pleasing

8. The preferred subjects for artwork for a medical office are
   a. Abstract
   b. Floral
   c. Landscapes
   d. *b* and *c* only

9. Most pediatricians' offices have
   a. A children's play area
   b. One large waiting area
   c. Separate areas for sick and well children
   d. *a* and *c* only

10. When speaking on the phone, *never*
    a. Chew gum
    b. Prop the headset on your shoulder
    c. Speak rapidly
    d. All of the above

2 Managing Appointments

CHAPTER COMPETENCIES

Review the information in your text that supports the following course objectives.

Learning Objectives

In this chapter, you'll learn:

1. To spell and define the key terms.
2. To describe the various systems for scheduling patient office visits, including manual and computerized scheduling.
3. To identify the factors that affect appointment scheduling.
4. To explain guidelines for scheduling appointments for new patients and return visits.
5. To list three ways to remind patients about appointments.
6. To describe how to triage patient emergencies, acutely ill patients, and walk-in patients.
7. To describe how to handle late patients and patients who miss their appointments.
8. To explain what to do if the physician is delayed.
9. To describe how to handle appointment cancellations made by the office or by the patient.
10. To schedule an appointment for a new patient.
11. To schedule a return appointment.
12. To schedule a referral following third-party guidelines.

CHAPTER OUTLINE	NOTES
Appointment Scheduling Systems	
Manual Appointment Scheduling	
The Appointment Book	
Establishing a Matrix	
Computerized Appointment Scheduling	
Types of Scheduling	
Structured Appointments	
Clustering	
Wave and Modified Wave	
Fixed Scheduling	
Streaming	
Double Booking	
Flexible Hours	
Open Hours	

CHAPTER OUTLINE *continued*	NOTES
Factors That Affect Scheduling	
Patients' Needs	
Providers' Preferences and Needs	
Physical Facilities	
Scheduling Guidelines	
New Patients	
Established Patients	
Preparing a Daily or Weekly Schedule	
Patient Reminders	
Appointment Cards	
Telephone Reminders	
Mailed Reminder Cards	
Adapting the Schedule	
Emergencies	
Patients Who Are Acutely Ill	
Walk-in Patients	
Late Patients	
Physician Delays	
Missed Appointments	
Cancellations	
Cancellations by the Office	
Cancellations by the Patient	
Making Appointments for Patients in Other Facilities	
Referrals and Consultations	
Diagnostic Testing	
Surgery	
When the Appointment Schedule Does Not Work	

LEARNING SELF-ASSESSMENT EXERCISES

Key Terms

Define the following key terms:

acute ______________________________

buffer ______________________________

chronic ______________________________

clustering ______________________________

constellation of symptoms ______________________________

consultation ______________________________

double booking ______________________________

matrix ______________________________

precertification ______________________________

providers ______________________________

referral ______________________________

STAT ______________________________

streaming ______________________________

tickler file ______________________________

wave scheduling system ______________________________

Matching

Match the definition in part 1 with the correct term in part 2.

PART 1

_____ 1. Each patient assigned a time

_____ 2. Greater range of appointment times available

_____ 3. Patients taken in order of arrival

_____ 4. More than one patient scheduled in a single time slot

_____ 5. Several patients scheduled in the first half hour and none in the second half-hour

PART 2

a. Double booking

b. Scheduled appointments

c. Wave scheduling system

d. Open scheduling

e. Flexible hours

Multiple Choice

1. Sign-in sheets are
   a. Used by many offices
   b. Legal documents
   c. Subject to subpoena
   d. All of the above

2. Before using the appointment book, you have to set up a
   a. Tickler file
   b. Matrix
   c. Staff schedule
   d. Color code system

3. Computerized scheduling
   a. Saves time
   b. Is time consuming
   c. Is difficult to learn
   d. None of the above

4. Before scheduling an appointment, you should
   a. Talk to the physician
   b. Ask about special transportation
   c. Know whether the patient has seen someone else for the condition
   d. All of the above

5. Office visitors other than patients include
   a. Other physicians
   b. Sales representatives
   c. Personal friends
   d. All of the above

6. Open time slots should be scheduled for any problems that arise. These slots are called
   a. Open time
   b. Flexible time
   c. Open blocks
   d. Flexible blocks

7. The issue of patient confidentiality *must* be considered in which of the following circumstances?
   a. Office sign-in sheets
   b. Home message machines
   c. Postcard appointment reminders
   d. All of the above

8. When making a series of appointments for a patient, it is helpful to
   a. Schedule appointments on the same day of the week
   b. Schedule appointments at the same time of day
   c. Give the patient a card for each visit
   d. *a* and *b* only

9. Preprinted appointment cards should
   a. Never be used
   b. Be used for annual examinations
   c. Include the reason for the visit
   d. Be used for all appointments

10. Patients who are more than 15 minutes late are
    a. Always rescheduled
    b. Always seen immediately
    c. Asked to explain
    d. Informed that they may have to wait

3 Written Communications

CHAPTER COMPETENCIES

Review the information in your text that supports the following course objectives.

Learning Objectives

In this chapter, you'll learn:

1. To spell and define the key terms.
2. To discuss the basic guidelines for grammar, punctuation, and spelling.
3. To describe six key guidelines for medical writing.
4. To discuss the eleven key components of a business letter.
5. To describe the three steps to writing a business letter.
6. To describe the process of writing a memorandum.
7. To discuss the various mailing options.
8. To identify the types of incoming written communication seen in a physician's office.
9. To list the items that must be included in an agenda.
10. To identify the items that must be included when typing minutes.

Performance Objectives

In this chapter, you'll learn:

1. To write a business letter.
2. To write a memorandum.
3. To address and send written communication.
4. To open and sort mail.

CHAPTER OUTLINE	NOTES
Professional Writing	
Basic Grammar and Punctuation Guidelines	
Basic Spelling Guidelines	
Guidelines for Medical Writing	
Accuracy	
Spelling	
Capitalization	
Abbreviations and Symbols	
Plural and Possessive	
Numbers	
Letter Development	
Components of a Letter	
Letter Formats	
Full Block	

CHAPTER OUTLINE *continued*	NOTES
Block	
Semiblock	
Writing a Business Letter	
Preparation	
Composition	
Editing	
Types of Business Letters	
Memorandum Development	
Components of a Memorandum	
Sending Written Communication	
Facsimile Machines	
Electronic Mail	
United States Postal Service	
Addressing Envelopes	
Affixing Postage	
USPS Mailing Options	
USPS Special Services	
Other Delivery Options	
Receiving and Handling Incoming Mail	
Types of Incoming Mail	
Opening and Sorting Mail	
Annotation	
Composing Agendas and Minutes	

LEARNING SELF-ASSESSMENT EXERCISES

Key Terms

Define the following key terms:

agenda ______________________________

annotation ______________________________

BiCaps ______________________________

block ______________________________

enclosure ______________________________

font ______________________________

full block ______________________________

intercaps ______________________________

margin ______________________________

memorandum ______________________________

proofread ______________________________

salutation ______________________________

semiblock ______________________________

template ______________________________

Matching

Match the definition in part 1 with the correct term in part 2.

PART 1

_____ 1. Greeting of the letter

_____ 2. Something included with a letter

_____ 3. Conclusion of the letter

_____ 4. Indication of who dictated the letter and who wrote it

_____ 5. Most formal format and most commonly used for professional letters

_____ 6. Same as block except first sentence of each paragraph is indented five spaces

_____ 7. Date, subject line, closing, and signature flush with the right margin

PART 2

a. Full block

b. Closing

c. Block

d. Enclosure

e. Identification line

f. Salutation

g. Semiblock

Multiple Choice

1. In letters to a physician, the salutation should
   a. Always be in capital letters
   b. Begin with "Dr."
   c. Be written out with the word "Doctor"
   d. Never use the first name

2. Which of the following items *can* be abbreviated in an inside address?
   a. City
   b. Town
   c. Business title
   d. State

3. The subject line of a letter is
   a. Placed five spaces below the inside address
   b. Mandatory
   c. Used to highlight the intent of a letter
   d. None of the above

4. Which of the following is *not* a step in writing a professional business letter?
   a. Mailing status
   b. Preparation
   c. Editing
   d. Composition

5. Facsimile machines allow transmission of
   a. Orders
   b. Test results
   c. Prescriptions
   d. All of the above

6. Electronic mail, or e-mail, allows for what type of communication?
   a. Computer to computer
   b. Computer to physician
   c. Physician to computer
   d. Physician to physician

7. The standard business envelope (No. 10) is
   a. 4×5 inches
   b. 3.5×5 inches
   c. 4×5.5 inches
   d. 4.125×9.5 inches

8. Which type of mailing option should be used to ensure the delivery of a letter or package by noon the next day?
   a. Priority mail
   b. Express mail
   c. First class mail
   d. Top priority mail

9. Carbon copies of letters are usually sent to
   a. The patient
   b. Managers
   c. The individual who requested that the given information be provided
   d. *b* and *c* only

10. Computer spell checks should be used
    a. With caution
    b. Only once
    c. To check grammar
    d. None of the above

4 Transcription

CHAPTER COMPETENCIES

Review the information in your text that supports the following course objectives.

Learning Objectives

In this chapter, you'll learn:

1. To explain the role of the medical assistant in performing medical transcription.
2. To explain the roles of the JCAHO and HIPAA on medical transcription.
3. To list the various reports generated in inpatient and outpatient medical facilities.
4. To list the rules of medical transcription as outlined by the AAMT.
5. To discuss the various medical transcription systems.

Performance Objectives

In this chapter, you'll learn:

1. To transcribe various medical reports from taped dictation.
2. To use proper punctuation, grammar, and spelling.

CHAPTER OUTLINE	NOTES
Medical Transcription	
The Transcription Process	
Off-site Transcription	
Report Formatting	
Types of Medical Reports	
History and Physical Examination Reports	
Consultation Reports	
Progress Reports	
SOAP Notes	
Hospital Reports	
Operative Report	
Pathology Report	
Autopsy Report	
Radiology Report	
Discharge Summary	
Transcription Rules	
Abbreviations	
Capitalization	

CHAPTER OUTLINE *continued*	NOTES
Numbers	
Punctuation	
Apostrophes	
Commas	
Semicolons	
Colons	
Periods	
Quotation Marks	
Slash Marks	
Hyphens	
Grammar	
Spelling	
Transcription Systems	
Traditional Tape Dictation Systems	
Digital Systems	
Voice Recognition Systems	
Transcription With Word Processing Software	

LEARNING SELF-ASSESSMENT EXERCISES

Key Terms

Define the following key terms:

analogue ____________________

digital ____________________

transcription ____________________

Matching

Match the description in part 1 with the correct term in part 2.

PART 1

_____ 1. Typing a previously dictated message

_____ 2. Controls play, rewind, and fast forward

_____ 3. Used between items in a series

_____ 4. Used after headings

_____ 5. To show titles of articles, short stories, subdivisions, and so on

PART 2

a. Foot pedal

b. Colon

c. Quotation marks

d. Comma

e. Transcription

Multiple Choice

1. When one provider refers a patient to a specialist, what does the consulting physician prepare to report the findings of the encounter?
   a. Outpatient procedural code
   b. Consultation report
   c. Progress report
   d. None of the above

2. Entries in the medical record must be
   a. Neat and in red ink
   b. In chronological order
   c. Progress sheets
   d. Can be on sticky notes

3. Information that cannot be detected or measured is
   a. Chief complaint data
   b. Objective data
   c. History data
   d. Subjective data

4. The patient's appearance, vital signs, rashes, and the results of a urinalysis are all
   a. Chief complaint data
   b. Objective data
   c. History data
   d. Subjective data

5. Hospital reports include all of the following *except*
   a. Consultation reports
   b. Discharge summaries
   c. Pathology reports
   d. Chief complaints

6. Which report outlines the findings of gross and microscopic examinations performed on organs and tissue samples?
   a. Autopsy report
   b. Pathology report
   c. History report
   d. Biopsy report

7. Which of the following is a concise report of the reason for a patient's admission, tests performed, treatments given, results of those treatments and tests, and the condition of the patient when being moved to another facility?
   a. Autopsy report
   b. Discharge summary
   c. Transfer summary
   d. History report

8. Every licensed medical facility is required to keep a list of approved abbreviations that should be updated yearly.
   a. True
   b. False

9. For balance and clarity a zero should be added
   a. Before and after a decimal
   b. Before a decimal
   c. After a decimal
   d. Neither; the number should be spelled out

10. One of the most important skills necessary to be an efficient and productive transcriptionist is the ability to
    a. Speak clearly
    b.Type 120 words per minute
    c. Do more that one transcription at a time
    d. Punctuate without direction

5 Management of the Medical Office Team

CHAPTER COMPETENCIES

Review the information in your text that supports the following course objectives.

Learning Objectives

In this chapter, you'll learn:

1. To spell and define the key terms.
2. To describe what is meant by organizational structure.
3. To list seven responsibilities of the medical office manager.
4. To explain the five staffing issues that a medical office manager will be responsible for handling.
5. To list the types of policies and procedures that should be included in a medical office's policy and procedure manual.
6. To list five types of promotional materials that a medical office may distribute.
7. To discuss three financial concerns that the medical office manager must be capable of addressing.
8. To discuss four legal issues that affect medical office management.

Performance Objectives

In this chapter, you'll learn:

1. To write a job description.
2. To create a policy and procedures manuals.

CHAPTER OUTLINE	NOTES
Overview of Medical Office Management	
Organizational Structure	
The Medical Office Manager	
Responsibilities of the Medical Office Manager	
Communication	
Communicating With Patients	
Communicating With Staff	
Communicating Electronically	
Staffing Issues	
Writing Job Descriptions	
Hiring and Interviewing Employees	
Evaluating Employees	
Taking Disciplinary Action	
Terminating Employees	
Scheduling	

CHAPTER OUTLINE *continued*	NOTES
Policy and Procedures Manuals	
Tips for Writing Personnel Manuals	
Developing Promotional Materials	
Financial Concerns	
Budgets	
Payroll	
Petty Cash	
Maintenance and Inventory of Supplies	
Service Contracts	
Inventory	
Education	
Staff Education	
Patient Education	
Manager Education	
Legal Issues Regarding Office Management	
Americans with Disabilities Act	
Sexual Harassment	
Family and Medical Leave Act	
Other Legal Considerations	

LEARNING SELF-ASSESSMENT EXERCISES

Key Terms

Define the following key terms:

Americans with Disabilities Act ______________________________

budget ______________________________

compliance officer ______________________________

Family and Medical Leave Act ______________________________

job description ______________________________

mission statement ______________________________

organizational chart ______________________________

policy ______________________________

procedure ______________________________

Matching

Match the definition in part 1 with the correct term in part 2.

PART 1

_____ 1. Up to 12 weeks (unpaid) leave to meet family needs

_____ 2. Contains specific rules and regulations regarding laboratory safety

_____ 3. Federal agency that sets standards for employee safety

_____ 4. Private organization that sets standards for health care administration

_____ 5. Regulations designed to meet the needs of people with physical and mental disabilities

_____ 6. Logical system to keep track of supplies

_____ 7. Large outlays of money for equipment, property management, and building maintenance

PART 2

a. Capital budget

b. Inventory

c. ADA

d. OSHA

e. Family and Medical Leave Act

f. CLIA

g. JCAHO

Multiple Choice

1. Staff meetings should
   a. Never be canceled
   b. Never be canceled except in an emergency
   c. Be canceled if there is no quorum
   d. Be canceled if the manager is not present

2. Staffing issues
   a. Take most of the office manager's time
   b. Are delegated to line staff
   c. Are the prerogative of the physician
   d. None of the above

3. Job descriptions
   a. Are written by employees only
   b. Can be written with help of employees
   c. Are never given to employees
   d. Are signed by the manager only

4. Which of the following topics is *not appropriate* on a job application?
   a. Years of experience
   b. Last employer
   c. Schools attended
   d. Physical or mental disabilities

5. Disciplinary actions may be
   a. Written
   b. Verbal
   c. Recorded in the employee's file
   d. All of the above

6. The primary goal of scheduling is to meet the needs of the
   a. Office
   b. Employees
   c. Manager
   d. Patients

7. Requests for time off should
   a. Always be granted
   b. Be in writing
   c. Be received by a given date
   d. All of the above

8. All policies and procedures should be
   a. Signed annually
   b. Reviewed annually
   c. Written annually
   d. *a* and *b* only

9. A practice's mission statement can be
   a. Included in the policy and procedures manual
   b. Framed and placed in the waiting room
   c. Printed in patient instruction booklets
   d. All of the above

10. Developing and writing a budget is done with instructions from
    a. The manager only
    b. The financial officer
    c. The physician
    d. *b* and *c* only

6

Credit and Collections

CHAPTER COMPETENCIES

Review the information in your text that supports the following course objectives.

Learning Objectives

In this chapter, you'll learn:

1. To spell and define the key terms.
2. To explain the physician fee schedule.
3. To discuss forms of payment.
4. To explain the legal considerations in extending credit.
5. To discuss the legal implications of credit collection.
6. To describe three methods of debt collection.

Performance Objectives

In this chapter, you'll learn:

1. To use an aging schedule.
2. To write a collection letter.

CHAPTER OUTLINE	NOTES
Fees	
Fee Schedules	
Discussing Fees in Advance	
Forms of Payment	
Payment by Insurance Companies	
Adjusting Fees	
Credit	
Extending Credit	
Legal Considerations	
Collections	
Legal Considerations	
Collecting a Debt	
Monthly Billings	
Aging Accounts	
Collecting Overdue Accounts	
Collection Alternatives	

LEARNING SELF-ASSESSMENT EXERCISES

Key Terms

Define the following key terms:

adjustment ____________________

aging schedule ____________________

collections ____________________

credit ____________________

installment ____________________

participating provider ____________________

patient co-payment ____________________

professional courtesy ____________________

write-off ____________________

Matching

Match the definition in part 1 with the correct term in part 2.

PART 1

_____ 1. List of unpaid accounts

_____ 2. Allowable unpaid balance on bill

_____ 3. Cancellation of an unpaid debt

_____ 4. Health care professionals are charged a reduced rate

_____ 5. Changes in a posted account

_____ 6. Acquiring funds that are due

PART 2

a. Professional courtesy

b. Aging schedule

c. Write-off

d. Sliding scale fees

e. Adjustments

f. Credit

Multiple Choice

1. Discussion of fees with a patient should be
   a. Done in advance
   b. Done by the physician
   c. In writing
   d. *a* and *c*

2. The fees for a patient new to the practice should be
   a. Reduced
   b. 50% of the usual fee
   c. Collected at the first visit
   d. 80% of the usual fee

3. The patient's insurance card should
   a. Never be copied
   b. Be put in the chart
   c. Be examined once a year
   d. Be copied and the copy put in the chart

4. Interest that may be charged to a patient account is determined by
   a. The physician
   b. The patient
   c. The insurance company
   d. The law

5. Monthly billing statements may be
   a. All sent at the same time
   b. Divided by alphabet
   c. Mailed at different times
   d. All of the above

6. If a billing cycle is to be changed, you are legally required to notify patients
   a. 3 months prior to the billing change
   b. 2 months prior to the billing change
   c. 1 month prior to the billing change
   d. None of the above

7. Aging of an account is calculated from the
   a. First office visit
   b. First date of billing
   c. Date the appointment is scheduled
   d. Procedure date

8. A practice's billing and collection procedures should be reviewed if the aging report shows what portion of fees are being collected 30 days or more after billing?
   a. 20%
   b. 23%
   c. 40%
   d. 50%

9. Fees paid to a medical practice may be paid for by
   a. A third party
   b. The patient
   c. An insurer
   d. Any of the above

10. When credit cards are accepted by a medical practice, the medical practice agrees to pay the credit card company
   a. 5.2%
   b. 1.8%
   c. 2.3%
   d. 3.1%

7

Bookkeeping and Banking

CHAPTER COMPETENCIES

Review the information in your text that supports the following course objectives.

Learning Objectives

In this chapter, you'll learn:

1. To spell and define the key terms.
2. To explain the concept of the pegboard bookkeeping system.
3. To describe the components of the pegboard system.
4. To identify and discuss the special features of the pegboard day sheet.
5. To describe the functions of a computer accounting system.
6. To list the uses and components of computer accounting reports.
7. To explain the services and procedures of the bank.

Performance Objectives

In this chapter, you'll learn:

1. To record financial transactions, such as charges, payments, credits, and adjustments to patient ledger cards.
2. To balance a day sheet.
3. To complete a bank deposit slip and make a deposit.
4. To reconcile a bank statement.
5. To write a check.
6. To maintain a petty cash account.

CHAPTER OUTLINE	NOTES
Daily Bookkeeping	
Manual Accounting	
Pegboard Bookkeeping System	
Day Sheet	
Ledger Cards	
Encounter Forms and Charge Slips	
Posting a Charge	
Posting a Payment	
Posting a Credit	
Posting a Credit Adjustment	
Posting a Debit Adjustment	
Posting to Cash-Paid-Out Section of Day Sheet	
Computer Accounting	
Posting to Computer Accounts	
Computer Accounting Reports	

CHAPTER OUTLINE *continued*	NOTES
Banking	
Banks and Their Services	
Checking Accounts	
Savings Accounts	
Money Market Accounts	
Bank Fees	
Monthly Service Fees	
Overdraft Protection	
Returned Check Fee	
Types of Checks	
Writing Checks for Accounts Payable	
Receiving Checks and Making Deposits	
Reconciling Bank Statements	
Petty Cash	

LEARNING SELF-ASSESSMENT EXERCISES

Key Terms

Define the following key terms:

accounts payable ____________________

accounts receivable ____________________

adjustment ____________________

balance ____________________

bookkeeping ____________________

charge slip ____________________

credit ____________________

day sheet ____________________

debit ____________________

encounter form ____________________

ledger card ____________________

posting ____________________

returned check fee ____________________

service charge ____________________

Matching

Match the definition in part 1 with the correct term in part 2.

PART 1

_____ 1. A book of accounts

_____ 2. Money owed *to* the practice

_____ 3. Money owed *by* the practice

_____ 4. Charge

_____ 5. Payment

_____ 6. Be equal

_____ 7. Indicates name and account number on back of check

_____ 8. Fee charged monthly for using bank account

PART 2

a. Service charge

b. Accounts payable

c. Ledger

d. Credit

e. Accounts receivable

f. Debit

g. Endorse

h. Balance

Multiple Choice

1. In a bookkeeping system, things of value relating to the practice are called
   a. Liabilities
   b. Assets
   c. Debits
   d. Credits

2. The amount of capital the physician has invested in the practice is referred to as
   a. Equity
   b. Credits
   c. Assets
   d. Liabilities

3. If an error is made when posting a charge, you
   a. May erase carefully
   b. Write the word "error" in red
   c. Neatly white-out the error
   d. Draw a single line through the error, then rewrite the transaction

4. A ledger card is a legal document and should be kept for
   a. 10 years
   b. 7 years
   c. 5 years
   d. 1 year

5. Overpayments under $5 are
   a. Sent back to the patient
   b. Placed in petty cash
   c. Left on the account as a credit
   d. Deposited in a special overpayment account

6. Computer bookkeeping systems
   a. Operate as expanded calculators
   b. Are faster than pegboards
   c. Easily generate a variety of reports
   d. All of the above

7. An impress account refers to
   a. Petty cash
   b. A special bank account
   c. Computerized software
   d. Insurance funds

8. Ledger cards are filed
   a. By patient number
   b. Under the physician's name
   c. By time order
   d. Alphabetically

9. In bookkeeping, when brackets are used around a number it means
   a. The same as
   b. The opposite of
   c. An error
   d. A deletion

10. Most facilities request that medical offices write off the balance of an account once it is sent to a collection agency, so that
    a. Books always balance
    b. It complies with tax law on accounts receivable
    c. There is better control
    d. None of the above

8 Accounts Payable and Payroll

CHAPTER COMPETENCIES

Review the information in your text that supports the following course objectives.

LEARNING OBJECTIVES

In this chapter, you'll learn:

1. To spell and define the key terms.
2. To describe the accounting cycle.
3. To describe the components of a record-keeping system.
4. To explain the process of ordering supplies and paying invoices.
5. To discuss the types of payroll records.
6. To explain which taxes are withheld from paychecks.

Performance Objectives

In this chapter, you'll learn:

1. To issue a payroll check, using the pegboard system.
2. To calculate the amount of an employee's payroll check for a given pay period.

CHAPTER OUTLINE	NOTES
Accounting Cycle	
Record-Keeping Components	
Accounts Payable	
Ordering Goods and Services	
Receiving Supplies	
Paying Invoices	
Manual Payment	
Pegboard Payment	
Computer Payment	
Payroll	
Types of Payroll Systems	
Manual Payroll Systems	
Pegboard Payroll Systems	
Computer Payroll Systems	
Employee Records	
Tax Withholdings	
Payment of Taxes	
W-2 Forms	
Preparation of Reports	
Assisting With Audits	

LEARNING SELF-ASSESSMENT EXERCISES

Key Terms

Define the following key terms:

accounting cycle ____________________
audit ____________________
check register ____________________
check stub ____________________
federal unemployment tax ____________________
FICA ____________________
gross income ____________________
Internal Revenue Service (IRS) ____________________
invoice ____________________
liabilities ____________________
net pay ____________________
packing slip ____________________
payroll ____________________
payroll journal ____________________
profit-and-loss statement ____________________
purchase order ____________________
summation report ____________________
withholding ____________________

Matching

Match the definition in part 1 with the correct term in part 2.

PART 1

_____ 1. Reviews of accounts

_____ 2. Back page of each check register

_____ 3. Amount of money earned before taxes

_____ 4. Pay to employees and taxes

_____ 5. Amount of money earned after taxes

_____ 6. Employer pays this for each employee based on the employee's gross income.

_____ 7. Federal and state taxes removed from employee's paycheck

PART 2

a. Payroll journal

b. Unemployment tax

c. Audit

d. Gross income

e. Net pay

f. Tax withholding

g. Payroll

Multiple Choice

1. The Internal Revenue Service examines a business's income statements for the amount of profit and the resulting owed fees
   a. Once per year
   b. Twice per year
   c. Four times per year
   d. None of the above
2. Records such as receipts should be retained for
   a. 5 years
   b. 7 years
   c. 10 years
   d. 2 years
3. It is preferable to pay for supplies by
   a. Check
   b. Cash
   c. Credit card
   d. *a* and *c*
4. A purchase order lists
   a. Supplies ordered
   b. Supply order numbers
   c. Previous purchases
   d. *a* and *b*
5. Bills can be paid
   a. Daily
   b. Weekly
   c. Biweekly
   d. All of the above
6. Corrections on facility checks
   a. May never be done
   b. May be carefully erased
   c. May be crossed out
   d. May be done carefully using Wite-Out
7. Computerized financial data should be recorded
   a. On the hard drive
   b. On a floppy disk
   c. On hard copy
   d. All of the above
8. Biweekly payroll checks are issued
   a. 52 times per year
   b. 26 times per year
   c. 12 times per year
   d. 24 times per year
9. The federally mandated taxes are
   a. Social Security
   b. Medicare
   c. Federal income tax
   d. All of the above
10. The compilation of a business's financial records is called
    a. Bookkeeping
    b. Accounting
    c. Ledger management
    d. Database tracking

9 Health Insurance

CHAPTER COMPETENCIES

Review the information in your text that supports the following course objectives.

Learning Objectives

In this chapter, you'll learn:

1. To spell and define the key terms.
2. To describe group, individual, and government-sponsored (public) health benefits and explain the differences between them.
3. To explain the differences between Medicare and Medicaid.
4. To list the information required on a medical claim form and explain why each piece of information is needed.
5. To name two legal issues affecting claims submissions.
6. To explain how managed care programs work.
7. To explain the differences between health maintenance organizations, preferred provider organizations, and physician hospital organizations.

Performance Objective

In this chapter, you'll learn:

1. To fill out a CMS-1500 claim form.

CHAPTER OUTLINE	NOTES
Health Benefits Plans	
Group Health Benefits	
Individual Health Benefits	
Government-Sponsored (Public) Health Benefits	
Medicare	
Medicaid	
TRICARE/CHAMPVA	
Managed Care	
Health Maintenance Organizations	
Preferred Provider Organizations	
Physician Hospital Organizations	
Other Managed Care Programs	
The Future of Managed Care	
Workers' Compensation	
Filing Claims	
Electronic Claims Submission	
Explanation of Benefits	
Policies in the Practice	

LEARNING SELF-ASSESSMENT EXERCISES

Key Terms

Define the following key terms:

assignment of benefits ______________________________
balance billing ______________________________
birthday rule ______________________________
capitation ______________________________
carrier ______________________________
claims ______________________________
claims administrator ______________________________
coinsurance ______________________________
coordination of benefits ______________________________
co-payments ______________________________
crossover claim ______________________________
deductible ______________________________
dependent ______________________________
eligibility ______________________________
employee ______________________________
explanation of benefits (EOB) ______________________________
fee-for-service ______________________________
fee schedule ______________________________
group member ______________________________
health maintenance organization (HMO) ______________________________
independent practice association (IPA) ______________________________
insurance ______________________________
insured ______________________________
managed care ______________________________
Medicare ______________________________
peer review organization ______________________________
physician hospital organization ______________________________
plan maximum ______________________________
preexisting condition ______________________________
preferred provider organization (PPO) ______________________________
third-party administrator ______________________________
unbundling ______________________________
usual, customary, and reasonable (UCR) ______________________________
utilization review ______________________________

Matching

Match the definition in part 1 with the correct term in part 2.

PART I

_____ 1. Provide medical care for the elderly

_____ 2. Medical program for uniformed services

_____ 3. Government-sponsored program providing health care to low-income individuals

_____ 4. Covers medical expenses for work-related injury or illness

_____ 5. Program administered by the area Veterans Administration

_____ 6. Kaiser Permanente Health Plan

_____ 7. Nongroup physicians organized into entities

PART 2

a. Workers' compensation

b. IPA

c. Medicare

d. HMO

e. CHAMPUS

f. CHAMPVA

g. Medicaid

Multiple Choice

1. Medicaid patients receive a new ID card
   a. Once every 3 months
   b. Once a month
   c. Once a year
   d. Once every 6 weeks

2. Health benefits are commonly referred to as
   a. Insurance
   b. Plans
   c. Insured
   d. Assets

3. Medicare provides benefits for all of the following individuals *except*
   a. Persons with end-stage renal disease
   b. Elderly persons age 65 or older
   c. All injured persons
   d. Disabled persons who have been receiving Social Security benefits for 24 months

4. Persons who are entitled to Social Security
   a. Are automatically enrolled in Medicare Part A
   b. Are automatically enrolled in Medicare Part B
   c. Are automatically enrolled in Medicare Parts A and B
   d. Are not automatically enrolled in Medicare

5. After the deductible has been met, what percentage of the approved charges does Medicare reimburse to the physician?
   a. 70
   b. 80
   c. 90
   d. 20

6. Medicare will accept original claims (no copies) filed on a
   a. CMS-1500
   b. CMA 1500
   c. CSM 1500
   d. HPCA 1500

7. When a patient gives written authorization for an insurance plan to reimburse the physician for billed charges, the patient has
   a. Relinquished benefits
   b. Determined benefits
   c. Assigned benefits
   d. The money sent to himself or herself, not the physician

8. Claims that are submitted electronically
   a. Are more accurate than others
   b. Are not rejected
   c. Cannot be corrected online
   d. Reduce the reimbursement cycle

9. Managed care programs often have a gatekeeper provision. A gatekeeper is
   a. A primary care physician
   b. A specialty physician
   c. A referring physician
   d. Any of the above

10. Balance billing is
    a. Illegal
    b. Practiced by HMOs
    c. Prohibited by managed care
    d. Practiced by IPS HMOs

10

Diagnostic Coding

CHAPTER COMPETENCIES

Review the information in your text that supports the following course objectives.

Learning Objectives

In this chapter, you'll learn:

1. To spell and define the key terms.
2. To name and describe the coding system used to describe diseases, injuries, and other reasons for encounters with a medical provider.
3. To give four examples of how diagnostic coding is used.
4. To describe the relationship between coding and reimbursement.
5. To explain the format of the ICD-9-CM.
6. To list the steps in identifying a proper code.
7. To name common errors in outpatient diagnostic coding.

CHAPTER OUTLINE	NOTES
Diagnostic Coding	
Inpatient Versus Outpatient Coding	
ICD-9-CM: The Code Book	
Volume 1: Tabular List of Diseases	
Supplementary Classifications	
Volume 2: Alphabetic Index to Diseases	
Volume 3: Inpatient Coding	
Locating the Appropriate Code	
Using ICD-9-CM Conventions	
Main Term	
Fourth and Fifth Digits	
Primary Codes	
When More Than One Code Is Used	
Late Effects	
Coding Suspected Conditions	
Documentation Requirements	
The Future of Diagnostic Coding: *International Classification of Diseases, Tenth Revision*	

LEARNING SELF-ASSESSMENT EXERCISES

Key Terms

Define the following key terms:

advance beneficiary notice ______________________

audits ______________________

conventions ______________________

cross-reference ______________________

E-codes ______________________

eponym ______________________

etiology ______________________

inpatient ______________________

International Classification of Diseases, Ninth Revision, Clinical Modification ______________________

late effects ______________________

main terms ______________________

medical necessity ______________________

outpatient ______________________

primary diagnosis ______________________

service ______________________

specificity ______________________

V-codes ______________________

Matching

Match the definition in part 1 with the correct term in part 2.

PART 1

_____ 1. The assignment of a number to a verbal statement or description

_____ 2. Used to report services and procedures

_____ 3. Ensures payment of treatments and procedures likely to be denied by Medicare

_____ 4. Alphabetic Index to Diseases

_____ 5. Include general notes using specific terms, cross-references, abbreviations, punctuation marks, symbols, typeface, and format

PART 2

a. Volume 2

b. Conventions

c. ABN

d. Coding

e. CPT

Multiple Choice

1. Which organization developed the ICD-9-CM statistical classification system?
   a. WHO
   b. CDC
   c. OSHA
   d. NCHS
2. Where can you purchase updates and addenda for ICD-9-CM coding books?
   a. AMA
   b. Local medical society
   c. Coding book publisher
   d. CMS
3. How many sections does the alphabetic index of the ICD-9-CM have?
   a. Six
   b. Three
   c. Four
   d. Ten
4. What is used to justify physician services, whether those services are provided in the hospital or the office?
   a. Volume 1
   b. Volume 2
   c. Volume 3
   d. Volumes 1 and 2
5. The daily visits the physician makes to the inpatient are billed and coded by
   a. The hospital
   b. The physician's office
   c. Medicare
   d. CMS
6. To become an expert coder you need general knowledge in all the following areas *except*
   a. Anatomy and physiology
   b. Medical terminology
   c. Pharmacology
   d. Using the code books
7. E-codes, which range from E800 to E999, are used to classify external causes of
   a. Injuries
   b. Diseases
   c. Poisonings
   d. *a* and *c* only
8. What is used to code live-born infants according to type of birth?
   a. E-codes
   b. B-codes
   c. V-codes
   d. E/M-codes
9. Which is organized by main terms printed in boldface type?
   a. Volume 1, section 2
   b. Volume 3, section 3
   c. Volume 2, section 1
   d. Volume 1, section 1
10. The patient's chief complaint or the reason the patient sought medical attention is
   a. The preliminary diagnosis
   b. The working diagnosis
   c. Listed last on the CMS-1500
   d. The primary diagnosis

11

Outpatient Procedural Coding

CHAPTER COMPETENCIES

Review the information in your text that supports the following course objectives.

Learning Objectives

In this chapter, you'll learn:

1. To spell and define the key terms.
2. To explain the format of Current Procedural Terminology (CPT-4) and its use.
3. To explain the Healthcare Common Procedure Coding System (HCPCS) and level 2 and 3 codes.
4. To explain what diagnostic related groups (DRGs) are and how they are used to determine Medicare payments.
5. To discuss the goals of resource-based relative value system (RBRVS).
6. To describe the relationship between coding and reimbursement.

CHAPTER OUTLINE	NOTES
Physician's Current Procedural Terminology	
Reading Descriptors	
Guidelines	
Unlisted Procedures and Special Reports	
Evaluation and Management Codes	
Anesthesia Codes	
Surgery Codes	
Unstarred Codes	
Starred Codes	
Integumentary System	
Repairs	
Cast Reapplication	
Multiple Procedures Furnished on the Same Day	
Radiology Codes	
Pathology and Laboratory Codes	
Medicine Codes	
CPT-4 Modifiers	

CHAPTER OUTLINE *continued*	NOTES
Healthcare Common Procedure Coding System	
HCPCS Level 1 Codes	
HCPCS Level 2 Codes: National Codes	
HCPCS Level 3 Codes: Local Codes	
Reimbursement	
Diagnostic Related Groups	
Resource-Based Relative Value Scale	
Fraud and Coding	

LEARNING SELF-ASSESSMENT EXERCISES

Key Terms

Define the following key terms:

Current Procedural Terminology ____________________

descriptor ____________________

diagnostic related group ____________________

Healthcare Common Procedure Coding System ____________________

key component ____________________

modifiers ____________________

outlier ____________________

procedure ____________________

resource-based relative value scale ____________________

upcoding ____________________

Matching

Match the definition in part 1 with the correct term in part 2.

PART 1	PART 2
_____ 1. Congress decided to use CPT-4 to code all physicians' procedures and services for Medicare patients	a. Unlisted
_____ 2. CPT-4 is divided into this many major sections	b. Six
_____ 3. A copy of the procedure must be submitted with the claim when the code is this	c. 1980
_____ 4. Five-digit numbers that begin with 9	d. Four
_____ 5. Classifications of histories and physical examinations	e. E/M

Multiple Choice

1. What organization established CPT coding?
   a. American Heart Association
   b. American Physicians Association
   c. American Association of Medical Assistants
   d. American Medical Association

2. CPT-4 coding allows insurance companies to do all of the following *except*
   a. Communicate easily with one another
   b. Speed claims processing
   c. Specify what the physician will be paid
   d. Compare reimbursement amounts

3. What five-digit numbers begin with 9?
   a. E/M codes
   b. Pathology and laboratory codes
   c. Surgery codes
   d. All CPT codes

4. Which of the following is not a classification of histories and physicals?
   a. Problem focused
   b. Counseling
   c. Expanded problem focused
   d. Detailed

5. What do codes that begin with 0 designate?
   a. Anesthesia
   b. Emergency
   c. Radiology
   d. Surgery

6. What do codes that begin with 8 designate?
   a. Pathology and laboratory
   b. Radiology
   c. Emergency
   d. Medicines

7. Cardiac diagnostic testing is covered under which section of the CPT codes?
   a. E/M codes
   b. Medicine codes
   c. History and physicals
   d. Surgery

8. A list of all CPT modifiers is found in
   a. Appendix B
   b. Appendix E
   c. Appendix C
   d. Appendix A

9. HCPCS is the acronym for
   a. Health Care Plans Control Services
   b. Health Care Physicians Centralized Services
   c. Health Care Procedure Control Systems
   d. Healthcare Common Procedure Coding System

10. Categories into which inpatients are placed according to similarity of their diagnoses, treatment, and length of hospital stay are
    a. Diagnostic related groups
    b. Diagnostic rules governing hospital stays
    c. Diagnostic procedures and treatment plans
    d. Diagnostic plans and follow-up of hospital admissions

Notes

Notes

Notes

Notes

Notes

Notes

Skill Drills

1. List seven duties of the medical office receptionist.

2. Describe the eleven types of incoming calls received by the medical office.

3. List the six items of information necessary to document a telephone message.

4. Identify six of the thirteen items that are found on a patient registration form.

Critical Thinking Practice

You receive a call from a patient who complains of being short of breath.

1. What questions will you ask this patient to determine whether this is an emergency?

2. What information will you ask for first?

3. Describe the different types of telephone services and special features that are available for medical offices.

4. In reviewing your tickler file, you discover that it is time to schedule a follow-up appointment for Mrs. Smith. You place an outgoing call to the patient. Explain the procedure or procedures you will use in making this call and patient appointment.

Charting Documentation

Using the information from critical thinking practice question 4, write a narrative chart note describing your interaction with the patient.

Date **Time**

 Name________________ Instructor ______________

Skill Drills

1. List three ways to remind patients about appointments.

2. Identify three factors that affect appointment scheduling.

Critical Thinking Practice

1. Compare and contrast guidelines for scheduling appointments for new patients and return visits.

2. Dr. Wong calls at 11:30 A.M. to say that he is delayed at the hospital and expects to be in the office by 2:30 P.M. Two patients are waiting in the office and three are on the schedule for 1:30 to 2:30 P.M. Describe how you will handle this delay and how you will handle the patients waiting to be seen.

3. Dr. Walters calls in ill and asks you to cancel her first morning appointment. You call Mrs. Steel and inform her of the situation. Write a script of your conversation with this patient.

Charting Documentation

1. With regard to critical thinking practice question 3, write a narrative chart note describing your interaction with the patient.

Date **Time**

Skill Drills

1. Name the six types of mailing options.

2. Name the 12 types of incoming written communication seen in the physician's office.

3. Name the nine items that must be included in minutes.

4. Name the five items that must be included in an agenda.

 Name________________ Instructor ______________

Critical Thinking Practice

1. The office manager has asked you to write an interoffice memorandum to explain the new policy regarding vacation scheduling. Describe the process of memorandum development.

2. Dr. Smith has asked you to assume responsibility for transcribing physical examination reports for the office. This is a new task for you. Discuss the transcription process, including the skills necessary to transcribe accurately and the basic parts of a transcription machine and their functions.

3. Dr. Adams has asked you to type a letter to Dr. Smith, an associate of Dr. Adams, to request Mrs. Jones' medical records. Dr. Adams would also like to know whether Dr. Smith considers Mrs. Jones an acceptable candidate for a new drug study for patients with chronic hypertension. As you prepare to compose this letter, you may envision yourself speaking to Dr. Smith. Explain how this would benefit composing this letter. Be specific.

4. The goal of composition of a letter is **clear, concise,** and **accurate** writing. Give an example of an **unclear** statement, a **wordy** statement, and an **inaccurate** statement. Next to each example **rewrite the messages** properly.

Unclear

Wordy

Inaccurate

Name__________________ Instructor ______________

Skill Drills

1. List the personal qualities needed to transcribe well.

2. List the five requirements of a professional document.

3. What is JCAHO?

4. List JCAHO's two requirements regarding history and physical examination reports.

Critical Thinking Practice

1. Define SOAP and state why the SOAP format for documentation is so vital to the medical record.

2. Using the punctuation rules of transcription and given a transcribed report, edit the report for possible errors.

3. List and state the use of each part of a transcription machine.

 Name__________________ Instructor ________________

Skill Drills

1. List the seven responsibilities of the medical office manager.

2. List the seven types of policies and procedures that should be included in a medical office's policy and procedures manual.

3. List five types of promotional material that a medical office may distribute.

4. Identify three ways that a manager can communicate with medical office staff.

Critical Thinking Practice

1. Dr. Abrams has asked you, the senior medical assistant, to assume the responsibility for staffing the office. What are the major issues to be considered? Identify one major focus for each issue.

2. Miss Young is a new medical assistant in the office. You have been asked to orient her to the operations of the clinic. One of the first items of discussion should be the organizational structure of the office. What will you explain to Miss Young when you describe the organizational structure?

3. Mrs. Jones is the office manager for a six-physician group orthopedic practice. The budget for this practice is large and complex, as there are two clinic sites for the practice and a staff of 30 individuals. Discuss three financial concerns that the medical office manager must be capable of addressing to maintain control of the budget.

4. Legal issues are an area of responsibility of the medical office manager. Discuss four legal issues for the manager that involve employees and/or regulations governing the medical practice.

Skill Drills

1. Describe three methods of debt collection.

2. Identify three forms of payment for services.

3. Identify five practices that a debt collector *may not* use to collect a debt from an individual.

Critical Thinking Practice

1. Mrs. Smith is seeing Dr. Jones for the first time and has asked the medical assistant to explain Dr. Jones' fees. Explain to Mrs. Smith how Dr. Jones establishes the fees he charges his patients.

2. Explain the legal considerations in extending credit.

3. Describe the legal implications of credit collections.

 Name_________________ Instructor _______________

Critical Thinking Practice

1. You are a newly hired administrative assistant responsible for ordering supplies. Explain all of the things you will need to consider to make sure you are getting quality supplies at a reasonable cost.

2. A large order of supplies has been delivered to your office. How can you be sure that you have received all of the items that were ordered?

3. Compare and contrast the manual payroll system with the pegboard payroll system.

Skill Drills

1. Explain the differences between Medicare and Medicaid.

2. List 10 of the 33 items of information required on a medical claim form and explain why each piece of information is needed.

3. Name two legal issues affecting claims submission.

4. List the six areas of health care covered by Medicaid.

Critical Thinking Practice

1. Explain how managed care programs work.

2. Describe group, individual, and government-sponsored (public) health benefits and explain the differences between each.

3. Explain the differences between HMOs, PPOs, and physician hospital organizations.

4. A patient may be covered by more than one health plan, such as by an employer while being a dependent on a spouse's plan. With regard to this situation, identify the primary plan and explain coordination of benefits.

Patient Education

1. Mrs. Smith is moving out of the area and is seeing Dr. Jones, her private practice physician, for the last time. After the move, Mrs. Smith will have to choose a new physician. Mrs. Smith has the choice of a HMO or a PPO. Mrs. Smith approaches Dr. Jones' medical assistant and asks her to explain the difference. How can you teach Mrs. Smith about the differences between a HMO and a PPO?

Skill Drills

1. List four reasons medical information is standardized by coding systems.

2. Summarize the CMS Diagnostic Coding Guidelines.

3. Compare and contrast inpatient and outpatient coding.

4. Discuss the purpose of the CMS-1500 and state the other name for this form.

Critical Thinking Practice

1. At a medical office staff meeting, you are asked to explain the relationship between coding and reimbursement. What can you tell this group?

2. What event in a medical office could trigger a chart audit? Discuss how this could be avoided.

3. List three key points to the future of diagnostic coding.

 Name_________________ Instructor _______________

Skill Drills

1. State the importance of key components in CPT coding.

2. What must the physician do to qualify for a decision-making level for an established patient? For a new patient?

3. State the two types of modifiers.

4. State the significance of the asterisk (*) in surgical codes.

5. Why do you have to pay special attention when coding automated multichannel tests?

Critical Thinking Practice

1. You are a medical assistant working in a family practice. The medical assistant who usually does the coding is on maternity leave. You have been assigned to take that position for 6 months. After 2 months you realize that many Medicare claims have been overcoded. What do you do? What might happen to this physician if this continues to occur?

2. How often does the CPT code book have to be replaced? What are the possible consequences if it is not replaced as indicated?

PROCEDURE 1-1: Handling Incoming Calls

Equipment/Supplies: Telephone, message pad, pen or pencil, headset (if applicable)

Standards: Given the needed equipment and a place to work the student will perform this skill with _____% accuracy in a total of _____ minutes. *(Your instructor will tell you what the percentage and time limits will be before you begin.)*

Key: 4 = Satisfactory 0 = Unsatisfactory NA = this step is not counted

Procedure Steps	Self	Partner	Instructor
1. Answer the phone within two rings.	☐	☐	☐
2. Greet the caller with your name and name of the office.	☐	☐	☐
3. Determine the nature of or reason for the call.	☐	☐	☐
4. Triage the call according to office policy.	☐	☐	☐
5. Record the message correctly on a message pad. Include name of the caller, date and time, telephone number where the caller can be reached, description of the caller's concerns, and the person to whom the message is routed. Clarify information as needed.	☐	☐	☐
6. Give the caller an approximate time frame for a return call.	☐	☐	☐
7. Ask the caller whether he or she has any additional questions or if they need any other help. Allow the caller to disconnect first.	☐	☐	☐
8. Place the message in an appropriate place or note any follow-up action necessary.	☐	☐	☐

Calculation

Total Possible Points: _____
Total Points Earned: _____ Multiplied by 100 = _____ Divided by Total Possible Points = _____%

Pass ☐ Fail ☐

Comments:

Student signature______________________________ Date______________
Partner signature______________________________ Date______________
Instructor's signature______________________________ Date______________

 Name_______________ Instructor _____________

PROCEDURE 1-2: Calling Emergency Medical Services

Equipment/Supplies: Telephone, patient information, pen or pencil

Standards: Given the needed equipment and a place to work the student will perform this skill with _____% accuracy in a total of _____ minutes. *(Your instructor will tell you what the percentage and time limits will be before you begin.)*

Key: 4 = Satisfactory 0 = Unsatisfactory NA = this step is not counted

Procedure Steps	Self	Partner	Instructor
1. Obtain the following information before dialing EMS: patient's name, age, sex, nature of medical condition, type of service the physician is requesting, any special instructions or requests by the physician, your location, and any special information for access.	☐	☐	☐
2. Dial 911 or other EMS number.	☐	☐	☐
3. Calmly provide the dispatcher with the information.	☐	☐	☐
4. Answer the dispatcher's questions calmly and professionally. Follow the dispatcher's instructions if applicable.	☐	☐	☐
5. End the call per the dispatcher's instructions.	☐	☐	☐

Calculation

Total Possible Points: _____
Total Points Earned: _____ Multiplied by 100 = _____ Divided by Total Possible Points = _____%

Pass ☐ Fail ☐

Comments:

Student signature_______________________________ Date_____________
Partner signature_______________________________ Date_____________
Instructor's signature_______________________________ Date_____________

PROCEDURE 2-1: Making an Appointment for a New Patient

Equipment/Supplies: Appointment book, telephone, pen or pencil

Standards: Given the needed equipment and a place to work the student will perform this skill with _____% accuracy in a total of _____ minutes. *(Your instructor will tell you what the percentage and time limits will be before you begin.)*

Key: 4 = Satisfactory 0 = Unsatisfactory NA = this step is not counted

Procedure Steps	Self	Partner	Instructor
1. Obtain as much information as possible from the patient: full name with correct spelling, mailing address, day and evening telephone numbers, reason for the visit, name of the referring physician or individual.	☐	☐	☐
2. Explain the payment policy of the practice. Most offices require full or partial payment at the time of an initial visit. Instruct patients to bring all pertinent insurance information.	☐	☐	☐
3. Ensure that the patient knows how to get to the office; if needed, give concise directions.	☐	☐	☐
4. Tell the patient approximately how long the office visit will be.	☐	☐	☐
5. To avoid violating confidentiality, ask the patient whether it is permissible to call at home or at work.	☐	☐	☐
6. Before ending the call, confirm the time and date of the appointment.	☐	☐	☐
7. Always check your appointment book to be sure that you have placed the appointment on the correct day in the right time slot.	☐	☐	☐

Calculation

Total Possible Points: _____
Total Points Earned: _____ Multiplied by 100 = _____ Divided by Total Possible Points = _____%

Pass ☐ Fail ☐

Comments:

Student signature_______________________________ Date_____________
Partner signature_______________________________ Date_____________
Instructor's signature_______________________________ Date_____________

 Name_________________ Instructor _______________

PROCEDURE 2-2: Making an Appointment for an Established Patient

Equipment/Supplies: Appointment book, telephone, pen or pencil, appointment cards

Standards: Given the needed equipment and a place to work the student will perform this skill with _____% accuracy in a total of _____ minutes. *(Your instructor will tell you what the percentage and time limits will be before you begin.)*

Key: 4 = Satisfactory 0 = Unsatisfactory NA = this step is not counted

Procedure Steps	Self	Partner	Instructor
1. Review the patient's chart to determine what will be done at the return visit. Carefully check your appointment book or computer system before offering an appointment.	☐	☐	☐
2. Offer the patient a specific time and date. Give the patient a choice and, if neither time is convenient, offer another specific time and date.	☐	☐	☐
3. Write the patient's name and telephone number in the appointment book.	☐	☐	☐
4. Transfer the pertinent information to an appointment card and give it to the patient.	☐	☐	☐
5. Repeat aloud the appointment day, date, and time to the patient as you hand over the card.	☐	☐	☐
6. Double-check your book to be sure you have not made an error.	☐	☐	☐
7. End your conversation with a pleasant word and a smile.	☐	☐	☐

Calculation

Total Possible Points: _____
Total Points Earned: _____ Multiplied by 100 = _____ Divided by Total Possible Points = _____%

Pass ☐ Fail ☐

Comments:

Student signature_______________________________ Date_______________
Partner signature_______________________________ Date_______________
Instructor's signature_______________________________ Date_______________

PROCEDURE 2-3: Making an Appointment for a Referral to Another Provider

Equipment/Supplies: Chart, preferred provider list, telephone, pen or pencil

Standards: Given the needed equipment and a place to work the student will perform this skill with _____% accuracy in a total of _____ minutes. *(Your instructor will tell you what the percentage and time limits will be before you begin.)*

Key: 4 = Satisfactory 0 = Unsatisfactory NA = this step is not counted

Procedure Steps	Self	Partner	Instructor
1. Review the patient's chart to determine what kind of appointment is needed. Make certain the requirements of any third-party payers are met.	❑	❑	❑
2. Refer to the preferred provider list for the patient's insurance company. Allow the patient to choose a provider from the list.	❑	❑	❑
3. Call the provider to schedule the appointment. Have the following information available when you make the call: ■ Physician's name and telephone number ■ Patient's name, address, and telephone number ■ Reason for the call ■ Degree of urgency ■ Whether the patient is being sent for consultation or referral	❑	❑	❑
4. Record in the patient's chart the time, date of the call, and person who received your call.	❑	❑	❑
5. Tell the person you are calling that you wish to be notified if your patient does not keep the appointment. If this occurs, be sure to tell your physician and enter this information in the patient's record.	❑	❑	❑
6. Write down the name, address, and telephone number of the doctor you are referring your patient to and include the date and time of the appointment. Give or mail this information to your patient.	❑	❑	❑

Calculation

Total Possible Points: _____

Total Points Earned: _____ Multiplied by 100 = _____ Divided by Total Possible Points = _____%

Pass ❑ Fail ❑

Comments:

Student signature________________________________ Date______________

Partner signature________________________________ Date______________

Instructor's signature________________________________ Date______________

 Name__________ Instructor __________

PROCEDURE 3-1: Writing a Business Letter

Equipment/Supplies: Paper, writing utensil, computer with word processing software, printer

Standards: Given the needed equipment and a place to work the student will perform this skill with _____% accuracy in a total of _____ minutes. *(Your instructor will tell you what the percentage and time limits will be before you begin.)*

Key: 4 = Satisfactory 0 = Unsatisfactory NA = this step is not counted

Procedure Steps	Self	Partner	Instructor
1. Prepare your message by determining who your reader is, what you want them to do, what you want to say, and how you want to organize your message.	☐	☐	☐
2. Select appropriate template or format, margin, and font for the letter.	☐	☐	☐
3. Create a letterhead.	☐	☐	☐
4. Type the date (include month, day, and year) two to four lines below the letterhead.	☐	☐	☐
5. Type the inside address four lines below the date.	☐	☐	☐
6. Type the salutation two lines below the inside address.	☐	☐	☐
7. Type the body of the letter using language that is clear, concise, and accurate.	☐	☐	☐
8. Type the closing two lines below the body of the letter.	☐	☐	☐
9. Leave three lines of space for the signature.	☐	☐	☐
10. Type the name of the person sending the document four lines below the closing.	☐	☐	☐
11. Type the identification line two lines below the typed name.	☐	☐	☐
12. Indicate enclosures, if applicable, two lines below the identification line.	☐	☐	☐
13. Check document for proper grammar, spelling, and punctuation.	☐	☐	☐
14. Check document for accuracy—be sure that all addresses and phone numbers are correct.	☐	☐	☐

15. Check that each paragraph is kept to one topic only. ☐ ☐ ☐
16. Save document with a proper file name. ☐ ☐ ☐
17. Print document. ☐ ☐ ☐

Calculation

Total Possible Points: _____
Total Points Earned: _____ Multiplied by 100 = _____ Divided by Total Possible Points = _____%

Pass ☐ Fail ☐

Comments:

Student signature______________________________ Date__________
Partner signature______________________________ Date__________
Instructor's signature______________________________ Date__________

PROCEDURE 5-2: Performing an Inventory of Supplies and Equipment

Equipment/Supplies: Computer with spreadsheet software, list of supplies, printer, paper

Standards: Given the needed equipment and a place to work the student will perform this skill with _____% accuracy in a total of _____ minutes. *(Your instructor will tell you what the percentage and time limits will be before you begin.)*

Key: 4 = Satisfactory 0 = Unsatisfactory NA = this step is not counted

Procedure Steps	Self	Partner	Instructor
1. Turn on the computer, monitor, and printer.	☐	☐	☐
2. Open the spreadsheet software program.	☐	☐	☐
3. Create a file called Supply Inventory.	☐	☐	☐
4. Type the title of the spreadsheet (e.g., Medical Office Supplies for Inventory) in the appropriate cell.	☐	☐	☐
5. Create a row for each type of supply, and columns to indicate the number of each supply available, the amount of each supply on hand during each month of the year (January through December), and how many supplies must be reordered each month.	☐	☐	☐
6. Create formulas in the appropriate cell that will allow automatic calculations for the amount on hand each month. Also create formulas to automatically calculate how many supplies will need to be ordered each month.	☐	☐	☐
7. Create a "total" amount column at the end of the spreadsheet and create a formula to automatically calculate the yearly total amount reordered.	☐	☐	☐
8. Save all work.	☐	☐	☐
9. Print the finished spreadsheet.	☐	☐	☐

Calculation

Total Possible Points: _____

Total Points Earned: _____ Multiplied by 100 = _____ Divided by Total Possible Points = _____%

Pass ☐ Fail ☐

Comments:

Student signature____ Date______________

Partner signature____ Date______________

Instructor's signature____________________________________ Date______________

PROCEDURE 7-1: Balancing the Day Sheet

Equipment/Supplies: Calculator, current day sheet with yesterday's balance total, carbon paper, all ledger cards with transactions on the day sheet, pencil, pen

Standards: Given the needed equipment and a place to work the student will perform this skill with _____% accuracy in a total of _____ minutes. *(Your instructor will tell you what the percentage and time limits will be before you begin.)*

Key: 4 = Satisfactory 0 = Unsatisfactory NA = this step is not counted

Procedure Steps	Self	Partner	Instructor
1. Determine whether all entries are complete.	☐	☐	☐
2. Add each column with a calculator and place the total in pencil in the appropriate column.	☐	☐	☐
3. Add the totals from the current day to the totals from the previous day sheet.	☐	☐	☐
4. To verify the accuracy of the entries, add the total of the previous balance column and the total of the current balance column.	☐	☐	☐
5. From this total, subtract the totals of the payment and adjustment columns. This amount will equal the current balance column total.	☐	☐	☐
6. When the totals are verified, go back over them in pen.	☐	☐	☐

Calculation

Total Possible Points: _____

Total Points Earned: _____ Multiplied by 100 = _____ Divided by Total Possible Points = _____%

Pass ☐ Fail ☐

Comments:

Student signature______________________________ Date______________

Partner signature______________________________ Date______________

Instructor's signature____________________________ Date______________

 Name________________ Instructor ______________

PROCEDURE 7-2: Posting Charges to the Patient's Account

Equipment/Supplies: Day sheet, carbon paper, pegboard, ledger card, charge slip and/or encounter form, calculator, form, pen

Standards: Given the needed equipment and a place to work the student will perform this skill with _____% accuracy in a total of _____ minutes. *(Your instructor will tell you what the percentage and time limits will be before you begin.)*

Key: 4 = Satisfactory 0 = Unsatisfactory NA = this step is not counted

Procedure Steps	Self	Partner	Instructor
1. Determine whether all entries are complete.	☐	☐	☐
2. Add each column with a calculator and place the total in pencil in the appropriate column.	☐	☐	☐
3. Add the totals from the current day to the totals from the previous day sheet.	☐	☐	☐
4. To verify the accuracy of the entries, add the total of the previous balance column and the total of the current balance column.	☐	☐	☐
5. From this total, subtract the totals of the payment and adjustment columns. This amount will equal the current balance column total.	☐	☐	☐
6. When the totals are verified, go back over them in pen.	☐	☐	☐

Calculation

Total Possible Points: _____
Total Points Earned: _____ Multiplied by 100 = _____ Divided by Total Possible Points = _____%

Pass ☐ Fail ☐

Comments:

Student signature_______________________________ Date______________
Partner signature_______________________________ Date______________
Instructor's signature_______________________________ Date______________

SKILL

PROCEDURE 7-3: Posting Payments to the Patient's Account

Equipment/Supplies: Day sheet, carbon paper, pegboard, ledger card, charge slip and/or encounter form, calculator, form, pen

Standards: Given the needed equipment and a place to work the student will perform this skill with _____% accuracy in a total of _____ minutes. *(Your instructor will tell you what the percentage and time limits will be before you begin.)*

Key: 4 = Satisfactory 0 = Unsatisfactory NA = this step is not counted

Procedure Steps	Self	Partner	Instructor
1. Align the patient's ledger card on the day sheet. If the patient is paying for services received by the physician today, the charge slip that shows today's charges should also be placed on the day sheet.	☐	☐	☐
2. Enter the patient's name and previous balance in the appropriate columns. If using a charge slip, make sure you enter the charge slip number in the receipt number column.	☐	☐	☐
3. Enter the posting date in the date column.	☐	☐	☐
4. Enter the type of payment in the description column, whether personal check (pers. ck.), money order (m. o.), credit card (MC, VISA), or insurance check (ins. ck.).	☐	☐	☐
5. Enter the amount of payment in the payment column.	☐	☐	☐
6. Enter the amount of payment on the deposit section of the day sheet in the cash or checks column.	☐	☐	☐
7. Subtract the payment amount from the previous balance and record the new balance in the new balance column.	☐	☐	☐

Calculation

Total Possible Points: _____

Total Points Earned: _____ Multiplied by 100 = _____ Divided by Total Possible Points = _____%

Pass ☐ Fail ☐

Comments:

Student signature______________________________ Date_______________

Partner signature______________________________ Date_______________

Instructor's signature____________________________ Date_______________

 Name__________ Instructor __________

PROCEDURE 7-4: Posting a Credit Adjustment

Equipment/Supplies: Day sheet, carbon, pegboard, ledger card, calculator, pen

Standards: Given the needed equipment and a place to work the student will perform this skill with _____% accuracy in a total of _____ minutes. *(Your instructor will tell you what the percentage and time limits will be before you begin.)*

Key: 4 = Satisfactory 0 = Unsatisfactory NA = this step is not counted

Procedure Steps	Self	Partner	Instructor
1. Align the patient's ledger card on the day sheet.	☐	☐	☐
2. Record the patient's name, previous balance, and the date in the appropriate columns.	☐	☐	☐
3. Record [in brackets] the amount of the adjustment in the adjustment column of the ledger card. Brackets indicate that the amount is subtracted.	☐	☐	☐
4. Enter a description of the adjustment in the professional service column (insurance adjustment or correction adjustment).	☐	☐	☐
5. Subtract the amount of the adjustment from the previous balance and record the new balance in the balance column.	☐	☐	☐

Calculation

Total Possible Points: _____
Total Points Earned: _____ Multiplied by 100 = _____ Divided by Total Possible Points = _____%

Pass ☐ Fail ☐

Comments:

Student signature__________ Date__________
Partner signature__________ Date__________
Instructor's signature__________ Date__________

PROCEDURE 7-5: Reconciling a Bank Statement

Equipment/Supplies: Monthly bank statement, check register, calculator, pen

Standards: Given the needed equipment and a place to work the student will perform this skill with _____% accuracy in a total of _____ minutes. *(Your instructor will tell you what the percentage and time limits will be before you begin.)*

Key: 4 = Satisfactory 0 = Unsatisfactory NA = this step is not counted

Procedure Steps	Self	Partner	Instructor
1. Determine which portion (dates and/or check numbers) of the checkbook is covered on this bank statement.	☐	☐	☐
2. Locate the ending balance and the list of checks and deposits on the bank statement.	☐	☐	☐
3. Check your check register or record of disbursements against the bank statement and check off each check and deposit on your record that has been recorded on the bank statement.	☐	☐	☐
4. Total all outstanding checks that are not listed on the bank statement. Write this total in the space provided on the worksheet on the back of the bank statement.	☐	☐	☐
5. Total all outstanding deposits that do no appear on the bank statement and write this total in the space provided on the worksheet.	☐	☐	☐
6. Note any additional charges, such as service charges, automatic teller machine charges, or charges for returned checks, that do not appear on the bank statement.	☐	☐	☐
7. Calculate the balance, using the worksheet provided on the back of the statement.	☐	☐	☐
8. Starting with the ending balance, add the total of outstanding deposits.	☐	☐	☐
9. Subtract the total of checks or withdrawals.	☐	☐	☐
10. Verify that the figure is the same as the ending balance on the bank statement.	☐	☐	☐
11. If the figures do not match, recheck your work. If the two numbers still do not match, contact the bank to check for possible bank errors.	☐	☐	☐

Calculation

Total Possible Points: _____
Total Points Earned: _____ Multiplied by 100 = _____ Divided by Total Possible Points = _____%

Pass ☐ Fail ☐

Comments:

Student signature____ Date________________
Partner signature____ Date________________
Instructor's signature_____________________________________ Date________________

Name_________________ Instructor ______________

PROCEDURE 7-6: Preparing a Bank Deposit

Equipment/Supplies: Calculator with tape, currency, coins, checks for deposit, deposit slip, endorsement stamp, deposit envelope

Standards: Given the needed equipment and a place to work the student will perform this skill with _____% accuracy in a total of _____ minutes. *(Your instructor will tell you what the percentage and time limits will be before you begin.)*

Key: 4 = Satisfactory 0 = Unsatisfactory NA = this step is not counted

Procedure Steps	Self	Partner	Instructor
1. Organize currency by arranging bills face up and sorting with the largest denomination on top.	☐	☐	☐
2. Count currency and coins and record the total in the cash block on the deposit slip.	☐	☐	☐
3. Endorse the back of each check with pre-printed stamp, "For Deposit Only."	☐	☐	☐
4. Record the amount of each check beside an identifying number on the deposit slip.	☐	☐	☐
5. Total the amount of checks and record in the total of checks line on the deposit slip.	☐	☐	☐
6. Total the amount of cash and the amount of checks and record in the total deposit line on the deposit slip.	☐	☐	☐
7. Record the total amount of the deposit in the office checkbook register.	☐	☐	☐
8. Make a copy of both sides of the deposit slip for office records.	☐	☐	☐
9. Place the cash, checks, and the completed deposit slip in a envelope or bank bag for transporting to the bank for deposit.	☐	☐	☐

Calculation

Total Possible Points: _____

Total Points Earned: _____ Multiplied by 100 = _____ Divided by Total Possible Points = _____%

Pass ☐ Fail ☐

Comments:

Student signature________________________________ Date_______________

Partner signature________________________________ Date_______________

Instructor's signature________________________________ Date_______________

PROCEDURE 7-7: Posting Payments Using a Pegboard System

Equipment/Supplies: Pen, pegboard, calculator, day sheet, encounter forms, ledger cards, previous day's balance, list of patients and charges, fee schedule

Standards: Given the needed equipment and a place to work the student will perform this skill with _____% accuracy in a total of _____ minutes. *(Your instructor will tell you what the percentage and time limits will be before you begin.)*

Key: 4 = Satisfactory 0 = Unsatisfactory NA = this step is not counted

Procedure Steps	Self	Partner	Instructor
1. Place a new day sheet on the pegboard and record the totals from the previous day sheet.	❑	❑	❑
2. Align the patient's ledger card with the first available line on the daysheet.	❑	❑	❑
3. Place receipt to align with the appropriate line on the ledger card.	❑	❑	❑
4. Record the number of the receipt in the appropriate column.	❑	❑	❑
5. Write the patient's name on the receipt.	❑	❑	❑
6. Record any existing balance the patient owes in the previous balance column of the daysheet.	❑	❑	❑
7. Record the source and type of the payment in the description line (e.g., Blue-Cross/Blue Shield (BC/BS) check for date of service (DOS) 5/28/05).	❑	❑	❑
8. Determine any discounts or adjustments and record in the adjustment column. a. Check the explanation of benefits (EOB) for any disallowed amounts from participating third-party payers. Record the difference in the charge and the allowed amount in the adjustment column. b. Record professional discounts, discounts for cash, etc. in the adjustment column.	❑	❑	❑
9. Record the total payment in the payment column on the receipt, pressing down firmly so that the writing will transfer to the ledger card and the day sheet.	❑	❑	❑
10. Subtract the payment and adjustments from the outstanding or previous balance, and record the current balance.	❑	❑	❑
11. Return the patient's ledger card to its storage area.	❑	❑	❑

Calculation

Total Possible Points: _____

Total Points Earned: _____ Multiplied by 100 = _____ Divided by Total Possible Points = _____%

Pass ❑ Fail ❑

Comments:

Student signature________________________________ Date______________

Partner signature________________________________ Date______________

Instructor's signature________________________________ Date______________

 Name__________________ Instructor _______________

PROCEDURE 7-8: Processing a Credit Balance

Equipment/Supplies: Pen, pegboard, calculator, day sheet, ledger card

Standards: Given the needed equipment and a place to work the student will perform this skill with _____% accuracy in a total of _____ minutes. *(Your instructor will tell you what the percentage and time limits will be before you begin.)*

Key: 4 = Satisfactory 0 = Unsatisfactory NA = this step is not counted

Procedure Steps	Self	Partner	Instructor
1. Determine the reason for the credit balance.	❑	❑	❑
2. Place brackets [ ] around the balance indicating that it is a negative number.	❑	❑	❑
3. Write a refund check following the steps in Procedure 7-9: Processing a Refund.	❑	❑	❑

Calculation

Total Possible Points: _____
Total Points Earned: _____ Multiplied by 100 = _____ Divided by Total Possible Points = _____%

Pass ❑ Fail ❑

Comments:

Student signature________________________________ Date__________
Partner signature________________________________ Date__________
Instructor's signature________________________________ Date__________

PROCEDURE 7-9: Processing a Refund

Equipment/Supplies: Pen, pegboard, calculator, day sheet, ledger card, checkbook, check register, word processor letterhead, envelope, postage,copy machine, patient's chart, refund file

Standards: Given the needed equipment and a place to work the student will perform this skill with _____% accuracy in a total of _____ minutes. *(Your instructor will tell you what the percentage and time limits will be before you begin.)*

Key: 4 = Satisfactory 0 = Unsatisfactory NA = this step is not counted

Procedure Steps	Self	Partner	Instructor
1. Determine who gets the refund, the patient or the insurance company.	❑	❑	❑
2. Pull patient's ledger card and place on current day sheet aligned with the first available line.	❑	❑	❑
3. Write the amount of the refund in the adjustment column [in brackets] indicating it is a debit, not a credit, adjustment.	❑	❑	❑
4. Write "Refund to Patient" or "Refund to _______" (name of insurance company) in the description column.	❑	❑	❑
5. Write a check for the credit amount made out to the appropriate party.	❑	❑	❑
6. Record the amount and name of payee in the check register.	❑	❑	❑
7. Mail the check with letter of explanation to the patient or insurance company.	❑	❑	❑
8. Place a copy of the check and the letter in the patient's record or in the refund file.	❑	❑	❑
9. Return the patient's ledger card to its storage area.	❑	❑	❑

Calculation

Total Possible Points: _____
Total Points Earned: _____ Multiplied by 100 = _____ Divided by Total Possible Points = _____%

Pass ❑ Fail ❑

Comments:

Student signature_____________________________ Date______________
Partner signature_____________________________ Date______________
Instructor's signature_____________________________ Date______________

 Name________________ Instructor ______________

PROCEDURE 9-1: Processing Insurance Claim Forms

Equipment/Supplies: CMS-1500 claim form, patient's file, dates and names of services performed, medical dictionary, CPT-4, ICD-9-CM Volumes 1 and 2, computer software for insurance processing

Standards: Given the needed equipment and a place to work the student will perform this skill with _____% accuracy in a total of _____ minutes. *(Your instructor will tell you what the percentage and time limits will be before you begin.)*

Key: 4 = Satisfactory 0 = Unsatisfactory NA = this step is not counted

Procedure Steps	Self	Partner	Instructor
1. Using the ICD-9-CM index, locate a code or code range for each service or procedure performed for the patient.	❑	❑	❑
2. Find that code or code range in the CPT-4 book.	❑	❑	❑
3. Read the descriptor up to the semi-colon for codes that are not stand alone codes.	❑	❑	❑
4. Review the documentation (operative report, x-ray report, lab report, etc.) to match the appropriate code.	❑	❑	❑
5. If necessary, confirm your choice with the provider who performed the service.	❑	❑	❑
5. Place the selected code in block 21of the CMS-1500 claim form.	❑	❑	❑

Calculation

Total Possible Points: _____
Total Points Earned: _____ Multiplied by 100 = _____ Divided by Total Possible Points = _____%

Pass ❑ Fail ❑

Comments:

Student signature________________________________ Date______________
Partner signature________________________________ Date______________
Instructor's signature________________________________ Date______________

SKILL

PROCEDURE 10-1: Locating a Diagnostic Code

Equipment/Supplies: Current code book, patient's medical record

Standards: Given the needed equipment and a place to work the student will perform this skill with _____% accuracy in a total of _____ minutes. *(Your instructor will tell you what the percentage and time limits will be before you begin.)*

Key: 4 = Satisfactory 0 = Unsatisfactory NA = this step is not counted

Procedure Steps	Self	Partner	Instructor
1. Choose the main term within the diagnostic statement.	☐	☐	☐
2. Locate the main term in Volume 2.	☐	☐	☐
3. Refer to all notes and conventions under the main term.	☐	☐	☐
4. Find the appropriate indented subordinate term.	☐	☐	☐
5. Follow any relevant instructional terms, such as "see also."	☐	☐	☐
6. Confirm the selected code by cross-referencing Volume 1. Make sure you have added any necessary fourth or fifth digits.	☐	☐	☐
7. Assign the code.	☐	☐	☐

Calculation

Total Possible Points: _____
Total Points Earned: _____ Multiplied by 100 = _____ Divided by Total Possible Points = _____%

Pass ☐ Fail ☐

Comments:

Student signature______________________________ Date______________
Partner signature______________________________ Date______________
Instructor's signature__________________________ Date______________

 Name________________ Instructor ______________

PROCEDURE 11-1: Locating a CPT code

Equipment/Supplies: Current CPT code book, patient's medical record

Standards: Given the needed equipment and a place to work the student will perform this skill with _____% accuracy in a total of _____ minutes. *(Your instructor will tell you what the percentage and time limits will be before you begin.)*

Key: 4 = Satisfactory 0 = Unsatisfactory NA = this step is not counted

Procedure Steps	Self	Partner	Instructor
1. Identify the type of procedure, service, or medical supplies provided to the patient.	☐	☐	☐
2. Select one of these sections and open the book to that section: ■ Evaluation and management (E/M) ■ Anesthesia ■ Surgery ■ Radiology ■ Pathology and laboratory ■ Medicine	☐	☐	☐
3. Review the section guidelines for any specific issues.	☐	☐	☐
4. If you are selecting an E/M code, check the medical record for documentation of the key components. Two of the three are required for established patients; three of three are required for new patients.	☐	☐	☐
5. Select the appropriate code based on the level of history, examination, and medical decision making.	☐	☐	☐
6. Attach the CPT modifier if the procedure or service requires additional clarification.	☐	☐	☐
7. Assign the CPT code.	☐	☐	☐

Calculation

Total Possible Points: _____
Total Points Earned: _____ Multiplied by 100 = _____ Divided by Total Possible Points = _____%

Pass ☐ Fail ☐

Comments:

Student signature________________________________ Date______________
Partner signature________________________________ Date______________
Instructor's signature________________________________ Date______________